Translational Ayurveda

Sanjeev Rastogi
Editor

Translational Ayurveda

Springer

Editor
Sanjeev Rastogi
Department of Kaya Chikitsa
State Ayurvedic College and Hospital, Lucknow University
Lucknow
India

ISBN 978-981-13-2061-3　　ISBN 978-981-13-2062-0 (eBook)
https://doi.org/10.1007/978-981-13-2062-0

Library of Congress Control Number: 2018958875

This Springer imprint is published by the registered company Springer Nature Singapore Pte Ltd.
The registered company address is: 152 Beach Road, #21-01/04 Gateway East, Singapore 189721, Singapore

Foreword

Translational medicine, translational science and now translational Ayurveda sound novel and innovative, but their practice is far from new. The Ayurvedic pioneers of the nineteenth century in Bengal and Kerala, for example, were faced with the problem of supplying ready-made, traditional formulations of proven quality to large numbers of patients who had no means to make them at home; nor did the physicians have the facilities and staff to produce them. The highly successful initiative to produce and supply traditional drugs to thousands of patients on the lines of drugs in modern medicine was the brainchild of Ayurvedic pioneers who faced no little opposition from their orthodox peers. Their initiative was a huge success which opened a new chapter in Ayurvedic pharmacy. In accomplishing this unprecedented feat, the pioneers adhered strictly to the directions in ancient texts but, at the same time, adopted whatever they felt was necessary and appropriate in the industrial production of modern drugs. Authentication of batches of raw materials, fixation of processing protocol, quality control and marketing found resonance in the manufacture of Ayurvedic formulations for the first time. The novel approach combined the resources, expertise and technologies from different disciplines to enhance the reach and quality of Ayurvedic formulations, which could legitimately claim to be the harbinger of translational Ayurveda.

Translational Ayurveda is of course not limited to the production of herbal formulations. The resources including techniques which Ayurveda would summon from different disciplines to become translational would vary depending on what is sought to be made translational. To develop herbal drugs for the global market, novel instruments to determine the constitutional type or prakriti of individuals or devices to study nādī in clinical practice would require in-depth collaboration with disciplines as diverse as medicinal chemistry, intellectual property, world trade, biomedical engineering and regulatory regime for instruments used in clinical practice across the world. As Ayurveda globalizes and its applications cross national and cultural frontiers, the process of translation would expand and become many-splendoured. This is inevitable as foreshadowed by the globalization of yoga.

Professor Rastogi has made a serious attempt to study translational Ayurveda and edited an interesting and enlightening volume. Divided into two parts, the first contains papers on the fundamentals and modalities of translational Ayurveda written by experts. The papers in this part deal with basic questions such as the translational potential of prakriti, translational concepts in Ayurvedic drug science and Ayurvedic

Rasayana therapy for mass benefit. Part II deals with translational Ayurveda in clinical practice and includes interesting discussions on the practice of integrative dermatology over 20 years in a hospital, sleep medicine, diabetes and cancer. Fittingly it concludes with a paper on 'Dreaming of Health for All' by Rastogi.

The book will be of interest to practitioners, investigators and friends of Ayurveda in India and foreign countries as it draws attention to an emerging frontier of Ayurveda. Professor Rastogi deserves our thanks for highlighting the translational aspect of Ayurveda which holds the key to extending the reach of Ayurvedic practice of high quality all across India and foreign countries.

M. S. Valiathan

Preface

Translational Ayurveda: From Book to Bedside is a documented cry of a distinct community of Ayurveda believers who want to be the judge for what their health care delivers and also wish to be judged essentially through their deliverables. There had been consistent and passionate arguments about the uniqueness of Ayurvedic fundamentals, principles, diagnostic methods, treatment approaches, procedures and formulations compared to contemporary biomedicine. Such arguments often begin in the backdrop of antiquity of Ayurveda and build up through limitations of biomedicine in terms of its limited understanding about diseases, treatment possibilities and adversities which might be an essential offshoot of a given medical intervention. These arguments also question about the reductionist approach of modern medicine dealing separately with every small section of the body and hence being unable to have a comprehensive view of the person as a whole having a disease. There had not been any doubts about the uniqueness and occasional superiority of traditional health-care wisdom over current health-care practices in a global context. Traditional health-care wisdom particularly Ayurveda and Traditional Chinese Medicine is actually the epitome of cumulated health-care knowledge which consistently kept the humanity alive much before the dawn of so-called modern medicine. Unfortunately, at the same time, many of these arguments favouring the former also look irrational, arbitrary, superficial, inconsistent and not withstandable against the word of evidence asking about the actual health-care benefits offered by such systems to the community having an access to a pluralistic health-care model with an equal opportunity to choose any system of health care for its individual needs.

Despite its literary excellence, the question of 'translational value of Ayurveda' remains the crux. How much of this science is there in real clinical practice as a help to its believers? There are number of studies which state that Ayurvedic physicians are poorly acquainted with the diagnostic and clinical examination methods as are dictated in their own classical texts. Such fundamental-based clinical practice of Ayurveda is missing even at Ayurvedic teaching institutions and is evident by finding the absence of crucial Ayurvedic clinical information on the prescriptions generated by qualified Ayurvedic physicians working at such institutions. Unfortunately, what is taught in classrooms as vital to the clinical practice of Ayurveda is hardly seen on prescriptions generated in the hospitals. There are commendable fundamentals with high appeal when discussed in classrooms, but how they appear at clinic?

Is it not strange to see that despite its much hype and galore among recent medical researchers, the concept like *prakriti* and its examination could not still find a place in routine Ayurvedic clinical practice? The same is true with number of other Ayurvedic fundamentals relevant to its clinical practice like *dashavidha pareeksha, anupana* (post-medication drink), *bhaishajya kala* (appropriate time of drug intake), disease diagnosis, selection of drugs and their doses in isolation or in combination. Contemporary Ayurvedic practice, on the contrary, has become patternised to a *vyadhi pratyanik* (disease focused) approach where the treatment is planned on the basis of disease without looking deep into many other aspects that might be crucial in determining a cure.

What deters us from using our fundamentals in real clinical settings? This is a question requiring an honest introspection of this science in terms of its intricacies and uniqueness looked at one point and the practical benefits it may offer on the other. If proposed benefits are tangible and heavier than the efforts, the scientific exercise is worth doing. If not, it would be hard to carry them forward merely on the basis of theoretical conceptualization.

A health-care science is required to be dynamic and resilient so as to accommodate ever renewing facts within its own pool of knowledge. It should be able to provide the best, consistent, reproducible, applicable, feasible and accessible solutions to existing and emerging health-care issues with a competitive edge over the other prevailing solutions. The solutions offered should also be timely and in tune with the current standards of living, economy and lifestyles. It should also be able to cater to the diversified needs of the population having a huge variability in terms of preference, age, vitality and affordability.

The health science shall be made simpler to the extent that its application shall not remain limited to high-tech tertiary health-care centers but can percolate down the stream to extend its benefits to the primary health-care services in the form of 'first-hand yet the best hand' health care within its own context.

Unfortunately, Ayurveda so far did not heed to a serious look at the vital issues of its translation and transformation as a health-care science meant for common people. Ironically, efforts made in the direction of bringing the Ayurveda down to common people have not added any good to the cause except adding indignity, dilution and inconsistency to the core of this science by presenting imprecise and inappropriate information at common platforms.

Throughout its ancient texts, Ayurveda is available in the forms of *sutras*, the compact capsular forms of knowledge having potential for further expansion as per the contextual need. Unfortunately, such exercises have also been rarely adopted in Ayurveda to make it really readable and applicable in a wider clinical spectrum. Such texts have remained limited to translations and commentaries which did not serve the purpose of expanding the sutras for their critical application in a real clinical setting where a decision about treatment plan is to be made in reference to the possible pathology and expected benefits.

Current researches adopted to prove the efficacy of Ayurvedic drug applications in various clinical conditions are also hard to be swallowed. The models adopted for such studies are often the ones where diseases are synthetically derived through introducing chemical or physical agents able to alter or destroy a tissue or organ function. Research interventions are subsequently initiated to restore the lost functions. This is ironical to apply these models on real diseases where a grossly different mechanism may apply to lead a disease. This issue is more pertinent to Ayurveda where the cause (*hetu*) of a disease has a direct bearing upon net treatment plan.

Ayurveda proposes a specific set of conditions causing a disease and while making efforts to correct the pathology primarily tries to correct the pathogenesis (*samprapti)* which might have occured due to the exposure of such *nidana* and its subsequent impact upon body functioning. Moreover, this is also a fundamental understanding that a disease manifests through multiple pathways, and therefore, an intervention may be effective only if it interrupts the particular pathway of disease production in a given case. Looking at this, the model for Ayurvedic drug studies essentially needs to come through the Ayurvedic way of disease production. Only then the real impact of an Ayurvedic intervention may be evaluated. This is why we argue that Ayurvedic researches require a different disease model for their studies and that the conventional models used in current pharmacological studies do not really fit into the ayurvedic context.

'Translational Ayurveda' primarily looks at Ayurvedic health-care wisdom in a wider perspective of its real-time applicability at bedside. While doing so, it also argues to look at difficulties, complexities and intricacies intertwined within this approach. It argues to look at existing gaps between classical and contemporary Ayurvedic health-care wisdom and the realistic health-care needs of the people. It further suggests finding ways to bridge the gaps through focused clinical, experimental, exploratory and observational researches. It essentially proposes utilizing the Ayurvedic propositions in various special health conditions and to determine what actually deters it to be used in its full strength. Doing so, it invites the medical scientists and biologists along with Ayurvedic experts to look collectively with extended arms to make a better and comprehensive understanding of Ayurveda for its most efficient use as a dependable health-care system.

We believe that this effort will be able to ignite the minds of young and senior scientists of the globe alike and will inspire them to come forward choosing their roles to make this noble science of health care more comprehensible. We don't know how this effort is going to be evaluated by the future generations but still have a strong feeling that this possibly is going to be a legacy thrust transition from our generation to the upcoming generations.

Lucknow, India Sanjeev Rastogi

Acknowledgement

This work *Translational Ayurveda: from Book to Bedside* is the outcome of a long process of progressive and forward thinking of a few contemporary leaders in Ayurveda having a global vision and outlook. This is my privilege to edit this exemplary volume which represents the worldview on the issue of taking Ayurveda forward to make its knowledge truly applicable in a wider spectrum of health care. This is universally admitted among Ayurveda believers that its wisdom represents the finest admixture of values, morality, ethics and behavior and eco preservation in the context of human health. It actually presents a compendium of complete balance between human and the nature in a mutually benefiting and supporting manner. This is surprising to see in Ayurveda the illustrious details about causes and manifestations of diseases and approaches to deal with them. In light of such descriptions, it is imperative to think of what actually is limiting the Ayurvedic science from its upscale utilization. This book is the result of serious brainstorming among thought leaders of Ayurveda and contemporary science trying to find the answers to this intricate question.

Whom shall we acknowledge for this book? The original legendary proponents of Ayurveda like Charaka, Sushruta and Vagbhata, for the legacy they have left behind; the believers of Ayurveda who stood by its principles despite all odds being faced historically; the patients who seek Ayurvedic interventions and hence giving an opportunity to test this science; or the researchers, practitioners and academicians of Ayurveda who are putting every inch of their effort to rekindle the fire of Ayurveda for the global benefit.

Factually, every stakeholder aiming to extend the benefit of Ayurveda to common people shall be acknowledged for their efforts made since long to make it possible. 'If I have seen a little further, it is by standing on the shoulder of the giants.' This saying of Sir Isaac Newton in 1676 has a bearing on Ayurveda for all we speak today is actually the wisdom assembled by the *apta* or the knowledge giants of their times. The truth is that if we need to look farther than what they have seen, we need to sit on their shoulders to be enabled. Unfortunately, contemporary Ayurveda has largely missed this progressive thrust and hence is just revolving around a pivot without a forward momentum.

I wish to acknowledge from the core of my heart, my teacher revered Prof. Ram Harsh Singh, Padma Shri, who happened to be a spiritual force for all I do for the benefit of Ayurveda and eventually for our own people. He is a live source of constant illumination, knowledge and wisdom which is not limited to Ayurveda but far and wide is extending to the science of value and humanity. I humbly and honestly admit that what I am today is only because I am blessed to have him as a teacher.

Prof. Francesco Chiappelli, UCLA, is my mentor in scientific research for the past 15 years. It is Prof. Chiappelli who actually pushed me deep into the fascinating field of scientific research methods and statistics and had shown their judicial application into Ayurveda. We together had produced many landmark research contributions, book chapters and a book on evidence-based Ayurveda already published by Springer. Prof. Chiappelli has contributed immensely to this book from its initial concept till it taking a final shape.

Our contributors to this book are doyens doing extraordinarily in their respective fields. This is highly admirable seeing a few of them although not directly linked with Ayurveda still taking pains to make Ayurveda better presented and utilized. What is presented in the book is actually the worldview of our time as the book contribution has a global representation. We acknowledge all our contributors for their time and efforts to make this book reaching a real benchmark standard.

Prof MS Valiathan, Padma Vibhushan, an all-time great cardiothoracic surgeon turned newage Ayurveda admirer, is a highly acclaimed name in the science academia. This is highly inspiring having him writing the foreword for this book. Prof Valiathan is the writer of few new age epics on Ayurveda, namely the legacy of Charaka, Sushruta and Vagbhata. He is the proponent of the concept of Ayurvedic biology stating that Ayurvedic understanding of human physiology is quite unique and is required to be respected in its own way. No one other than him could have been a better writer of a foreword for a book on translational Ayurveda.

My family deserves big thanks for allowing me to work for long hours on computer in order to complete the task. My wife Dr. Ranjana and son Shashwat need all the praise for granting me the time needed to accomplish the book in the present form.

Dr Naren Agrawal and Kumar Athiappan from the team Springer deserve a big mention for them being supportive to the whole project from its inception till completion. We had been associated with Springer for the past few years and had been able to produce three books from the house so far. Working with Springer has always been a fascinating experience.

I finally wish to acknowledge all my patients who have permitted me to experiment upon them and eventually allowing me to experience the power of Ayurveda. It is only with their support, I could really feel what Ayurveda is and how much it can help the humanity. It is with their help, I could learn the real meaning and the need of translational Ayurveda.

Contents

Part I Translational Ayurveda: Fundamentals and Modalities

1 **Translational Ayurveda: Befitting into the Context of Translational Research and Translational Effectiveness** 3
Sanjeev Rastogi and Francesco Chiappelli

2 **Translational Studies on Fundamental Principles of Ayurveda from Book to Bedside** 13
Ram H. Singh

3 **Translational Potential of Ayurveda *Prakriti*: Concepts in the Area of Personalized Medicine** 21
J. Douglas Coffin, Rammohan Rao, and Diana I. Lurie

4 **Ayurvedic Pharmaceutics, Manufacturing Processes and Novel Drug Delivery Systems in Ayurveda** 33
Chandra Kant Katiyar

5 **Pharmacological and Pharmaceutical Principles of Ayurvedic Drugs: A Concurrent Appraisal** 53
K. Nishteswar

6 **Ayurvedic *Rasayana* Therapy: A Rational Understanding Necessary for Mass Benefits** 77
Sanjeev Rastogi, Subhash C. Lakhotia, and Ram H. Singh

Part II Translational Ayurveda: Clinical Practice

7 **Understanding Cancer: Expanding the Horizon Through Applying the Collective Wisdom of Ayurveda and Conventional Medicine** 103
Sanjeev Rastogi, Sen Pathak, and Ram Harsh Singh

8 **Understanding Diabetes: Uncovering the Leads from Ayurveda** 123
Sanjeev Rastogi

9 Integrative Dermatology: Applying Knowledge of Ayurvedic Skin Care and Experience of the Past 20 Years at the Bedside 141
S. R. Narahari, M. G. Aggithaya, and T. J. Ryan

10 Sleep Medicine: What Can Ayurveda Contribute to the Contemporary Health Care? 161
Sanjeev Rastogi and Rajiv Rastogi

11 Ayurveda Abroad: Non-native Perspectives and Needs for Translating It to Western Settings 183
Christian Sumith Kessler

12 Dreaming of Health for All in an Unequal World: Finding a Fit for Traditional Health Care Exemplified Through Ayurveda 199
Sanjeev Rastogi and Arindam Bhattacharya

About the Editor

Sanjeev Rastogi is MD in Ayurvedic Medicine from Banaras Hindu University, Varanasi, and PhD from Lucknow University. He was Director of Rashtriya Ayurveda Vidyapeeth, an autonomous organization under the Ministry of Ayush, Government of India. Currently, he is working as Professor at the Post Graduate Department of Kaya Chikitsa, State Ayurvedic College and Hospital, Lucknow. Dr Rastogi is widely known for his research on Ayurveda. He is also on the editorial board of many scientific journals and is senior editor for *Annals of Ayurvedic Medicine*, a peer-reviewed, quarterly journal owned by the Association of Ayurvedic Physicians of India.

Part I

Translational Ayurveda: Fundamentals and Modalities

Translational Ayurveda: Befitting into the Context of Translational Research and Translational Effectiveness

1

Sanjeev Rastogi and Francesco Chiappelli

1.1 Introduction

1.1.1 Translational Research and Translational Effectiveness: Current Scenario and the Contextual Relevance

Translational research largely implies to the research in basic sciences having a possible application and subsequent bearing upon human health. Such research may aim at finding the practical, feasible, and realistic ways of applying the knowledge obtained in the laboratory or through other methods of research, experimental or observational, upon human beings. Translational effectiveness, in the same spirit, makes the translational research more relevant in terms of its effectiveness in a real clinical setting contrasting to the idealistically controlled environment of the laboratory or strictly controlled clinical trials [1]. Effectiveness research has a special bearing here differentiating it from the efficacy research by finding the former more close to real life compared to the latter representing a controlled situation. For a clinician sometimes the inferences obtained through high-end researches like that of randomized clinical trials do not have a practical utility because of differences in the research conditions and real-life clinical situations. In real life, a human and his functions are net sum of multiple interdependent factors mutually affecting each other and eventually the overall functions of the body. A RCT don't consider all such confounding factors and hence may not be verbatim applicable to the clinical

S. Rastogi (✉)
Department of Kaya Chikitsa, State Ayurvedic College and Hospital, Lucknow University, Lucknow, India

F. Chiappelli
UCLA School of Dentistry, Los Angeles, CA, USA
e-mail: fchiappelli@dentistry.ucla.edu

S. Rastogi (ed.), *Translational Ayurveda*, https://doi.org/10.1007/978-981-13-2062-0_1

practice. Translational research following translational effectiveness research matters in this regard for its being almost ready-to-use recipe having an instant utility.

Translational research is relatively a new entrant in medical research world. The word is used as early as in 1990 referring to variety of researches done in the field of cancer management [2]. The term however is variously defined until recently. NIH in 2010 defined translational research as:

> *Translational research includes two areas of translation. One is the process of applying discoveries generated during research in the laboratory, and in preclinical studies, to the development of trials and studies in humans. The second area of translation concerns research aimed at enhancing the adoption of best practices in the community. Cost-effectiveness of prevention and treatment strategies is also an important part of translational science* [3].

Although the term is used differently by different people in different contexts, the basic idea of translational research is to make quick applications of clinical or basic researches for the actual patient management. This is largely seen that the benefits of laboratory or basic researches or even the clinical researches are not effectively transferred to the actual patient management and hence the benefits of huge investments of time and money made in context of research do not sufficiently reach to the end users.

Seeing the practical relevance of translational research, various organizations have been established focusing solely upon such strategic approach. National Center for Advancing Translational Sciences (NCATS) is one such institute established by NIH aiming to transform and accelerate the translational research process [4]. India also has taken up many initiatives to establish translational research particularly in the field of modern medical science. Infrastructure for translational research and translational clinical trials in India comprises of UNESCO Regional Centre for Biotechnology (RCB) and Translational Health Science and Technology Institute (THSTI) incorporating Vaccine and Infectious Disease Research Centre (VIDRC) and Clinical Development Services Agency (CDSA). Institute for Stem Cell Biology and Regenerative Medicine (inSTEM) and Centre for Cellular and Molecular Platforms (C-CAMP) are two more institutions with similar objectives that started at Bangalore. To work in toxicology, there are two key institutions, namely, Indian Institute of Toxicology Research (IITR), Lucknow, and Indian Institute of Toxicology (IIT), Pune.

The National Institute of Biologicals at NOIDA and Central Drug Research Institute at Lucknow offer a drug testing facility. The Primate Research Center at National Institute of Immunology, New Delhi; National Institute of Nutrition, Hyderabad; National Center for Nonhuman Primate Breeding and Research, Susnavgarh, Genome Valley, Hyderabad; and National Institute of Cholera and Enteric Diseases, Kolkata, provide national animal research facilities.

Many biotech parks have also been set in India to bring the clustered research facilities to help industry and academician. The Indian Institutes of Science Education and Research (IISER) and National Institute of Pharmaceutical Education and Research (NIPER) focus, respectively, in area of science and pharmaceutical education and research. There are many institutes and schools related with public health. There are many central and state universities and medical colleges which are individually engaged in translational research in India. Seeing the difficulty of amalgamating the researches done at basic sciences and clinical sciences separately to create a meaningful mix for patient benefit, now the charge is on translational research comprising of a multidisciplinary team from various disciplines working together for the ultimate goal of patient benefit [5].

Although translational research in health care is a global phenomenon, not much of it is shared by traditional, alternative, and complementary medicine. India, despite being a unique country for officially adopting a pluralistic health-care strategy [6], is nowhere in the scene when it comes to translational research in alternative health care.

Translational research in Ayurveda seems a little awry from its conventional concept. Ayurveda in view of its own biology to understand health and diseases has beautifully laid its novel health-care principles and proposes explicit methods for their practice. Much of the Ayurveda wisdom is generated through a continuous process of observations and experimentations emerging as an outcome of an ongoing interaction between man and the environment. Not much of traditional Ayurveda therefore is researched in laboratory contrasting to the conventional medicine where wisdom evolves through the laboratory experimentations. The translation research question in Ayurveda (or any other traditional health-care system), having an inheritance of thousands of years, therefore should focus upon the contextual and contemporary revalidation of its theories, principles, and practices initially evolved centuries ago. Once it is revalidated through routine researches, the next question is to make such revalidated information user-friendly, i.e., to find the practical ways of applying such knowledge in the context of real patient management in a clinical setting.

Hence, one large part of translational research in Ayurveda belongs to the reinterpretation of its classical wisdom as contemporary knowledge essentially in a practically usable format. This reinterpretation of Ayurvedic classical native text is however not limited to its translation into other languages but essentially mean for its transformation into the language of science through creation of adequate bridges in between to facilitate the cross talk between the duo [7]. The objective of the whole exercise however remains the same, to bring all health-care knowledge at a common platform where this can effectively and collectively be utilized for human well-being.

On health-related issues, we find the knowledge available to us through multiple resources. Of all the plethora of knowledge, only that which is meaningful and is available for its instant application is a translatable knowledge. Sometimes, a complex knowledge piece is required to be fragmented into simpler, comprehensible forms to make it applicable, and similarly, on the other side, some simple knowledge from multiple sources is required to be assembled together to find the solution of a complex problem by looking at it from multiple angles of views. Problems are required to be thought for their solutions by exploring, experimenting, and applying the existing knowledge to find some novel clues. Sometimes an existing knowledge

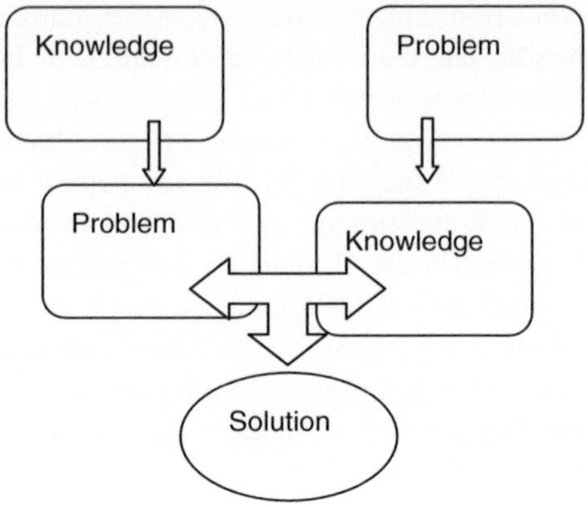

Fig. 1.1 Top to bottom and bottom to top translational approach

may give the clue to some unresolved problem which was not initially looked at from that angle. These problem first or "top to bottom" and the knowledge first or the "bottom to top" approaches are eventually complimentary to each other in looking at the same issue but with a different perspective requiring different expertise and resources [8]. These approaches however essentially converge at a common goal of easing out the life of the people through producing the effective solutions to the existing problems (Fig. 1.1). It is for this reason, translational research is having its absolute applicability in almost every field of life although its applicability in health care seems more pronounced [9].

1.2 Translational Perspectives of Current Research in Ayurveda: Had We Missed the Bus?

Manohar PR (2014) in one of his thought-provoking article unearthed a bitter truth about conventional Ayurveda research. The truth is that so far Ayurveda has been consistently tried to get evaluated without actually understanding it [10]. Evaluating without understanding is derogatory to the whole Ayurveda wisdom without being credited for how it has served the humanity for centuries before the arrival of evidence-based medicine of today. This evaluation without understanding sometimes led to the methodological errors in research planning eventually causing erratic or false inference generation. There are plenty of such examples in the published literature where the essence of Ayurveda was ignored in research planning and eventually resulted in wrong interpretations, often undermining the role of Ayurveda in certain conditions. Researches on *Guggulu* set a good case to exemplify such errors which have been made in scientific research due to the ignorance of Ayurvedic science. This may be noted that the claims of *Guggulu* for it being a hypolipidemic agent [11] have remained shrouded in mystery owing to the contrary reporting in many subsequent clinical and experimental studies [12] without taking a note that Ayurveda proposed hypolipidemic (*lekhana*) property to aged *Guggulu* resin alone and not to the freshly collected resin [13].[1]

Without taking a note of what qualitative change might occur through aging of *Guggulu* resin and how it differs pharmacologically from the fresh *Guggulu* resin, Guggulu resin was evaluated without noticing its age and inferred for absence of its lipid-lowering effects claimed earlier.

The same is about the controversy emerging on toxicity related with herbo-metallic compound of Ayurveda. With contrary claims on safety and toxicity of such compounds [14–16], this has not yet been studied on priority, how Ayurvedic classical drug preparation methods might be offering a cutting-edge advantage to Ayurvedic herbo-mineral preparations making them less toxic yet more effective.

Researches done in Ayurveda so far have neither been done with an intention to understand Ayurveda for its better application subsequently nor been done in a translational mode in order to solve a clinical riddle on the issues directly mattering to the end beneficiary. Such issues are cost, effectiveness, dose forms, duration of the therapy, primary and secondary end points of the therapy, and comparing single herbs with combination therapies and comparing *samshamana* with *samshodhana* therapy. This is important to note that Ayurvedic biology has largely been ignored while planning the researches in Ayurveda and the efforts were solely to prove Ayurveda on the grounds of modern tools and technology with justifying if they are suited to reply the questions of Ayurveda or not. This has largely been stressed that Ayurveda requires its own research methodology backed up with modern tools of research as per its own requirement [17]. Unfortunately such calls have not been heeded so far.

Although huge infrastructure is found dedicated to translational research in conventional medicine in India, very little is actually done to translate the wisdom of ancient clinical science available in Ayurveda and other alternative systems of healing prevailing in India and other parts of the world. Similarly, very little has been done so far to recognize and to adopt the best clinical practices in Ayurveda on the ground in order to reveal the science behind such practices for their subsequent use in improving the health-care outcomes. Translational research in Ayurveda is translated and interpreted variously in different spheres of Ayurveda. There had been a few isolated sparse activities in the field, and often the word "translational" is used more in tune to development in modern science rather than its real connotation to Ayurveda. All India Institute of Ayurveda (AIIA), a premier institute of education and research in Ayurveda in India, places on record having a Department of Translational Research and Biomedical Research. Although the objectives and modus operandi of the department are not yet clear, this looks to be an extension of biomedical research alone with no clear road map of what is meant by translational research adopted by them and how they wish to achieve the goals [18]. Translational Research and Innovative Science ThRough Ayurgenomics (TRISUTRA)

---

[1] स नवो वृंहणो वृष्य: पुराणस्त्वति लेखन: । भाव प्रकाश निघन्टु, कर्पूरादि वर्ग , गुग्गुलु प्रकरण ४१.

New (fresh) *Guggulu* promotes weight gain and is aphrodisiac, whereas old (aged) *Guggulu* promotes weight loss (*Bhavaprakasha nighantu*, *karpuraadi varga*, *guggulu prakaran* 41).

established by Council of Scientific and Industrial Research (CSIR), at CSIR-Institute of Genomics and Integrative Biology, New Delhi, is another ambitious organization working with the objectives of developing affordable health-care solutions based on traditional knowledge of Ayurveda and modern genomics. This is an interdisciplinary network center aiming to enable cross talk between Ayurveda, modern medicine, and genomic science [19]. Further defining its objectives, TRISUTRA aims at conducting research for validation and providing scientific evidence to principles/concepts described in Ayurveda for predictive, personalized, and preemptive approach toward health and diseased conditions; developing data and sample repositories for prospective research studies; developing interdisciplinary human resources; and undertaking and coordinating translational research for developing affordable health-care solutions for diseases of national priority based on Ayurveda literature. This unit is told to strive toward providing scientific credence and global acceptability to Ayurveda and new leads to genomics, creates interdisciplinary expertise, and would also provide marketable leads that would be beneficial to health, nutrition, and Ayurveda industry.

The Central Council for Research in Ayurvedic Sciences (CCRAS), an apex organization for research in Ayurveda in India, also performs research in Ayurveda through its 30 centers spread throughout the country and also through Extra Mural Research (EMR) model where the people from various expertise areas are invited to propose their research ideas aiming to enrich Ayurveda and its understanding. CCRAS has set its priority list of research through EMR, and this is surprising to see that translational research is not in the priority of the apex research organization of Ayurveda in India [20].

Catching the T1 momentum of translational research emphasizing on the requirement of a physician to be groomed as a scientist by entering into the nitty-gritty of research technology, a conceptually similar, though on smaller scale, 2-year vaidya—scientist fellowship program with support from the Ministry of AYUSH, Government of India, was launched at FRLHT, Bangalore [21]. After running successfully for 2 years, the program failed to find the funds and hence was compelled to see a premature termination.

Current Ayurveda researches conducted globally and particularly in India continue to be of poor quality and hence of poor impact. As one important reason, this has seriously dented and damaged the clinical practice standards in Ayurveda during the past half century [22] for not being of much help to improve it. There are soaring gaps between what people expect from Ayurveda and what is being served. Such gaps often fail to find a place in research priorities set for Ayurveda in a global or Indian scenario. In India, because of its failure in perceiving the health-care needs of the people, Ayurveda popularity is found declining recently [23]. The National Sample Survey Organization (NSSO) report 2015, in this regard, is an eye-opener saying that over 90% of Indians now prefer allopathic system of health care comparing to Ayurveda [24]. What global renaissance Ayurveda is observing now should not essentially be equated to regained faith in Ayurveda but, up to some extent, may be a reflection of repeated failures from other health-care approaches, forcing the people to wander at all other possible alternatives [25].

This is noticed that above 85% of health researches lack a translational component and therefore remain practically of no use to the end users hence avoidably wasted [26]. Ayurvedic research, although does not have any such comparable data, seems that it might be poorer than what is being observed in conventional health research. Unfortunately any concern about this lack of translatability and avoidable wastage of public money on Ayurvedic health researches is not apparent in the zone of near sight.

1.3 Translational Research and Translational Effectiveness Research: Road Map for Ayurveda

Translational research differs from the conventional research in one fundamental aspect that it focuses primarily on the immediate utility of the research for human welfare, whereas the latter may look at any aspect of science having an immediate or a remote utility. It is for this reason, a translational research seems focused, multidisciplinary, and goal-oriented aiming to find a solution to a prevailing question related to health care. Conventional research may involve the aspects of translational research along with many other areas of research which may not be of immediate importance but may help in understanding the underlying science better. Translational research therefore is largely patient centric where the problems being faced by every individual frame important research questions and the research methods and protocols are being designed around such questions in order to find their practical solutions. Such problems may be pervasive belonging to a large population or limited belonging to a subpopulation, community, cohort, or an individual. Although it may be affecting a large population, the problem is equally important even if it is affecting a single person.

In Ayurveda, such translational research is needed to be enacted in two essential and complementary manners. One of this is to understand what Ayurvedic classical texts are preaching for. Such approach is required to understand Ayurvedic biology and its various components like essentials of health and disease, methods of remaining away from disease, impact of food in health promotion and disease causation, methods of dealing with a disease, prognostic factors related with a disease, individual susceptibility of disease, etc. Extending the quest further, the enquiry can also be about Ayurvedic pharmacology, methods of dose determination, methods of knowing about pharmacological actions of herbal drug and compound, various formulations, their shelf life, Ayurvedic methods of drug preparation, toxicity, methods of choosing a composition to make a formulation, and methods of large production of a drug required for mass consumption.

Within the purview of drug, herb cultivation, harvest, storage, and processing shall also be evaluated in order to keep the traditionally recommended best practices alive. Similarly, much can further be explored in various other clinical and basic disciplines of Ayurveda. Some important areas among these are *rasayana*, Ayurvedic methods of improving progeny, Ayurvedic toxicology, Ayurvedic geriatrics, and reproductive medicine. Ayurvedic *shalya* and *shalakya* (surgery and ophthalmology) also form an important area for exploration. This textual translational exploration should mean to understand what and how of the elaborations along with a clear understanding of the achievable end point if the protocols are followed religiously as are described in texts. While determining the protocols for practical application of knowledge imbibed in the texts, the textual gaps are also required to be carefully and intelligently identified and researched for the appropriate answers to complete the protocol.

The other part of translational research in Ayurveda is relating to the best practices referring to solve a clinical riddle. This is common observation to Ayurvedic clinical practice that if a patient is identified on the basis of modern diagnostic tools and labeled with modern diagnosis, it becomes difficult to treat him from Ayurvedic perspectives comparing to the situation where he is examined through Ayurvedic principles and prescribed with the drugs on the basis of such examination. This is highly interesting to note that despite similarity of pathogenesis, these different approaches of disease understanding and treatment pay differently. There are a number of case reports in the published literature, referring to the conditions intractable to modern medicine, responding well to Ayurvedic approach of disease understanding and treatments tailored on the basis of such understanding [15, 16, 27–30]. Such clinical success however should act as a lead to subsequent translational research from observation to the exploration of its underlying science so that such success may be repeated on similar cases. This would eventually be the T2 phase of translational research in Ayurveda.

Translational effectiveness research in Ayurveda extends one step ahead of translational research by seeing the intensity of effectiveness having a potential to be translated as a meaningful improvement in patient's life. There can be proven effectiveness in a treatment modality referring to a set of clinical condition although such effectiveness is meaningful only if it brings qualitative changes in the life. Such qualitative changes may come in many forms of which a cost, duration, and dependence reduction may also matter besides real meaningful clinical improvements in a patient. This could be a Patient-Centered Outcomes Research (PCOR) focusing upon what outcome is actually deliverable at the end of the therapy.

Conclusion

Translational research and translational effectiveness research in Ayurveda are probably needed now more than any other time in the history. One important reason for this is that the current model of research in Ayurveda has not done any good to the elevation of the practice standards of Ayurveda. For over a half century of active research in Ayurveda, its clinical practice has not become more dependable, reproducible, and reliable. The clinical observations and subsequent decision making at Ayurveda bedside are still physician-based and not evidence-based with well-defined guidelines. Lack of clarity and protocols in Ayurvedic decision making eventually makes the whole science vulnerable to individual strengths and weaknesses [31]. The results of clinical interventions are therefore largely unpredictable and uncertain. A clearly focused, patient-centric, and well-defined outcome-based research is highly required in Ayurveda to make it user-friendly and dependable. Translational research and translational effectiveness research could be the way forward to this in the near future.

References

1. Chiappelli F. Translational effectiveness in practice-based patient-centered outcomes research. In: Fundamentals of evidence-based health care and translational science. Berlin: Springer; 2014.
2. Rubio DM, et al. Defining translational research: implications for training. Acad Med. 2010;85(3):470–5. https://doi.org/10.1097/ACM.0b013e3181ccd618.
3. National Institutes of Health. Definitions under Subsection 1 (Research Objectives), Section I (Funding Opportunity Description), Part II (Full Text of Announcement), of RFA-RM-07-007: Institutional Clinical and Translational Science Award (U54). Mar 2007. http://grants.nih.gov/grants/guide/rfa-files/RFA-RM-07-007.html. Accessed 25 Mar 2018.
4. National Center for Advancing Translational Science. https://ncats.nih.gov/about.html.
5. Kelkar D, Galwankar S, Kelkar S. Need for encouraging translational research in India. J Emerg Trauma Shock. 2012;5(1):107. https://doi.org/10.4103/0974-2700.93105.
6. National Health Policy 2017. https://mohfw.gov.in/sites/default/files/9147562941489753121.pdf. Last Accessed 12 Apr 2018.
7. Rastogi S. Building bridges between Ayurveda and modern science. Int J Ayurveda Res. 2010;1(1):41–6. https://doi.org/10.4103/0974-7788.59943.
8. Anand A, Rao MRS. Recipe for translational research in India: MD-PhD or PhD-MD. Ann Neurosci. 2013;20(3):85.
9. Gourie-Devi M. Translational research: basic science to health care. Way forward. Ann Indian Acad Neurol. 2013;16:135–6.
10. Ram Manohar P. Research for understanding as opposed to evaluating Ayurveda. Anc Sci Life. 2014;34(2):61–3. https://doi.org/10.4103/0257-7941.153456.
11. Das S, Datta A, Bagchi C, Chakraborty S, Mitra A, Tripathi SK. A comparative study of lipid-lowering effects of guggul and atorvastatin monotherapy in comparison to their combination in high cholesterol diet-induced hyperlipidemia in rabbits. J Diet Suppl. 2016;13(5):495–504. https://doi.org/10.3109/19390211.2015.1118654. Epub 2016 Jan 6.
12. Szapary PO, Wolfe ML, Bloedon LT, Cucchiara AJ, DerMarderosian AH, Cirigliano MD, Rader DJ. Guggulipid for the treatment of hypercholesterolemia: a randomized controlled trial. JAMA. 2003;290(6):765–72.
13. Dwivedi VN. Bhava prakasha nighantu. New Delhi: Moti Lal Banarasi Das; 1988. p. 107.
14. Devarbhavi H. Ayurvedic and herbal medicine-induced liver injury: it is time to wake up and take notice. Indian J Gastroenterol. 2018;37:5. https://doi.org/10.1007/s12664-018-0820-6.
15. Rastogi S, Srivastav PS. Ayurveda in critical care: illustrating ayurvedic intervention in a case of hepatic encephalopathy. Ayu. 2011;32(3):345–8.
16. Rastogi S, Rastogi R. Ayurvedic intervention in Metastatic Liver Disease. J Altern Complement Med. 2012;18(7):719–22.
17. Singh RH. Exploring issues in the development of Ayurvedic research methodology. J Ayurveda Integr Med. 2010;1(2):91–5. https://doi.org/10.4103/0975-9476.65067.
18. Department of Translational Research and Biomedical Research. http://aiia.co.in/department_staff.html. Last Accessed 2 Oct 2017.
19. **T**ranslational **R**esearch and **I**nnovative **S**cience **ThR**ough **A**yurgenomics. http://www.trisutra.in/.
20. Extra Mural Research, Ministry of AYUSH, Govt. of India. http://ayush.gov.in/schemes/extra-mural-research.
21. Patwardhan BK, Jogelkar V, Pathak N, Vaidya ADB. Vaidya-scientists: catalysing the Ayurveda renaissance. Curr Sci. 2011;100(4):476–83.

22. Rastogi S. Looking at prescription quality in Ayurveda: developing, validating and pilot testing a prescription quality index for Ayurveda. J Ayurveda Integr Med. 2017. https://doi.org/10.1016/j.jaim.2017.02.008. pii: S0975-9476(17)30003-7. [Epub ahead of print].
23. Singh M. Times News Network. The Times of India. Jul 8 2015. http://www.timesofindia.indiatimes.com/india/90-of-Indiansprefer-allopathy-over-AYUSH/articleshow/47981441.cms. Last Accessed 10 Apr 2018.
24. Singh RH. Declining popularity of AYUSH, the recent report of National Sample Survey Organisation. Ann Ayurvedic Med. 2015;4(1–2):2–4.
25. Rastogi S. Principle and practice of Ayurvedic rheumatology. Delhi: Chaukhambha Sanskrit Pratishthan; 2010.
26. Chalmers I, Glasziou P. Avoidable waste in the production and reporting of research evidence. Lancet. 2009;374(9683):86–9.
27. Rastogi S. Rehabilitative potential of Ayurveda upon neurological deficits caused by traumatic spinal cord injury (SCI): a case report. J Ayurveda Integr Med. 2014;5(1):56–9.
28. Rastogi S, Chaudhari P. Pigment reduction in nevus of Ota following leech therapy. J Ayurveda Integr Med. 2014;5:125–8.
29. Rastogi S, Chaudhari P. Ayurvedic management of achalasia. J Ayurveda Integr Med. 2015;6:41–4.
30. Rastogi S. Low pressure low flow voiding dysfunction in an elderly male treated through ayurveda: a case report. J Evid Based Complementary Altern Med. 2017;22(4):846–50.
31. Rastogi S, Chiappelli F, Ramchandani MH, Singh RH, editors. Evidence-based practice in complementary and alternative medicine: perspectives, protocols, problems and potential in Ayurveda. Berlin: Springer; 2012.

Translational Studies on Fundamental Principles of Ayurveda from Book to Bedside

2

Ram H. Singh

2.1 Introduction

Ayurveda is the oldest system of life science and health care based on its own fundamental principles originating from India. It was the world view of its time, but it shrank to India alone due to rapid emergence of European medicine in colonial India [1]. Now it is re-globalizing again because of its potential to enrich the mainstream of world medicine. This upsurge is faced with a global demand of evidence-based practice of Ayurvedic medicine. This can happen only if Ayurveda is subjected to intensive translational studies on its different aspects specially the fundamental principles bringing it down to the practice settings [2].

Ayurveda is to be studied for its science and therapeutics simultaneously. Science of Ayurveda is to be viewed from both angles, i.e., its physics and biology, explaining their meaning and understanding of the applications in professional sector, hence the connotation "from book to bedside of a patient [3]."

Ayurvedic physics begins with the concept of *Ayurvedavataran* and *Sristikrama*, i.e., evolution of the universe. The sequence of events to be traced are the *Mula Prakriti*, the *Trigunas (sattva, raja, tama)*, the evoluting Five *Tanmatras*, and the grossifying *Panchmahabhutas* through the ancient technology of *Panch-panchikaran*. All these can be explained and understood by application of *Tantrayuktis*. The *Tantrayukti* is the linguistic technology to reach the real meaning of classical textual descriptions [4]. There are 12 *Tantrayuktis*, viz., (1) *Adhikarana*, (2) *Yoga*, (3) *Hetwartha*, (4) *Padarth*, (5) *Pradesha*, (6) *Uddesha*, (7) *Nirdesha*, (8) *Wakyashesha*, (9) *Prayojana*, (10) *Upadesha*, (11) *Apadesha*, and (12) *Atidesha.*

But the *Tantrayukti* technology is largely used to understand the textual meaning of classical statements. For further translational studies, the outcome of *Tantrayukti* exercise needs more newer scientific methodology of material and biomedical

R. H. Singh
Department of Kaya Chikitsa, Faculty of Ayurveda, Institute of Medical Sciences, Banaras Hindu University, Varanasi, India

S. Rastogi (ed.), *Translational Ayurveda*, https://doi.org/10.1007/978-981-13-2062-0_2

sciences. The current trend is to use rating scales of the functions of the body and the symptoms of a disease to translate the subjective observations into mathematical mode [5]. Later in this chapter, I shall illustrate this point with some simple experimental observations. Besides rating scales a range of indicators and biomarkers are to be developed for each of the major biofactors described in Ayurvedic classics.

2.2 Translational Studies

Research is the prime need of Ayurveda today to bring it in the mainstream of evidence-based generic medical knowledge system. There has been long drawn controversy about the mode of research as whether it should be done with classical or with contemporary methods. The current medical research is largely biomechanical and measurement based using statistical designs and tools. Measurement and mathematical database is the characteristic need of current research with potential to lead to practical applications. Consensus is that classical methodology unless lashed with scientific measurement tools is of mere historical significance and is not dynamic and is unproductive. On the other hand, many experts believe that insistence on using mere modern medical research tools in Ayurveda as also other traditional knowledge systems is a major postcolonial conspiracy against traditional wisdom like Ayurveda and is an attempt to wind up traditional systems by pooling all the good and easily viable wisdom into the mainstream contemporary sciences leaving behind static philosophic principles which may not be suitable for useful translational studies and reverse innovation [6]. To me the mid way deem appropriate meaning that the base line and the goal of research have to be classical and the methodological tools have to be contemporary and science based. This idea is reflected in the very emblem of Banaras Hindu University.

Ayurveda is characterized by three important features which make it a very special system of medicine. These are (1) *pronature* approach, (2) comprehensive *holistic* approach, and (3) *personalized* care approach based on *Prakriti-Vikriti* considerations. The clinical research methodology has to be tuned with this trio approach [7]. The following is the scheme of ancient classical research methodology.

The Classical Methods

1. *Structure and function of the body* is studied by cadaver dissection as described by Susruta in *Sharira Sthana* in big details to identify the organs and structures of the body and their connections forming systems of physiology [8]. Caraka describes 13 such major systems or *Sthula Srotamsi*, viz., *Annavaha*, etc. The measurements were done by *Angul praman*, and the fluids were measured in *Anjali/Ardhanjali* or *astabindu pramana* besides *Chaturvidh Praman Vijnan—Pratyaksa* (direct observation), *Anuman* (inference), *Aptopadesha* (textual testimony), and *Yukti Praman* (experimental evidence) [9].
2. *The functions of the body were* studied in terms of the regulated and the regulator factors such as *Tridosha, viz., Vata, Pitta, and Kapha; Sapta dhatus, viz., rasa,*

rakta, mamsa, meda, asthi, majja, and shukra; the *Ojas* and the *Ojabala*, viz., *sahaja, kalaj, and yuktikrit;* and the *Baladoshas—vyapat, visransha,* and *kshaya*. The *Tridosha* are the regulators, while the rest of the other components of biol ogy are the relatively passive regulated factors. Equally important is the concept of *Agni* and *Agnibala bheda, Amadosha.* The *Srotamsi* or the inner transport system of the living body forms another important component of human biology. The *Shastra* is interpreted by appropriately applying the 12 *Tantrayuktis* which are essentially the classical linguistic technology designed for this subtle matter.

3. *The biomarkers* are quantified applying the relative pattern of 20 *Gurvadi Gunas* (physical properties) in relation to the theory of *Samanya and visesa ie* homology vs heterology—*Sarvada sarva bhawanam samanyam vriddhi karananm, Hrasa heturvisesah, Ubhayastu ubhayarth krit* (Caraka su. chapter 1) [10].
4. *Clinical methods and diagnostics* It comprise of 1. *Rogi-Roga Pariksa* methods including *Rogi* (patient) *Pariksa/*examination, viz., (1) *Prakriti*, (2) *Vikriti*, (3) *Sara*, (4) *Samhanan*, (5) *Pramana*, (6) *Sattva*, (7) *Satmya*, (8) *Ahara Sakti*, (9) *Vyayama Sakti*, and (10) *Vaya/Vayikarana* or aging and *Roga* (disease) *Pariksa/*examination through *Asthvidh Pariksa*, viz., (1) *Nadi*, (2) *Mutra*, (3) *Mala*, (4) *Jihwa*, (5) *Shabda*, (6) *Sparsha*, (7) *Drik*, (8) *Akriti* besides *Trayodashavidha (13) Srotas Pariksa/*examination.
5. *Chikitsa* through *Samshodhan* and *Sanshaman* and *Shadupakrama*, viz., (1) *Ruksana*, (2) *Snehan*, (3) *Svedana*, (4) *Stambhan*, (5) *Langhan*, and (6) *rimhana—all these biofactors* are studied interfacing 20 *Gurvadi Gunas* relative to the doctrine of *Samanya snd Visesa*, i.e., homology vs heterology or similarity vs dissimilarity.
6. *Pharmacology and materia medica*—Ayurveda uses the materia medica drawn from nature, i.e., plant kingdom, minerals, animal products, and marine products suitably processed in special dosage forms such as *Saras*, *Kalka*, *Churna*, *Putpaka*, *Phant*, *Kwath*, *Ghana*, *Vati*, *Gutika*, *Avaleha*, *Khand*, *Modaka*, *Ashava-Arista*, *Bhasma*, *Pisti*, etc. singly or in combinations, pure herbal, herbomineral, etc. There is mention of sophisticated system of pharmaceutics, posology, and toxicity assessment of products. The pharmacology is tested through *Rasa*, *Guns*, *Virya*, *Vipaka*, and *Prabhava* of the constituent ingredients largely on subjective and qualitative basis warranting modernization now.

The Contemporary Integrative Trends—The Contemporary trend is to follow the broad principles of Ayurveda and lash it with suitable modern tools, indicators, and biomarkers as well as symptom/function rating scales to measure the changes occurring under the impact of a pathology or the effect of a trial treatment administered [11]. Because of time and space constraint, only some examples based on my own study are reproduced below.

Prakriti and Nadi Pariksa—*Dosha Prakriti* and *Nadi* are the two most important components of Ayurvedic diagnostics. *Dosha Prakriti* is the sum total of physique, physiology, and psychology of an individual expressed in terms of the range of proportion of the three *doshas—vata*, *pitta*, *kapha*—in the genetic format of the

Table 2.1 The traits of *Doṣa Prakṛti* (psychophysical constitution)

	Vāta type	*Pitta* type	*Kapha* type
Physique	Small body frame Lean and thin	Medium body frame Muscular body	Big body frame Obese body
Physiology	Weak and sickly Unstable physiology Pulse: fast rate, low volume, low pitch	Good appetite, digestion Dynamic Pulse: high pitch, medium rate, medium volume	Stable, strong Good immunity Pulse: high volume, medium pitch, slow rate
Psyche	Nervous, irritable Talkative	Sharp, intelligent, dynamic, hot temper	Jovial, friendly, slow, comfortable

The mixed constitutions will have mixed features

Table 2.2 The *Tridoshic* rhythm in *Nadi* (pulse)

Determining *Doṣa*	Rate/ rhythm	Amplitude	Volume	Simile	Rhythm form
Vāta	Markedly rapid	Very low	Very low	Crawling pulse *Sarpagati*	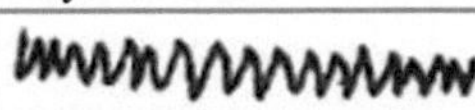
Pitta	Moderately rapid	Maximum	Medium	Jumping pulse *Manḍukagati*	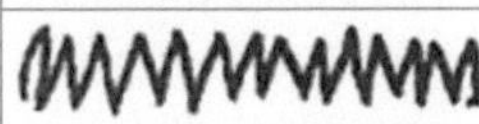
Kapha	Slow	Medium	High	Walking pulse *Hamsa gati*	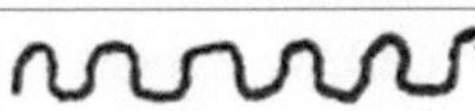

individual representing his genetically determined psychophysical personality as shown in the following table. *Nadi Pariksa* is done to examine the *tridoshic* rhythm of the *three gatis* of the *Nadi*, i.e., the pulse of an individual. The characteristic features are displayed in graphic below (Tables 2.1 and 2.2).

2.2.1 Measuring the *Agni* and the *Ojas* Status

A precise evaluation of *Ojas* status/*Oja Bala* is an important component of clinical assessment in Ayurvedic practice. The exact measurement of *Oja Bala* is difficult. Often it is measured in terms of the rate of *Ojas* depletion with negative scoring. With the spirit of examining Ayurvedic biology as it is the author of this communication is inclined to suggest that a semi-objective rating scale should be developed on the basis of classical descriptions of the functions of *Ojas*. The most appropriate such description is found in Susruta Samhita Sutra Sthana chapter 15 which is quoted below. These verses have been converted into rating scales for this purpose.

तत्र बलेन स्थिरोपचितमांसता सर्वचेष्टास्वप्रतिघातः स्वरवर्णप्रसादो बाह्यानामाभ्यन्तराणां च
करणानामात्मकार्यप्रतिपत्तिर्भवति ।।

Susruta Samhita. Sutra Sthana15:20

A rating scale based on this statement by the author is presented below along with a sample data which was generated to validate the rating scale. The sample data is reproduced below for ready reference.

The *Agni status* is the next important aspect of Ayurvedic biology which is often taken into account in the study of the quality of health and in the assessment of the therapeutic efficacy of the medication. The concept of *Agni* is very complex, and it is difficult to identify a real biomarker for its assessment. Hence the author is inclined to suggest developing a rating scale on the basis of the negative and positive functions of *Agni* as described in Ayurvedic texts. In our assessment the following statement of Caraka Samhita occurring in Caraka Vimana Sthana Chapter 8 verse 89 is most relevant. A tentative rating scale developed on the basis of this classical description is reproduced below along with a sample data in clinical settings generated over a series of patient of diabetes mellitus before and after treatment with an Ayurvedic formulation as an effort to validate the rating scale for its suitability (Tables 2.3, 2.4, and 2.5). However, both these scales need to be standardized further before they are accepted as a standard measure of assessment of *Oja Bala* and *Agni Bala*, respectively.

कार्यं धातुसाम्यं, तस्य लक्षणं विकारोपशमः। परीक्षा त्वस्य-रुगुपशमनं, स्वरवर्णयोगः, शरीरोपचयः, बलवृद्धिः, अभ्यवहार्याभिलाषः, रुचिराहारकाले, अभ्यवहृतस्य चाहारस्य काले सम्यग्जरणं, निद्रालाभो यथाकालं, वैकारिणां च स्वप्नानामदर्शनं, सुखेन च प्रतिबोधनं, वातमूत्रपुरीषरेतसां मुक्तिः, सर्वाकारैर्मनोबुद्धीन्द्रियाणां चाव्यापत्तिरिति ।।८९।।

Caraka Samhita Vimana Sthana 8:89

Table 2.3 *Ojas* status rating scale (1-2-3-4)

S. no.	Grading of features of *Ojas* status	Scores
1.	*Sthiropacita Mamsata* (stable strong muscles)	1-2-3-4
2.	*Svara Prasada* (graseous voice)	1-2-3-4
3.	*Varna Prasada* (Luster of skin)	1-2-3-4
4.	*Tvak* (Sense of touch)	1-2-3-4
5.	*Caksu* (Power of vision)	1-2-3-4
6.	*Srotra* (Sense of hearing)	1-2-3-4
7.	*Jihva* (Sense of taste)	1-2-3-4
8.	*Ghrana* (Sense of smell)	1-2-3-4
9.	*Payu* (Bowel function)	1-2-3-4
10.	*Upastha* (Mutrendriya function)	1-2-3-4
11.	*Upastha* (Jananendriya function)	1-2-3-4
12.	*Mana* and *Buddhi* (Psychological status)	1-2-3-4
13.	*Bala* (Physical strength)	1-2-3-4
14.	*Vyadhi* (Disease propensity)	1-2-3-4

Table 2.4 *Agni* status rating scale (0–3)

S. no.	Grading of features of *Agni* status	Scores
1.	Appearance of normal voice	0-1-2-3
2.	Appearance of normal complexion	0-1-2-3
3.	Nourishment of the body	0-1-2-3
4.	Physical strength	0-1-2-3
5.	Desire for taking food	0-1-2-3
6.	Appetite for food during meal time	0-1-2-3
7.	Proper digestion of food	0-1-2-3
8.	Normal and regular sleep	0-1-2-3
9.	Feeling of well-being	0-1-2-3
10.	Proper and timely evacuation of *Vāta*	0-1-2-3
11.	Proper and timely evacuation of *Mūtra*	0-1-2-3
12.	Proper and timely evacuation of *Purīṣa*	0-1-2-3
13.	Proper and timely evacuation of *Retas* (Libido)	0-1-2-3
14.	Status of mind and intellect	0-1-2-3

Table 2.5 Impact of an Ayurvedic medication on blood sugar PP and *Ojas* and *Agni* status in diabetics

	Blood sugar PP mean ± SD		Negative Ojas score mean ± SD		Agni status score mean ± SD	
Groups	BT	AT	BT	AT	BT	AT
Group A ($n = 33$) only Ay. drug	266.40 ± 71.77	209.40 ± 52.12	10.07 ± 8.45	6.07 ± 6.09	4.94 ± 3.27	0.55 ± 0.62
Group B ($n = 23$) add Ay. Drug	242.90 ± 41.38	178.07 ± 24.97	8.21 ± 6.21	5.42 ± 5.37	4.61 ± 4.36	1.09 ± 1.44
Group C ($n = 28$) control	237.60 ± 29.00	225.40 ± 31.32	9.50 ± 7.90	9.15 ± 7.34	5.11 ± 3.47	3.39 ± 2.33

2.3 The *Srotovijnan* and Inner Transport System

Besides the *Tridosha*, *Saptdhatus*, *Ojas*, and *Agni*, another major component of Ayurvedic biology is the *Srotas* system which denotes the entire inner transport system of the body. According to Ayurveda there are innumerable micro channels in the body which are called *Srotas* [12]. According to Caraka, besides the micro channels there are 13 gross channels which represent different physiological systems as also known today. These channels need periodical cleansing and biopurification which is done through selective *Panchkarma* therapy though every cell of the body is washed to restore their integrity. The major risk factor for integrity of *Srotas* system is the *Ama Dosha* present in the body due to depletion of *Agni*. The other risk factors are pollution with ingested and inhaled toxic substances besides the debris of daily wear and tear in the body due to disease, infection, and aging process. As these events are frequent, we do need frequent periodical cleansing; hence the science of *Samshodhan* and *Panchkarma* therapy was designed [13]. These procedures

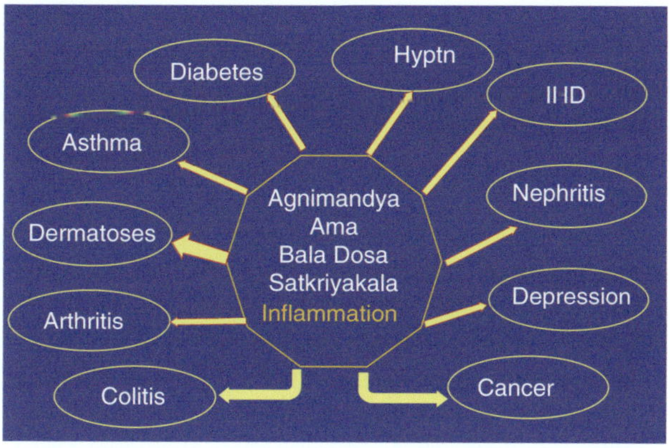

Fig. 2.1 Proposing Ayurvedic fundamental of pathogenesis for modern diagnosis

are useful even in modern therapy of patients. Therefore many Allopathic doctors also practice *Panchkarma* therapy today.

2.4 *Shatkriyakal*: The Unified Single Pathways of All Diseases

The Ayurvedic concept of *Shatkriyakal* or six stages of evolution of a disease denotes the single unified multiphasic pathway of all diseases (Fig. 2.1). Ayurveda describes these six phases in terms of *Tridoshic* response to diurnal and seasonal variations as well as the variety of aetiological factors of different diseases. Accordingly the *Kriyakalas* are considered to be of two kinds, viz., (1) *Ritu Kriyakala* and (2) *Vyadhi Kriyakala*. This ancient concept is very similar to the recent understanding in modern medicine that all diseases are basically a kind of inflammation. In other words inflammation is the single unified pathway of all pathologies.

2.5 Structure and Function of the Body

In ancient times the structure of the human body was studied by systematic cadaver dissection. Susruta was the first in the history who did cadaver dissection and who identified the relations and interconnections of different organs and systems. Subsequently, 13 gross channels/*Srotamsi* were identified by Caraka simulating different physiological systems of the living body known today as the digestive system, circulatory system, etc. Susruta did not use a knife and scalpel to dissect the cadaver; he used fine brush to dissect the structures layer by layer and identified fine structures more precisely [14]. I wonder if such techniques are used today too. Ayurveda besides organic anatomy believed more on humoral approach bridging the gap between structure and function. The main humors were the three *Doshas*, namely, *vata*, *pitta*, and *kapha*, the seven *Dhatus*, or the primordial tissues, both liquid and solid. Ayurveda also identified the quint essence of all *Dhatus* called *Ojas* which is responsible for the biostrength and immune strength of the body. Thirteen kinds of *Agni* or bio-fire system were described to deliberate on the entire process of digestion and metabolism.

Conclusion

Translational studies are necessary to reduce the gap between traditional and contemporary sciences and practices. Ayurveda conceives of many elegant theories and concepts which are often seen running parallel to the practice of medicine and have not remained much dynamic to the applied field of medical practice [15]. This gap between theory and practice causes loss of credibility of so sound theories, and hence many youngsters are tempted to replace the core Ayurvedic methodology with relatively weaker pure modern methods. This is a situation of a showdown, and there is a risk of complete loss of the so valuable ancient wisdom. Hence the present attempt of translational studies and reverse innovation is worth. The present study indicates that there is a rich scope of such studies. Pilot experimental studies on *Prakriti*, *Nadi*, *Agni*, *Ojas*, and *Rasayana* will reveal the fact.

References

1. Bala P. Knowing Ayurveda: historical and cultural reflections. Ann Ayurvedic Med. 2014;3(3–4):69–71.
2. Singh RH. Perspectives in innovation in the AYUSH sector. J Ayurveda Integr Med. 2011;2(2):52–4. https://doi.org/10.4103/0975-9476.82516.
3. Rastogi S. From book to bedside: challenges of translating Ayurvedic science of food and nutrition for the common benefits. In: Rastogi S, editor. Ayurvedic science of food and nutrition. New York: Springer; 2014.
4. Singh RH. In: Proceeding of National conference on Ancient Research Methodology. Bharat Adhyayan Kendra, B.H.U, Varanasi; 2017.
5. Singh RH. Exploring issues in the development of Ayurvedic research methodology. J Ayurveda Integr Med. 2010;1(2):91–5. https://doi.org/10.4103/0975-9476.65067.
6. Kessler CS. Internationalizing Ayurveda research: wash me but don't get me wet. Ann Ayurvedic Med. 2015;4(1–2):5–7.
7. Singh RH. Holistic principles of Ayurvedic medicine. Varanasi: Chaukhamba Surbharti Prakashan; 2003.
8. Sharma PV, editor. Sushruta Samhita. 1st ed. Varanasi: Chaukhamba Vishvabharati, Oriental Publishers and Distributors; 2015.
9. Sharma PV, editor. Charaka Samhita of Agnivesh, vol. 1-4. Varanasi/Delhi: Chaukhamba Orientalia Publication; 2015.
10. Bashist G, et al. Charaka Samhita, Online edition. Orlando: Spirit of India Publication; 2017.
11. Patwardhan B. Bridging Ayurveda with evidence-based scientific approaches in medicine. EPMA J. 2014;5(1):19.
12. Valiathan MS. Ayurvedic biology: a decadal vision document. Bengaluru: Indian Academy of Science; 2006.
13. Singh RH. Panchkarma therapy. Varanasi/Delhi: Chaukhamba Publications; 1992.
14. Loukas M, Lanteri A, Ferrauiola J, et al. Anatomy in ancient India: a focus on the Susruta Samhita. J Anat. 2010;217(6):646–50. https://doi.org/10.1111/j.1469-7580.2010.01294.x.
15. Singh RH. Ayurveda in India today. In: WHO Publication Proc. Symposium of traditional Medicine. Japan: WHO; 2002.

Translational Potential of Ayurveda *Prakriti*: Concepts in the Area of Personalized Medicine

3

J. Douglas Coffin, Rammohan Rao, and Diana I. Lurie

3.1 The Ayurvedic Approach as Personalized Medicine

Ayurveda was founded in ancient Hindu spiritual and medicinal paradigms that encompass all aspects of human existence integrated with nature. Five thousand years ago, or even five hundred years ago, humans had no concept of cells, proteins, DNA, or chromosomes. However, over those millennia, the Hindu culture had powerful means of observation and for recording both their philosophy and their observations of human behavior and biology. Hence, the *Charaka Samhita* (ancient Sanskrit Ayurvedic text) was developed, describing a system of medicine, Ayurveda, that was founded on inheritance of traits as (www.yinyoga.com [23]) *doshas* (the three types of energies that define each person) through *prakriti* in a spiritual sense that incorporated the Hindu philosophies of self, nature, procreation, and reincarnation (www.charaksamitaayurveda.com [22]).

Ayurveda focuses on the individual and the natural progression of a healthy existence in this life. The inherited *doshic* properties prescribe a unique Ayurvedic approach to health, wellness, and longevity (*Rasayana*). A positive, integrated interaction with nature is inherent in life and lifestyle. Based on their *doshic* constitution or *prakriti* as *Vata*, *Pitta*, or *Kapha*, the individual makes daily, weekly, seasonal and even life-stage adjustments to their food consumption, behavior, and environment. The goal is to cleanse the body of toxins and return it to its optimal, natural state through constitution-specific: diet, exercise, lifestyle practices, mantras, and natural product-based medications [1, 2]. The emphasis is on wellness and disease prevention for the individual as they progress through life [3].

J. D. Coffin (✉) · D. I. Lurie
Skaggs School of Pharmacy, The University of Montana, Missoula, MT, USA
e-mail: douglas.coffin@umontana.edu

R. Rao
Faculty, California College of Ayurveda, Nevada City, CA, USA

S. Rastogi (ed.), *Translational Ayurveda*, https://doi.org/10.1007/978-981-13-2062-0_3

Ayurveda incorporates the six philosophies of *Shad Darshan* for the healing of mankind. *Sankhya* philosophy (that deals with the material world) describes the principles of creation and the evolution of consciousness into matter. The first concept in *Sankhya* philosophy details *purusha* and *prakriti*. *Purusha* is considered to be pure consciousness, energy, and ultimate enlightenment. *Prakriti* is primordial matter, will, and creative potential [4]. *Prakriti* cannot exist without *purusha*, and *prakriti* is considered to be the feminine energy out of which the entire universe is born. Hence, the ancient philosophers ascribed the male as *purusha* and the female as *prakriti*. These were not biological but spiritual and abstract terms. The *prakriti* female is viewed as "mother earth" endowed with maternal characteristics as an agent of procreation in a changing domain. The *purusha* male is one who endures, creates, and endows as the masculine agent of physical strength and power (www.yinyoga.com).

The Hindu religion is hardly monolithic, so there are numerous interpretations, but these descriptions are fairly common and have the most biological relevance. *Prakriti* is described as the female component of sexual reproduction in humans. Thus, *prakriti* represents the superior female power and force—*Shakti*. *Prakriti* is dormant yet dynamic and is the primordial seed potential that evolves into all material forms—*Pravritti*. The observant Hindus knew nothing of physical chromosomes or genes, but they intuitively recognized that traits were passed from parents to their offspring. Likewise, they understood that sexual intercourse between males and females resulted in pregnancy. Thus, we can begin to make connections between *Sankhya* philosophy and modern genetics.

Out of *purusha* and *prakriti* evolves *Mahat* (creative intelligence). *Mahat* is supreme intelligence, that inner and innate wisdom and intelligence that permeates all things. This innate intelligence is a set of cosmic rules, regulations, and laws that govern the process of evolution. The relevance here is the idea that even a single cell has intelligence and its own unique function. This defines the unique function of each cell analogous to a cellular phenotype. One could pursue that interpretation from a genetic perspective, *Mahat* could translate into "genomics" akin to the "cellular intelligence" of our DNA and those proteins that are transcribed to give each cell its individualized function.

From *Mahat*, *Ahamkara* evolves as the ego, the sense of self [5] consistent with the genotypic and phenotypic variations or polymorphisms at the individual level. Hindu philosophers invoked *Ahamkara* to explain an individual's physical and mental behavior, daily dispositions, likes, dislikes, desires, and temperament. *Ahamkara* manifests a cell's basic identity (phenotype) that remains relatively constant, but is subjected to metabolic variations through lifestyle modifications and transformations.

Sankhya philosophy ascribes the human constitution to consciousness that breaks into three *gunas* (universal qualities) of *sattva* (pure essence of light, spirituality, right actions) *rajas* (principle of movement and change), and *tamas* (inertia and darkness). Our mind and bodies are influenced by these three universal qualities, and these *gunas* are present in all things and at the basic cellular level [5]. Through their potential qualities, the *gunas* (traits) shape the basic behavior of the cell, providing it with a specific identity and purity (*sattva)*; governing metabolism, movement, and cellular transformation (*rajas*); and enabling them to enter a quiescent state (*tamas*) when needed.

Furthermore, Ayurvedic philosophy attributes human existence and spirituality to an entire cosmos based on interacting energies of five elements: ether, air, fire, water, and earth. Different combinations of one or more of these elements constitute all material manifestations. Every cell in the body has all five elements, albeit in different proportions. These five elements manifest into three *dosha*s, basic types of energies that are found in everyone and everything. The *dosha*s represent different regulatory aspects within an organism including metabolic pathways involving numerous enzymes. Thus, if genes are inherited, then so are metabolic pathways with multiple enzymes.

Although the inheritance of enzymes and complex metabolic pathways is difficult to comprehend, the concept of *prakriti* has made it easy to identify pathways and genes that regulate certain diseases [1]. From a physiological and genetic perspective, one could say that all three *dosha*s and *gunas* are present in everyone, but how they are expressed individually is dependent on both DNA polymorphisms and protein expression. Overall, without knowledge of cells and molecular biology, the rudimentary concepts of human biology, form, and function are recognizable in the ancient foundations of Ayurveda and Hindu philosophy.

While Ayurveda recognizes inheritance of traits and characteristics, it also provides for how they are manifest in a lifestyle and life-span. The *prakriti* or constitution is evaluated by the Ayurvedic practitioner using an examination with algorithms that lead to a final diagnosis. The determination of *prakriti* in Ayurveda is at the core of personalized medicine since *prakriti*-based medicine has the potential to offer remedies for adverse health issues including severe drug reactions, drug withdrawal, and drug-induced complications. This approach can also be used to predict the effectiveness of drugs on the individual akin to western pharmacogenetics [6].

Therefore, Ayurveda holds promise whereby *prakriti* exams can be used to correlate behavior and physiology with genomic polymorphisms [7, 8]. As correlations between polymorphisms and the *dosha*s become valid, so can these constitutional exams be refined to improve those physiological-genomic connections. This suggests a bright future for Ayurveda and "Ayurgenetics" [9] whereby the personalized medicine embedded in Ayurveda by the Hindu culture over thousands of years can be merged with western genomics. This approach could optimize natural health and wellness, but also provide diagnostic and therapeutic regimens that are unique to the individual as east meets west [10].

3.2 Traditional "Western" Medical Approach

The natural history of western culture regarding health and medicine is profoundly different from Ayurveda. From the ancient western civilizations forward, western medicine began with technology development and a focus on understanding the form and function of the human body. Western scholastics that focused on learning the anatomical basis and physiological function of the human body are founded in Greek philosophy and expanded in the scholarly approaches to learning in a socioeconomic environment that was profoundly different from the eastern Hindu and Buddhist cultures. The great plagues that swept through Europe dictated that those technologies must be directed toward understanding the biological basis for the dread diseases and developing cures for them to the benefit of the human race.

Hippocrates is considered the "Father of Medicine" in the west based on his practice, school, and writings on clinical medicine. Indeed, the "Hippocratic oath" remains a foundation of modern western medicine. This contextual history often mentions the practice of medicine by the Egyptians and Chinese, but rarely includes the ancient Hindu medical history and Ayurveda.

Further insights into western medical history provide a context for its evolution with an approach that focuses on treatment by disease classification, a pathocentric approach. First is the societal context of medicine as a discipline, taught in schools as a philosophical approach toward advancing medical knowledge for the benefit of the society at large. Second came the rise of the Holy Roman Empire that stifled much of that scientific advance by placing church doctrine above either science or medicine.

Third came the plagues of the middle ages and the epidemics including cholera, small pox, malaria, and other dread diseases that presented pressing public health challenges to the scientific and medical establishments at the technologically oriented western medical universities. As city-states grew through the Renaissance, the dense populations and the opening of trade routes from Europe to Asia and Africa brought about the spread of new viral, parasitic and bacterial public health challenges. These placed public health at the forefront in western society, over personalized medicine.

The term "doctor" in the west literally means "teacher" as one who studies the science of medicine, teaches students in schools, spreads medical/scientific knowledge for the public, and practices medicine for public health. The Ayurvedic equivalent is and always has been a "practitioner" who administers personalized medicine to individuals [3] on a local level. The western doctors were often institutionalized, associated with churches, hospital, and universities. However, the more rural physicians, particularly in the United States through the mid-twentieth century, served as "family doctors" who made house calls and often practiced a more personalized medicine, closer to Ayurveda. The rural family doctor concept later faded in favor of the institutional approach that is prevelant in western medicine today.

The study of western medicine and public health from academic, scientific foundations and the advance of western academic medical centers led to huge technological breakthroughs to treat the dread diseases that plagued the city-states. One of first great breakthroughs was the microscope (c1600) that allowed both identification of microscopic pathogens and descriptions of the cellular, microscopic ultrastructure of the human body. This was followed by vaccines and antibiotics. Pesticides and public health advances with sewage treatment, fresh drinking water, and food safety have controlled the disease vectors. These public health improvements led to a dramatic increase in life-spans for the technologically advanced countries (www.ourworldindata.org [24]). The life expectancy of pre-eighteenth-century humans was less than 40 years. Then, both clinical and public health advances expanded life expectancy to nearly 50 years at the turn of the twentieth century.

Bacterial infection was still the greatest cause of early death in the early twentieth century populations, that was later mitigated with the advent of antibiotics. The antibiotic breakthrough expanded life-spans to nearly 70 years by the 1950s as further advances in public health and occupational safety continued. The post-World War II era brought about remarkable breakthroughs in molecular biology, diagnostics, pharmacology, and therapeutics.

The evolution of western medicine in a scientific and technological milieu is understandable given the juxtaposition of its Greek foundation, its home in university medical schools, and the continuous public health challenges presented by the spread of pathogens as plagues. Non-western medicine, such as Ayurveda, Chinese medicine, and medical practices in hunter-gatherer or local agricultural, non-city-state settings evolved differently. The cultural emphasis was on personal treatment of the individual who became sick or injured. The practitioners passed down medicine for diagnostics, therapeutics, and pharmacology through generations as apprenticeships for individual learning from person to person. Schools in nations such as India (and China) were not often aligned with the technological universities. Hence, the emphasis on tradition and personalized medicine remained with a foundation in Hindu philosophy and Indian culture.

Human life expectancy in many "underdeveloped nations" has not advanced at the western pace. Indeed, the life-span in "third world" underdeveloped nations remains at pre-World War II levels compared to the "developed" nations of the "west." A lack of fresh drinking water from poor public health facilities still present dysentery, brought about by inadequate sewage disposal, as the major public health problem. Vaccines and pharmaceuticals are often unavailable to prevent and treat infection. Poor food safety combined with the lack of comprehensive public health and health care strategies is the greatest challenge (www.ourworldindata.org).

The twenty-first-century march in technology-based western medicine continues with fact-based intellectual medical science that utilizes hypothesis testing. There is an intentional exclusion of anything spiritual or religious for diagnostics and therapeutics. Information from study of the human body and physical condition is continuously compiled, as it was from its ancient beginnings by brilliant biomedical scientists. New advances are continuously integrated into modern western medicine that constitutes a seemingly miraculous infinite drive toward unlocking the infinitesimal and comprehensive secrets of human physiology and pathology.

However, that technological revolution has brought western health care into the personalized medicine domain. First, there is the recognition that each individual person has a predisposition to a subset of the major diseases. Second, pharmacogenetics is based on individual efficacy for drugs that were previously believed to work uniformly across the population. Then, individual diet, lifestyle, and behavioral and occupational influences are found to have a profound impact on the individual and, hence, public health and welfare. Ayurveda recognized this from the start [11], bringing eastern and western medicine to a nexus where the traditional Ayurvedic philosophy can benefit western medicine and the western technologies can be applied to Ayurveda through the scope of personalized medicine.

3.3 Genetics in Medicine, Health, and Wellness

Personalized medicine [3] is based on heredity that is, in turn, based on genetics with principles that are illustrated in Fig. 3.1. The human life cycle is at the core of this paradigm. Hindus, like many other cultures, observed that sexual intercourse produced human offspring that have characteristics of, but are not identical to their parents. The Hindus adopted and adapted by accepting the biological reality of embryology and human development both *in utero* and post-partition, combined with genetics and inheritance of traits. *Purusha* and *prakriti* represent the union of gametes and *Mahat*; the cellular intelligence in DNA is analogous to the informational genome. The resulting *Ahamkara* as the offspring "self" equates to an individual phenotype with unique combinations of *gunas* and energetic elements as traits [2, 12].

Thus, the term *prakriti* has evolved to describe heredity in the context of the Ayurvedic human life cycle where *prakriti* transfers *dosha*s and *gunas* as traits to offspring that provide each individual with a unique *doshic* combination. *Prakriti* has unique behavioral and physiological characteristics that constitute the individual, and also cohorts in the population, based on the "universality" in the spiritual connotations for the terms.

However, the biological central dogma provides that those behavioral and physiological characteristics are encoded by the individual's unique genome. This brings us right to the frontiers of Ayurgenetics (or Ayurgenomics; [6, 9]) whereby heredity—*prakriti*—transfers/encodes a *doshic* combination. Several studies have now demonstrated the link of the *tridoshic* theory with various metabolic systems and biomarkers as genomic linkages [13, 14].

Within the context of the Hindu religion, *prakriti* and *tridoshic* inheritance became the core of their medical philosophy and the foundation of Ayurveda. Personalized, western medicine emerged with the genetic revolution of the late twentieth century. Western medical and biological technology found the physiological foundation for the human life cycle in cells, chromosomes, genes, and DNA. This knowledge is now the foundation of the newly minted twenty-first-century medicinal practice of Clinical Medical Genetics.

The genetic revolution is really a recent event grounded in the technological advances of the last 150 years. It began much like the ancient Hindu observations of heredity, with observations on traits passing through generations. The monk, Gregor Mendel, studied peas in his garden where he observed that traits or characteristics (color and texture) were transferable between generations based on fixed ratios.

The next great advancement was attributed to Thomas Hunt Morgan in his studies with fruit flies that identified the physical vehicle, the chromosome, for transmission of traits and genes through generations. Considerable research efforts then focused on the molecular structure of chromosomes that was revealed as deoxyribonucleic acid (DNA) with a double-helical structure in the 1950s. To Ayurveda, these western technological advances provided a physical and molecular basis for *prakriti*, the physical transference of traits for individual constitution, somewhat like *gunas* that loosely translate to inherited properties across generations, consistent with heredity in *prakriti*.

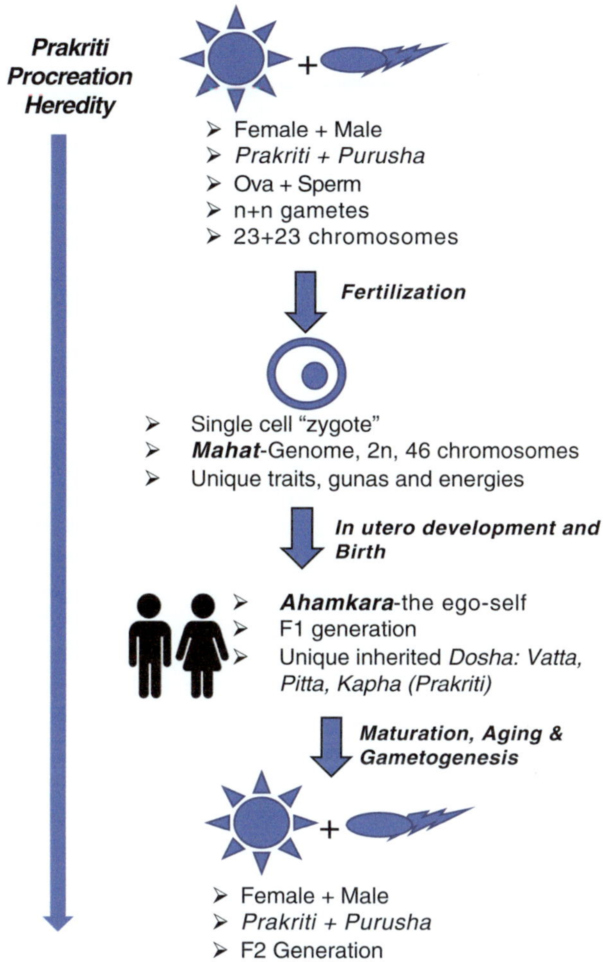

Fig. 3.1 *Prakriti* and *tridosha* in the Ayurvedic human life cycle. The *Charaka Samhita* for Ayurveda recognized the basic components of procreation and heredity in the human life cycle. Sexual intercourse resulted in new individuals with similar, but unique traits derived from the parental generation that were also present in the population at large. From *Shad Darshan* they attributed these traits to *gunas* and energies that were universal but also hereditary. *Purusha* the male ethos (and gamete) engenders power, strength, longevity, and survival. The female-endowed *prakriti* engenders all of the maternal propagation of the species, the female gamete, and the resulting individual's inherited *tridoshic* physiological constitution. *Prakriti* and inheritance of a unique dosha are, therefore, the basis for Ayurgenetics and Ayurvedic personalized medicine. Note how *Mahat* the concept of cellular knowledge energy that flows from *prakriti* corresponds with the informational genome, and then *Ahamkara* is akin to the individual ego-self as a unique combination of universal *gunas* and energies (traits). Overall, the western scientific descriptions (gametes, fertilization, chromosomes, genomes, etc.) correspond to the ancient Hindu philosophical concepts (*prakriti, Mahat, Ahamkara*) in modern Ayurveda that incorporates western technology while preserving Hindu philosophies and practices in personalized medicine

Once DNA was characterized as the molecular basis for genetic heredity, the central dogma was constructed whereby DNA coded for mRNA that was translated into the amino acid sequences for proteins. This provided the molecular basis for "polymorphsims" or "many looks" whereby the proteins that constitute the physical human are the product of genetics and heredity in the human life cycle. The variation of these traits results from mutations in DNA that become fixed in the population and transmitted through pedigrees, describing generations of families and ethnicities. Hence, there is a nexus between eastern and western medicine with a technological and molecular confirmation of the Ayurvedic principles for *dosha*s, whereby *prakriti* (heredity) endows each person with a unique physical and behavioral constitution, or *dosha*.

These incredible advancements in human biology have recently revolutionized clinical medicine. Ayurveda has long recognized that *dosha*s are not only the basis of individual health and wellness but also predisposition for diseases and inherited physiological disorders. Once again, western genomics, the study of differences in DNA sequences across populations, provides scientific confirmation of the traditional Ayurvedic observation. "Cloning," that is, isolation and characterization of DNA, and experimental genetics allow scientists to predictably and specifically alter the genome in test animals (mice) and link genomic function to DNA structure, physiological characteristics and pathologies. As *dosha*s are ascribed to individuals by the Ayurvedic practitioner, they are also recognized as inherent characteristics of the human population. Ayurveda has a very solid scientific foundation where all persons are classified with a *dosha* that is linked to epidemiology and pathogenesis individually, in cohorts, and in the population overall.

3.4 Intersection Between Genetics and Medicine

The genetic revolution has spawned a new discipline as Clinical Medical Genetics and personalized medicine along with it. Clinical genetics actually had its foundation in obstetrics and pediatrics. Physicians had always recognized the nature of mutations as teratology that later made distinctions between genetic and nongenetic causes. Medical schools collected and studied aborted fetuses and then published the results for centuries from the European and American academic hospitals. Advances in genetics, particularly karyotyping in the twentieth century, allowed linkage mapping of disorders through populations and pedigrees. That was the standard for the genetic basis of disease and its clinical applications to human health for decades, until the turn of the twenty-first century.

Advances in genomics (study of the genome, i.e. chromosomes and DNA) have exploded with unique applications for western medicine and huge implications for Ayurveda. Rapid and advanced information processing has had nearly as great an impact on genomics as the discoveries in biology proper. Modern DNA sequencing has progressed from the point where 20 years ago it required a month to sequence 1000 base pairs to the current state where "next-generation sequencing" allows deciphering of all three billion base pairs for the entire human genome in a matter of days (www.bitesizedbio/nextgenerationsequncing [25]). Moreover, advances in bioinformatics that entails processing of the sequence information to diagnose and predict pathologies both individually, but also in cohorts and entire populations represent the greatest breakthrough.

These genomic technologies are applied to screening newborns for inherited genetic disorders, diagnostics for adult diseases such as cancer, and for the health and wellness domain that intersects particularly well with Ayurveda. Consider the ability to diagnose an inherited generic disorder such as congenital heart disease before birth. Upon partition, the pediatricians and surgeons can be prepared to intervene immediately. This example and many others such as phenylketonuria, immunodeficiency, and neurological disorders can be treated both immediately and strategically, mitigating damage to the newborn. Likewise, applied cancer genomics allows genotyping of biopsies that dictates selection of highly effective anticancer drugs. These advanced therapeutics provide far more effective treatments, but avoid the toxic side effects of traditional, broad-spectrum chemotherapies.

The shortcoming in western medicine has been adopting the practitioner's culture and practices to personalized medicine, which is Ayurveda's strength. Western medicine relies on ethnicity to classify individuals for personalized medicine. While ethnicity could correlate with some parameters such as diet and cultural habits, the classification is based on physical characteristics such as skin color or stature that don't correlate well with health or disease. In genetic terms, ethnicity is confounded by outbreeding to the point where it provides little scientific basis for genetic conclusions and, therefore, little guidance for personalized medicine.

Ayurveda's *dosha* analysis takes a more scientifically sound approach by testing and *de novo* classifying each person individually with algorithms. Each person is viewed from *prakriti* as an individual with a personalized medicine perspective, rather than a member of a cohort based on appearance. Now, we can integrate the best components of the two systems approaches and arrive at Ayurgenetics.

3.5 Ayurgenetics

The concept is relatively simple: Ayurveda plus Clinical Medical Genetics yields Ayurgenetics as a modernized form of the traditional, ancient Ayurvedic approach [15–17]. This is personalized western medicine that combines millennia of accumulated knowledge utilizing the *tridosha* system based on the individual's *prakriti* for *de novo* assessment. The resulting Ayurvedic prescription is a unique combination of spiritual and physical approaches to health, wellness, and disease prevention. Ayurgenetics has been used to provide a genomic-based *dosha* analysis and then feedback from the resulting lifestyle wellness analysis that may also optimize some of the Ayurvedic prescriptions and practices. A more refined *dosha* analysis, combined with more research on the traditional Ayurvedic procedures, may reveal new and improved recommendations for specific *dosha*s.

Specifically, this applies to pharmacogenetics and diet. Pharmacogenetics is a rapidly evolving system for personalized medicine in the west that is also finding rapid application in the *tridosha* system [18, 19]. Specific alleles for both metabolism of drugs (pharmacokinetics) and the drug-ligand interaction (pharmacodynamics) have been found to be *dosha* associated with *Pitta* as rapid metabolizers, *Vata* as intermediate metabolizers, and *Kapha* as slow metabolizers of certain drugs [9].

In terms of diet, the dietary carbohydrate/protein ratios are often different for someone who is *Pitta* versus *Kapha*; therefore, Ayurvedic dietary recommendations would focus on specific types of carbohydrates and proteins for *Pitta* versus *Kapha*. These could change and be further refined during specific seasons, during a year and over a lifetime as the individual ages. The same is true of exercise, medication and sleep habits that are also *dosha* specific. Western medicine has nothing similar to this approach.

Indeed, western medicine can benefit from Ayurgenetics by jettisoning the traditional ethnicity-based classification of patients that is used for western personalized medicine recommendations. Several current western disease prevention algorithms use ethnicity as a major component. While data exist to link a cohort with greater risk for a given disease, e.g., hypertension, there is little or no solid physiological or genetic data to correlate skin color, stature, or facial features with the disease or disorder on an individual basis. Cultural or other nonphysiological risk factors could play a larger role to increase risk. The western system needs a system similar to the Ayurvedic *prakriti* and the *tridosha* process that assigns health and risk on and individual basis *de novo*, rather than utilizing cohorts and making assumptions.

Both western medicine and Ayurveda could progress in drug development by using a genetic-bioinformatic approach to medicinal chemistry. Indian herbalists are using genetics to analyze medicinal plants to find active compounds [20, 21]. The Ayurvedic practitioners are able to refine their herbal and medicinal plant therapies based on better scientific and pharmacological information in the context of their existing personalized Ayurvedic practices. Likewise, western physicians are now using individual genetic tests to refine their pharmacology and therapeutics while incorporating more traditional herbal compounds.

3.6 Summary

The twenty-first-century expression "the world is smaller" applies to so many issues, but it is certainly true for the juxtaposition of cultures and medical practices that we are witnessing in Ayurveda and Ayurgenetics. The profound influences of the Hindu religion and culture ingrained personalized medicine into Ayurveda. Meanwhile, the Euro-American separation of religion from science after the bitter experiences of the dark ages, combined with a socioeconomic technology boom, resulted in an explosion of medicinal science through the twenty-first century that is unparalleled in human history. However, the challenge for the west has been to incorporate personalized medicine brought by Clinical Medical Genetics into their engrained systematic approaches. The challenge for the east is to transform some cherished religious dogmas into modern medicine while preserving valuable spiritual and cultural traditions. Consequently "East meets West" in a grand cultural, medicinal, and scientific transformation that could have profound results for both cultures.

References

1. Dey S, Pahwa P. *Prakriti* and its associations with metabolism, chronic diseases, and genotypes: possibilities of new born screening and a lifetime of personalized prevention. J Ayurveda Integr Med. 2014;5(1):15–24. https://doi.org/10.4103/0975-9476.128848.
2. Prasher B, Gibson G, Mukerji M. Genomic insights into ayurvedic and western approaches to personalized medicine. J Genet. 2016;95(1):209–28. https://doi.org/10.1007/s12041-015-0607-9.
3. Rastogi S. Building bridges between Ayurveda and modern science. Int J Ayurveda Res. 2010;1(1):41–6. https://doi.org/10.4103/0974-7788.59943.
4. Gupta D, Pandy A, Kar AC. Concept of *Prakriti*: an Ayurvedic review. World J Pharm Pharm Sci. 2015;4(9):284–90.
5. Lad V. Textbook of Ayurveda: fundamental principles. Albuquerque: Ayurvedic Press; 2002.
6. Gupta PD. Pharmacogenetics, pharmacogenomics and ayurgenomics for personalized medicine: a paradigm shift. Indian J Pharm Sci. 2015;77(2):135–41.
7. Patwardhan B. Time for evidence-based Ayurveda: a clarion call for action. J Ayurveda Integr Med. 2013;4(2):63–6. https://doi.org/10.4103/0975-9476.113860.
8. Prasher B, Negi S, Aggarwal S, et al. Whole genome expression and biochemical correlates of extreme constitutional types defined in Ayurveda. J Transl Med. 2008;6:48. https://doi.org/10.1186/1479-5876-6-48.
9. Prasher B, Varma B, Kumar A, et al. Ayurgenomics for stratified medicine: TRISUTRA consortium initiative across ethnically and geographically diverse Indian populations. J Ethnopharmacol. 2017;197(Suppl C):274–93.
10. Chatterjee B, Pancholi J. *Prakriti*-based medicine: a step towards personalized medicine. Ayu. 2011;32(2):141–6. https://doi.org/10.4103/0974-8520.92539.
11. Tripathi YB. Molecular approach to ayurveda. Indian J Exp Biol. 2000;38(5):409–14.
12. Corcos AF. Reproduction and heredity beliefs of the Hindus based on their sacred books. J Hered. 1984;75(2):152–4.
13. Aggarwal S, Gheware A, Agrawal A, et al. Combined genetic effects of EGLN1 and VWF modulate thrombotic outcome in hypoxia revealed by Ayurgenomics approach. J Transl Med. 2015;13:9. https://doi.org/10.1186/s12967-015-0542-9.
14. Bhushan P, Kalpana J, Arvind C. Classification of human population based on HLA gene polymorphism and the concept of *Prakriti* in Ayurveda. J Altern Complement Med. 2005;11(2):349–53. https://doi.org/10.1089/acm.2005.11.349.
15. Patwardhan B, Bodeker G. Ayurvedic genomics: establishing a genetic basis for mind-body typologies. J Altern Complement Med. 2008;14(5):571–6. https://doi.org/10.1089/acm.2007.0515.
16. Rizzo-Sierra CV. Ayurvedic genomics, constitutional psychology, and endocrinology: the missing connection. J Altern Complement Med. 2011;17(5):465–8. https://doi.org/10.1089/acm.2010.0412.
17. Sethi TP, Prasher B, Mukerji M. Ayurgenomics: a new way of threading molecular variability for stratified medicine. ACS Chem Biol. 2011;6(9):875–80. https://doi.org/10.1021/cb2003016.
18. Coffin D, Lurie D. Ayurgenetics: East meets West in modern health, wellness, and medicine. Ayurveda J Health. 2016;14(4):17–23.
19. Lurie D. Ayurveda and pharmacogenomics. Ann Ayurvedic Med. 2012;1(4):126–8.
20. Khatoon S, Rai V, Rawat AK, et al. Comparative pharmacognostic studies of three Phyllanthus species. J Ethnopharmacol. 2006;104(1–2):79–86. S0378-8741(05)00587-8 [pii].
21. Rastogi S, Kalra A, Gupta V, et al. Unravelling the genome of Holy basil: an "incomparable" "elixir of life" of traditional Indian medicine. BMC Genomics. 2015;16:413. https://doi.org/10.1186/s12864-015-1640-z.
22. Charaka Samhita Ayurveda. Charaka Samhita. http://www.charakasamhita.com/. Accessed Nov 2017.

23. Clark B. Yin Yoga. Yinyoga.com. http://www.yinyoga.com/ys1_4.1.1_purusha_*prakriti*.php. Accessed Nov 2017.
24. Ortiz-Ospina E. "Life Expectancy"—what does this actually mean? 2017. www.ourworldindata.org.
25. Science Squared. Next generation sequencing. Bitesize Bio. 2017. https://bitesizebio.com/21193/a-beginners-guide-to-next-generation-sequencing-ngs-technology/. Accessed Nov 2017.

Ayurvedic Pharmaceutics, Manufacturing Processes and Novel Drug Delivery Systems in Ayurveda

4

Chandra Kant Katiyar

4.1 Ayurvedic Pharmaceutics

Charaka Samhita [1] has mentioned four components of treatment which include physicians, drugs, attendants and patients, and all of them need to be endowed with four qualities each, and only then they can lead to the alleviation of disorders (*Ch. Su-9/3*). If any of these components is absent, treatment remains incomplete. Drug is one of the important components of this treatment matrix. Further, *Charaka Samhita* (*Ch.Su.-9/7*) has propagated four qualities of ideal drug which include the following: abundance (availability in plenty), efficacy (of optimum quality having full potency), should be able to be prepared and presented in various dosage forms (should be able to deliver through multiple delivery formats), and should be with normal composition (meeting proper standards of quality).

These should be considered as directive principles of Ayurvedic pharmaceutics.

- In current context it may be interpreted as ensuring that raw material is available in plenty and there is no shortage. All measures of sustainable use are to be followed to ensure the same.
- Enough data either exist or need to be generated to prove efficacy.
- The raw material should have flexibility of being used on various formats and should meet quality specifications.

The medicine, therefore, should be formulated for administration to patients keeping in mind the need of consumers, property and quality of ingredients to ensure delivering desirable efficacy and safety if used properly.

Charaka Samhita further sermonises as below.

Even poison may become an effective drug if used judiciously, whereas improper use of even elixir may be harmful (*Ch.Su.1/126*).

C. K. Katiyar
Emami Ltd, Kolkata, India

S. Rastogi (ed.), *Translational Ayurveda*, https://doi.org/10.1007/978-981-13-2062-0_4

Use of unknown drug may prove injurious to health of the patients and is like poison or fire.

There is not a single substance on Earth which does not have medicinal value (*Ch.Su.26/12*) expanding the base of source of drugs, therefore.

4.2 Bhaisajya Kalpana

Ayurvedic medicines may be manufactured from herbs and ingredients of mineral or metallic origin or of animal origin; however, they are broadly categorised into two:

(a) *Kashtha aushadhi* (predominantly of herbal origin)
(b) *Rasa aushadhi* (predominantly mineral or metallic origin)

Plants, minerals, metals and ingredients of animal origin are naturally occurring basic sources of drugs and could not be used as such for medicinal purposes. They need to undergo certain processing to make them suitable for ingestion or local application, and this is called *Bhaisajya Kalpana* or Ayurvedic pharmaceutics.

Historically Ayurvedic pharmaceutics can be divided into two periods, pre-*Nagarjuna* and post-*Nagarjuna*, which are also called *Aarsha* and *Siddha*. Major sources of drugs in the pre-Nagarjuna period were plants and sometimes animals and rarely minerals or metals. However, raw materials for Ayurvedic medicines became predominantly minerals and metals, and plants played supportive role in post-*Nagarjuna* period, and this particular development gave rise to a new Ayurvedic discipline called *Rasa Shastra*, where *Rasa* means mercury.

The word *Bhaisajya Kalpana* is mostly used in relation to the preparation of plant-based drugs, while *Rasa Shastra* is used for metallic or mineral formulations. However, for the purpose of convenience in this article, we will use the term Ayurvedic pharmaceutics to include both.

4.3 Dosage Forms of Ayurveda

Ayurveda has recommended food also as medium to treat disease, and therefore, it does not discriminate between food and medicines when it comes to formats of delivery systems. Precisely for this reason, more than 100 dosage forms have been mentioned in ancient Ayurvedic texts as in Table 4.1 below.

Table 4.1 Number of dosage forms

Charaka Samhita (12th BC)	128 dosage forms
Sushruta Samhita (10th BC)	129 dosage forms
Ashtanga Hridaya (6th AD)	90 dosage forms
Chakradutta (9th AD)	90 dosage forms
Sharangadhara (14th AD)	75 dosage forms
Bhaishajya Ratnavali (18th AD)	98 dosage forms

Table 4.2 Category of Ayurvedic dosage forms

Solid	Liquids	Semisolids	Fumes
Churna	*Taila*	*Upanaha* (poultice)	*Dhumrapana*
Anjana	*Asav/Arishta*	*Ghrita*	*Dhupana*
Mansa Potti	*Ark*	*Ashchyotana*	
Utkarika	*Kwatha*	Avaleha	
Khsar	*Takra*	*Manda*	
Vati	*Phanta*	Mansa rasa	
Gutika	*Hima*	*Patrasveda*	
Modak	*Swarasa*	*Madhucchishta (bees wax)*	
Guda	*Madya*	*Tilapishta*	
Dhumravarti	*Mansarasa*	*Odana (rice preparation)*	
Puplika	*Madhu* (honey)	*Vesavara*	
Prithuka	*Khsirapak*	*Vilepi*	
Mandoor	*Peya*	*Krishara*	
Rasakriya	*Yusha*	*Kalka*	
Varti	*Karna purana*		
Shashkuli			
Ghanasatva			
Saktu			
Pottali			
Bhasmas/Rasaushadhis			

These Ayurvedic dosage forms are categorised as solid, semi-solid, liquid and fumes in Table 4.2 for easy understanding.

For all the dosage forms, Ayurveda recommended five basic dosage forms which are:

1. *Swarasa* (expressed Juice)
2. *Kalka* (paste)
3. *Shrita* (decoction)
4. *Hima* (cold infusion)
5. *Phanta* (hot infusion)

4.3.1 Important Ayurvedic Dosage Forms

Given below are the major dosage forms of Ayurvedic formulations. Details of these preparations may be seen in Ayurvedic Formulary of India [2].

4.3.1.1 *Churna*

Churna is a fine powder of one or more than one herb with mesh size of approximately 80. This is the simplest dosage form but, however, poses a big challenge of containing microbial load. Shelf life of Churna product is about 2 years if kept in the packaging having good moisture barrier property.

4.3.1.2 *Asava* and *Arishta*

Asava and *Arishta* are unique contributions of Ayurveda and can be broadly likened with medicated wine. These products are self-fermented using *Woodfordia fruticosa* flowers as fermentation agent.

When cold percolation product is fermented, it is called *Asava*, and when decoction of multiple herbs is subjected to fermentation, it is called *Arishta*. Earlier earthen pots were used to manufacture *Asava Arishta*, but nowadays modern fermenters are used to control the process to ensure batch-to-batch consistency. Its shelf life is indefinite, and its efficacy improves as per the age, that is, "older it is better it is".

4.3.1.3 *Arka*

Certain drugs are distilled after being soaked in water and are called *Arka*. They mostly constitute of volatile matter.

4.3.1.4 *Avaleha* or *Leha* and *Paka*

Avaleha are semi-solid preparations. Decoction of multiple herbs is filtered; sugar is added and boiled to form a thick pasty material. Desired spices are added, and the product is kept for cooling. Final product is semi-solid in appearance. In certain products *Bhasmas* are also added. In products like *Chyawanprash*, pulp of Amla is fried with *ghee* or oil, and, hence, *Avaleha* may contain fat also. The colour and the smell depend on the herbs and ingredients used to make the product. Normally they are stable for 2–3 years.

4.3.1.5 *Kvatha Churna*

Single or combination of herbs is converted to coarse powder which is used to prepare decoction after boiling in water and is known as *Kvatha* or *Kasayas*.

4.3.1.6 *Guggulu*

Guggulu is a category of products where Commiphora mukul exudate is used as major ingredient and also acts as binding agent. Before being used as therapeutic agent, it is subjected to *Shodhana* process involving liquids like *Gomutra* or *Triphala* decoction. *Guggulu*-based products are normally converted into pills and have shelf life of about 2–3 years.

4.3.1.7 *Ghrita* and *Taila*

These are medications prepared by processing *Ghrita* and *Taila* with herbs. The process involves adding one-fourth quantity of herbs and four to eight times liquid like water or decoction of herbs to one part of *Ghrita* or oil and boiled till total water is evaporated. They are mostly used for external application; however, sometimes internal use is also recommended.

4.3.1.8 *Lepa*

Powder of herbs used as paste for external application is called *Lepa*.

4.3.1.9 *Vati* and *Gutika*

Ayurvedic ingredients prepared in the form of pills or tablets are called *Vati* or *Gutika*. They may contain active ingredients of plant or mineral or animal origins. Normally they are stable for 2 years.

4.3.1.10 *Sattva*

Dried water extract is called as Sattva of a herbal drug. It may be prepared using cold or hot process.

4.3.1.11 *Kupipakva Rasayana*

This is a unique dosage form of Ayurveda involving the process of sublimation of mixture of metal, minerals or herbs with mercury. Most of the time, mercury is triturated with sulphur and is subjected to the process of sublimation in glass flask. Their shelf life is indefinite.

4.3.1.12 *Bhasma*

Powder of metals or mineral obtained through the process of calcination is called *Bhasmas*. Temperature required to convert various metals to *Bhasmas* is decided through the size of pit and the number of cow dung it can accommodate. Usual process of manufacturing *Bhasmas* involve three steps knows as *Shodhana*, *Marana* and in certain cases specific treatment. Currently computerised furnaces are also used to manufacture *Bhasmas*.

4.4 Evolution of Ayurvedic Dosage Forms

Initially Ayurveda recommended five basic dosage forms which were:

1. *Swarasa* (expressed juices)
2. *Kalka* (bolus)
3. *Kwath* (decoction)
4. *Him* (cold infusion)
5. *Phanta* (hot infusion)

Besides the above *Churna* was the most elementary dosage form. Journey of the evolution of Ayurvedic dosage forms is a beautiful depiction of need-gap-led innovation in ancient times.

Initial dosage forms were in practice by the physicians, but all of them had issues of short shelf life, unpalatable taste and larger doses required to exhibit desired effect. This need-gap led to advanced dosage forms like *Vati*, *Gutika* and *Avaleha* which had better shelf life and were more palatable.

Kwath Kalpana was very effective, but the taste was bad and shelf life short. Ancient sages enhanced shelf life and improved palatability of these decoctions by introducing fermentation technology to develope new dosage form called *Asava* or

Aristha. When decoction was fermented, it was called *Aristha*, and when cold infusion was fermented, it was called *Asava*, though there were few exceptions also to this rule. Fermentations process produced low percentage of alcohol (6–8%) which not only helped in improving palatability but also helped in faster activity helping in faster absorption of active compounds.

Novelty of this dosage form lies in the fact that since it was self-fermented, it had unlimited shelf life. Besides self-generated alcohol also acted as self-preservatives.

As discussed earlier, origin of lot of Ayurvedic dosage forms can be traced to food formats. One such dosage form is *Avaleha* or semi-solid. Use of sugar or jaggery to produce *Avaleha* not only helped in masking the bitter taste to make them palatable but also helped provide them longer shelf life since high content of sugar acts as preservative.

Medicated oils and medicated ghee are novel dosage forms of Ayurveda to provide lipophilic compounds in convenient dosage forms. Products like *Brahmi Ghrita* are used to enhance memory. But to import memory-enhancing property, its active compounds need to cross the blood-brain barrier (BBB). Its lipophilic dosage form makes it possible to push actives across the same in lipophilic medium.

Lipophilic dosage forms of *Ghrita* and *Taila* are remarkable examples of the application of food formats to deliver the drugs.

While these developments were going on one side, there was parallel development of a new science called alchemy. Alchemy was used to convert lower metals like copper (Cu) into higher metals liked gold (Au) or lower metals like tin (Sn) into higher metals like silver (Ag). Alchemists were using mercury for this purpose.

Few intelligent *Vaidyas* were probably keeping close watch on this development and thought that when mercury can convert lower metal into higher metal, why can't we use them on human beings to alleviate the disease? The great science of mercurials called *Rasa Shastra* thus evolved. It introduced use of mercury and sulphur besides other metals in ancient Ayurvedic medicine.

In the pre-*Nagarjuna* period, botanicals were the only options for therapeutic armamentarium, but they had their own problems like requirement of high doses, poor palatability, short shelf life and inconvenient to use besides each patient also required customised treatment due to his unique psychosomatic constituents also known as *Prakriti* and stage of disease.

Introduction of *Rasaushadhies* (mercurial and metallic preparations) in approximately eleventh century AD created the same revolution in Ayurvedic medicines with the discovery of penicillin as an antibiotic created for modern medicine much later.

Mercury-based products also called *Rasaushadhis* were effective in small doses (mostly 125–250 mg), were quicker in actions and were *Prakriti* natural, meaning the *Vaidyas* need not consider the *Prakriti* of the patient while administering *Rasaushadhis* to him. Ancient sages were also highly conscious of toxic effects on mercury and their products and, therefore, recommended various dos and don'ts for their administration. They paid special emphasis on various manufacturing processes to ensure that mercury or metal becomes non-toxic before it is administered. A fact that has now been proven by various toxicity studies conducted by Central Council for Research in Ayurveda Sciences (CCRAS), Ministry of Ayush, government of India, and published in the book *Evidence Based Safety of Ayurvedic Medicines* [3].

Currently most of the proprietary Ayurvedic medicines are manufactured on contemporary dosage forms like tablet, capsule, gel, syrup, etc. for which principles of *Modern Pharmaceutics* are applied while developing the same.

4.5 Wisdom in Designing Ayurvedic Formulations

The perusal of *Charak Samhita* Vol-II [4] provides original composition of very popular Ayurvedic recipe *Chyawanprash*. The critical analysis of the same leads to a very interesting observation which appears to have escaped the attention of several scholars of Ayurveda.

Composition of *Chyawanprash* in *Charaka Samhita* mentions all other ingredients by weight except Amla which has been recommended to be used 500 by number. This is very interesting. Since weight and measurement were fairly developed in those times and all other ingredients were mentioned in particular quantity in terms of weight, then why is Amla recommended by number?

The author tried to investigate this mystery during his industry career, and observations were astounding. Currently there are two varieties of Amla available in the market:

(a) Forest origin or *Junglee* which is smaller in size
(b) Cultivated or *Kalami* which is bigger in size

If 1 kg of *Amla* is weighed and *Amla* counted by numbers, forest origin *Amla* (weighing approximately 15 g) would be 65 in number and if cultivated *Amla* is taken weighing approximately 25 g per *Amla*, their number would be 40. Therefore, the number of *Amla* per kg is more for smaller and less for bigger variety. Laboratory experiments revealed that fibre content in both the varieties of *Amla* was the same irrespective of their size. Bigger size *Amla* had higher water content than smaller one.

It does not take rocket science to understand the importance of this experiment. If *Amla* is used by weight fibre, content of *Amla* would vary depending upon the variety used, leading to batch-to-batch inconsistency as well as difference in therapeutic benefits and product efficacy since it is the major ingredient of *Chyawanprash*. Therefore, if *Amla* is used by count of 500, its fibre content would remain constant the same from batch-to-batch ensuring same efficacy.

Such wisdom and contribution of such ancient sages to *Bhaishajya Kalpana* need to be highly appreciated.

4.6 Concepts of New Drug Delivery System

New drug delivery system has an approach of modern pharmaceutical sciences to develop innovative methods and dosage forms to deliver the drugs in targeted manner.

A careful study of *Bhaisajya Kalpana* of Ayurveda reveals that concepts of new drug delivery system were incorporated in it by two means:

(a) Adjunct route: by suggesting various *Anupanas*
(b) Formulation design: by suggesting various dosage forms keeping targets in consideration

Ayurveda is replete with instances where same drug has been recommended for different indications by changing only *Anupana*. One commonly known example is *Icchabhedi Rasa* which taken with cold water relieves constipation and taken with hot water acts as antidiarrhoeal agent.

As discussed elsewhere in this chapter, the development of *Ghrita* to deliver lipophilic active ingredients of medicinal plants to targeted organs like the brain to improve cognitive functions (crossing blood-brain barriers) is a simple yet innovative approach of *Ayurveda* towards delivery system.

Asava Aristha is an another unique dosage form providing the following benefits:

(a) Faster absorption of active phytochemicals.
(b) Faster activity ensured due to the presence of alcohol which acts as carrier medium.
(c) To convert prodrugs into drugs by chemical transformation during slow fermentation process. Vidhu Aeri et al. [5] have demonstrated that during lab-scale manufacture of *Ashokaristha*, gallic acid and kaempferol were quantified in the fermented product. Quantity of gallic acid was found to be increased up to 3.24 times higher than decoction which indicated occurrence of hydrolysis of flavonol glycosides during the fermentation process.
(d) Nikhil Kumar Singh et al. [6] demonstrated the presence of water-soluble vitamins B_1, B_2, B_3 and B_6 in *Drakshaya*, *Ashokarishta*, *Lauhasava*, *Arjunarishta* and *Ashagaurishta*. Presence of vitamin B_9 (folic acid) has also been reported to be responsible for the improvement in anaemic conditions without additional supplementation of iron. The production of these vitamins further enhances the biological activity of *Asava Arishtas*.
(e) Provide excellent shelf life to the product (unlimited).
(f) Introduction of mercurial and metallic *Rasaushadhis* after eleventh century AD revolutionalised Ayurvedic therapeutics.

Recently *Bhasma* preparations of metals have been compared with nanotechnology-based formulations. Nanoparticles are currently a very hot topic of research related to targeted drug delivery systems. Indian contemporary scientists are very well aware of the existence of this technology in Ayurveda long ago in terms of *Bhasmas*.

In a recent publication, Daniel et al. [7] conducted a comparative study of incinerated ancient gold particles (*Swarna Bhasma*) and chemically synthesised gold particles on the mechanism of their cellular entry in human cells. They observed much better absorption of *Swarna Bhasma* in the cell through defined mechanism as compared to synthetic one.

Ancient Ayurvedic *Bhaisajya Kalpana* or Ayurvedic pharmaceutics is replete with practical applications of new drug delivery systems.

4.7 Quality Specifications of Raw Materials and Finished Products as per *Ayurvedic Pharmacopoeia of India*

India is one of the very few countries rich in traditional systems of medicine. India is also one of the few countries which have their own pharmacopoeia providing quality standards of raw material, suggesting methods of manufacture and also recommending quality specifications of the finished products.

Ayurvedic Pharmacopoeia of India Part 1 (*Vol. I to vol. VIII*) [8–10] has provided quality specifications of various raw materials used in the manufacture of Ayurvedic drugs. These raw materials include herbs, minerals, metals, etc.

Ayurvedic Pharmacopoeia of India Part 2 (*Vol. I and II*) [11, 12] has provided quality specifications of the dosage forms. Their quality parameters are also mentioned below for the information of the readers.

Given below are the parameters of their quality which need to be tested mandatorily as per the Standard Test Procedures (STPs) mentioned in their volumes. Readers may refer to original pharmacopoeia to see the testing procedures.

4.7.1 Raw Materials

Sl no	Quality parameters
A. **Herbal raw material** [8]	
1	Macroscopic description
2	Microscopic description
3	Foreign matter (% w/w)
4	Total ash (% w/w)
5	Acid-insoluble ash (% w/w)
6	Alcohol-soluble extractive
7	Identification by thin-layer chromatography
8	Assay (% w/w)
9	Heavy metal content (ppm): (a) Lead (b) Arsenic (c) Cadmium (d) Mercury

(continued)

Sl no	Quality parameters
10	Microbiological contamination: A. Total plate count (CFU/g) B. Total yeast and mould count (CFU/g) C. Presence of pathogen (a) *E. coli* (b) *S. aureus* (c) *Salmonella* sp. (d) *P. aeruginosa*
11	Pesticide residues
12	Aflatoxins
B. Herbal extracts [10]	
1	Description
2	Total ash (% w/w)
3	Acid-insoluble ash (% w/w)
4	pH
5	Identification by thin-layer chromatography
6	Assay (% w/w)
7	Total soluble solids (% w/w)
8	Heavy metal content (ppm): (a) Lead (b) Arsenic (c) Cadmium (d) Mercury
9	Microbiological contamination: A. Total plate count (CFU/g) B. Total yeast and mould count (CFU/g) C. Presence of pathogen (a) *E. coli* (b) *S. aureus* (c) *Salmonella* sp. (d) *P. aeruginosa*
10	Pesticide residues
11	Aflatoxins
C. Metals [9]	
1	Physical properties
2	Hardness
3	Specific gravity
4	Reaction with acids
5	Assay (% w/w)
6	Heavy metal and arsenic (ppm)
7	Other elements (ppm)
8	Microbiological contamination: A. Total plate count (CFU/g) B. Total yeast and mould count (CFU/g) C. Presence of pathogen (a) *E. coli* (b) *S. aureus* (c) *Salmonella* sp. (d) *P. aeruginosa*

Sl no	Quality parameters
D. Minerals [9]	
1	Physical properties
2	Hardness
3	Hardness
4	Specific gravity
	Optical properties
5	Effect of heat
6	Solubility
7	Assay (% w/w)
8	Heavy metal and arsenic (ppm)
9	Other elements
10	Microbiological contamination: A. Total plate count (CFU/g) B. Total yeast and mould count (CFU/g) C. Presence of pathogen (a) *E. coli* (b) *S. aureus* (c) *Salmonella* sp. (d) *P. aeruginosa*

4.7.2 Finished Products

Sl no	Quality parameters
A. *Avaleha*: [11]	
1	Description
2	Identification by microscopy
3	Identification by thin-layer chromatography
4	Loss on drying (% w/w)
5	Total ash (% w/w)
6	Acid-insoluble ash (% w/w)
7	Alcohol-soluble extractive (% w/w)
8	Water-soluble extractive (% w/w)
9	pH (of 1% aqueous solution)
10	Assay (% w/w)
11	Test for heavy metals (ppm)
12	Microbiological contamination: A. Total plate count (CFU/g) B. Total yeast and mould count (CFU/g) C. Presence of pathogen (a) *E. coli* (b) *S. aureus* (c) *Salmonella* sp. (d) *P. aeruginosa*
13	Pesticide residues
14	Aflatoxins (ppm)

(continued)

Sl no	Quality parameters
B. *Churna* (powder) [11]	
1	Description
2	Identification by thin-layer chromatography
3	Test for chloride
4	Loss on drying (% w/w)
5	Total ash (% w/w)
6	Acid insoluble ash (% w/w)
7	Alcohol-soluble extractive (% w/w)
8	Water-soluble extractive (% w/w)
9	pH (of 10% aqueous solution)
10	Assay (% w/w)
11	Test for heavy metals (ppm)
12	Microbiological contamination: A. Total plate count (CFU/g) B. Total yeast and mould count (CFU/g) C. Presence of pathogen (a) *E. coli* (b) *S. aureus* (c) *Salmonella* sp. (d) *P. aeruginosa*
13	Pesticide residues
14	Aflatoxins (ppm)
C. *Ghrita* [11]	
1	Description
2	Identification by thin-layer chromatography
3	Refractive index at 40°
4	Weigh per mL at 40° (g)
5	Saponification value
6	Iodine value
7	Acid value
8	Peroxide value
9	Congealing point (degree centigrade)
10	Mineral oil
	Test for heavy metals (ppm)
11	Microbiological contamination: A. Total plate count (CFU/g) B. Total yeast and mould count (CFU/g) C. Presence of pathogen (a) *E. coli* (b) *S. aureus* (c) *Salmonella* sp. (d) *P. aeruginosa*
12	Pesticide residues
13	Aflatoxins (ppm)

Sl no	Quality parameters
D. *Guggulu* [11]	
1	Description
2	Identification by microscopy
3	Identification by thin-layer chromatography
4	Loss on drying (% w/w)
5	Total ash (% w/w)
6	Acid-insoluble ash (% w/w)
7	Alcohol-soluble extractive (% w/w)
8	Water-soluble extractive (% w/w)
9	pH (of 1% aqueous solution)
10	Test for heavy metals (ppm)
11	Microbiological contamination: A. Total plate count (CFU/g) B. Total yeast and mould count (CFU/g) C. Presence of pathogen (a) *E. coli* (b) *S. aureus* (c) *Salmonella* sp. (d) *P. aeruginosa*
12	Pesticide residues
13	Aflatoxins (ppm)
E. *Vati/Gutika* (Tablet) [11]	
1	Description
2	Identification by microscopy
3	Identification by thin-layer chromatography
4	Loss on drying (% w/w)
5	Total ash (% w/w)
6	Acid-insoluble ash (% w/w)
7	Alcohol-soluble extractive (% w/w)
8	Water-soluble extractive (% w/w)
9	Assay (% w/w)
10	Test for heavy metals (ppm)
11	Microbiological contamination: A. Total plate count (CFU/g) B. Total yeast and mould count (CFU/g) C. Presence of pathogen (a) *E. coli* (b) *S. aureus* (c) *Salmonella* sp. (d) *P. aeruginosa*
12	Pesticide residues
13	Aflatoxins (ppm)

(continued)

Sl no	Quality parameters
F. *Kshara* [11]	
1	Description
2	Identification
3	Loss on drying (% w/w)
4	pH (of 10% aqueous solution)
5	Acid-insoluble ash (% w/w)
6	Sodium content (% w/w)
7	Potassium content (% w/w)
8	Iron content (% w/w)
9	Test for heavy metals (ppm)
10	Microbiological contamination: A. Total plate count (CFU/g) B. Total yeast and mould count (CFU/g) C. Presence of pathogen (a) *E. coli* (b) *S. aureus* (c) *Salmonella* sp. (d) *P. aeruginosa*
11	Pesticide residues
12	Aflatoxins (ppm)
G. *Taila* [11]	
1	Description
2	Identification by thin-layer chromatography
3	Refractive index at 40°
4	Weigh per mL at 40° (g)
5	Saponification value
6	Iodine value
7	Acid value
8	Peroxide value
9	Mineral oil
10	Test for heavy metals (ppm)
11	Microbiological contamination: A. Total plate count (CFU/g) B. Total yeast and mould count (CFU/g) C. Presence of pathogen (a) *E. coli* (b) *S. aureus* (c) *Salmonella* sp. (d) *P. aeruginosa*
12	Pesticide residues
13	Aflatoxins (ppm)
H. *Lepa* [11]	
1	Description
2	Identification
3	pH (5% aqueous solution)
4	Assay (% w/w)
5	Test for heavy metals (ppm)

Sl no	Quality parameters
6	Microbiological contamination: A. Total plate count (CFU/g) B. Total yeast and mould count (CFU/g) C. Presence of pathogen (a) *E. coli* (b) *S. aureus* (c) *Salmonella* sp. (d) *P. aeruginosa*
7	Pesticide residues
8	Aflatoxins (ppm)
I. ***Asava Arishta*** [12]	
1	Description
2	Identification by thin-layer chromatography
3	Total solids (% w/v)
4	Specific gravity at 25 °C
5	pH
6	Reducing sugars (% w/v)
7	Non-reducing sugars (% w/v)
8	Alcohol content (% v/v)
9	Methanol
10	Assay (% w/v)
11	Test for heavy metals (ppm)
12	Microbiological contamination: A. Total plate count (CFU/g) B. Total yeast and mould count (CFU/g) C. Presence of pathogen (a) *E. coli* (b) *S. aureus* (c) *Salmonella* sp. (d) *P. aeruginosa*
13	Pesticide residues
14	Aflatoxins (ppm)
J. ***Arka*** [12]	
1	Description
2	Identification (by thin-layer chromatography, gas chromatography)
3	Specific gravity at 20 °C
4	Test for heavy metals (ppm)
5	Microbiological contamination: A. Total plate count (CFU/g) B. Total yeast and mould count (CFU/g) C. Presence of pathogen (a) *E. coli* (b) *S. aureus* (c) *Salmonella* sp. (d) *P. aeruginosa*
6	Pesticide residues
7	Aflatoxins (ppm)

4.8 Contemporary Ayurvedic/Herbal Drug Development Process

Application of modern pharmacopoeial parameters of quality and manufacturing technology to produce Ayurvedic dosage forms has always been a challenge. Basic dosage forms of *Bhaisajya Kalpana* were conceptualised for small-scale production to meet the day-to-day requirement of limited number of patients during practice by Ayurvedic physicians in the ancient times. Feasibility of commercial production of large scale was not even considered at that time. Few companies started the application of modern manufacturing technologies using custom-made manufacturing equipments for Ayurvedic medicines. In the absence of any earlier experience either in practice or through curriculum, the graduate and post-graduate of pharmacy and chemical and mechanical engineers interacted with Ayurvedic physicians and designed the custom-made engineering equipments. Applications of fermenters, large-scale extractors, grinders, etc. are contributions of Ayurvedic industry. Industry-led need for mechanisation of *Bhasma* manufacturing process has resulted in the development of computerised electric furnaces designed to provide temperature pattern similar to *Gaja Put*, *Maha Puta*, *Kapota Puta*, etc. through interaction of *Rasa Shastra* specialists with mechanical engineers. Few companies and practitioners are already using it. Even the Ayurvedic Pharmacopoeia Committee has extended its recognition to this novel development.

Since pharmaceutics courses across India were mostly focussed on solution to problems of pharmaceutical industry, scientists with pharma background initially tried to learn Ayurvedic processes and then tried to apply them for the development of Ayurvedic products.

Drugs and Cosmetics Act of India provides guidance on manufacture and sale of Ayurvedic medicines which is implemented through states in federal structure.

Modern looking Ayurvedic companies typically have the following internal divisions/departments for smooth transition from concept to market:

Research and development
Marketing and sales
Corporate quality control
Centralised operations to control multiple manufacturing units
Centralised purchase
Centralised regulatory affairs

The following areas of expertise are required for contemporary Ayurvedic drug industry:

- Pharmaceutical technology
- Bio-resource management—agronomist
- Taxonomist
- Phytochemistry

Table 4.3 Depicting steps of Ayurvedic medicine development and capacities required to achieve the same

Steps	Expertise required
Literature search	Literature search using modern tools
Ingredient selection	Taxonomy, pharmacognosy, traditional medicine
Analysis of raw materials	Taxonomy, phytochemistry, analytical chemistry
Pre-formulation work	Pharmaceutics, pharmacognosy
Development of standards and specifications	Analytical chemistry, pharmaceutics, pharmacognosy
Microbiological testing	Microbiology
Formulation of product	Pharmaceutics, pharmacognosy
Accelerated stability studies	Pharmaceutics, pharmacognosy
Finished product specification	Analytical chemistry, pharmaceutics, pharmacognosy
Claim substantiation studies	Pharmacology, traditional medicine, clinical pharmacology
Toxicology and safety study	Pharmacology
Clinical evaluation	Ayurvedic medicine, modern medicine
Technology transfer	Pharmaceutics, pharmacognosy, analytical chemistry

- Analytical experts
- Pharmacologists
- Ayurvedic expert
- Formulation experts
- Regulatory experts
- Toxicologist
- Clinical pharmacologist

Activity-wise expertise required is depicted in Table 4.3 below.

Given below is currently followed typical Ayurvedic drug development process followed by the industry, though mostly for proprietary formulations.

4.8.1 Product Development Stages

1. **Product Brief**

   Normally companies use the preset proforma before product development. Proforma includes market information, need-gap, requirement of the dosage forms, the benchmark product, shape, colour of the product, packaging details, etc. The brief on development of product is shared by the customer which may be internal or external based on need-gap area. Most of the time, it is based upon some kind of market research.
2. **Identification of Active Ingredients and Their Doses**

   Experts of Ayurveda and pharmacology identify the ingredient based on similar classical Ayurvedic formulations or expertise or published researches and suggest their ratios in the product to deliver pre-decided dosage per day.

3. **Development of 3–4 Prototypes**

   Prototypes of the products are developed basis data on ingredients to pick up the most effective of them.
4. **Subjecting All the Prototypes to Primary Pharmacological Experimental Screening to Identify One Most Active Formulation**

   In vitro, cell-based bioassays for primary screening or in vivo experiments are conducted to identify most effective composition of the three to four prototypes for their further development.

4.8.1.1 Stage I activities

5. **Procurement of Active RMs or Active Botanical Ingredients (ABIs)**

   Raw material can be either crude herb or extracts going into the formulations as per the above. In case of metallic, mostly *Bhasmas* are prepared separately and used.
6. **Identification of Markers**

   Identification of marker compounds in herbs or extracts is done based on pharmacopoeial standards or literature. Good companies normally have their own library of marker compounds. Alternatively fingerprint thin-layer chromatography (TLC) plates are used to ensure quality.
7. **Complete Analysis of ABIs**

   Raw materials need to undergo complete analysis based on pharmacopoeial standards. In case pharmacopoeia has not prescribed the standards, in-house parameters can be used, and limits can be fixed basis data of few lots.
8. **Procurement of Excipients**

   Suitable excipients are identified and procured for the formulation and dosage.
9. **Analysis of Excipients**

   The excipients are analysed for quality based on pharmacopoeial standards.
10. **Stability of ABIs (for Extracts)**

    If the raw material is extracted, they are subjected to proper stability studies to decide their shelf life. Normally extracts are found to be stable up to 6 months.
11. **Excipient Compatibility Studies**

    Excipient compatibility study is a very important step in formulation development specially for tablet or capsules. This is required to ensure that the extracts once absorbed on the excipients should be released also. There are certain excipients having affinity for fatty ingredients which are not released to the body and thrown out as such. Excipient compatibility study, therefore, is a very important step in formulation development.
12. **Hygroscopicity Studies**

    Most of the herbal extracts and products are very hygroscopic in nature. This has an implication on the selection of right packaging material and depiction of shelf life.

4.8.1.2 Stage II Activities

13. **Lab-Scale Trials**

    These trials are taken inside the lab for feasibility studies.

14. **Tentative Specification of ABIs**

    Tentative quality specifications are fixed for active botanical ingredients.

15. **Specification of Excipients**

    Pharmaceutical quality standards are used for excipients.

16. **Selection of Packing Material**

    Selection of packing material is very critical and depends on several factors including dosage forms, nature of product, hygroscopicity of the product, presence and absence of volatile compounds, susceptibility for microbial load, etc.

17. **Preservative Efficacy Test**

    In certain products, preservatives are required to enhance their shelf life. Preservative efficacy test should always be conducted to evaluate their efficacy to prevent the growth of microorganisms.

18. **Stage II Batches**

    Stage II batches are taken.

19. **Stability Protocol**

    Stability protocol need to be decided depending upon geographical location of the market. For Indian market usually stability studies are conducted at temperature of 40 °C and humidity 75°. Shelf life of 2 years as assigned if product is stable for 6 months under these accelerated stability conditions.

20. **Observational Studies/Clinical Trials/Toxicity Studies**

    Requirement of clinical trials or toxicity study depends upon regulatory requirement as well as company's internal policies on the same. Drugs and Cosmetics Act of India Rule 158 B has provided guidance in this regard.

4.8.1.3 Stage III Activities

21. **Finalization of Packing Material**

    Packing material for commercial use is finalised based on stability studies.

22. **Label Claim and Medical Rationale**

    Label claim is decided based on literature, studies conducted, and keeping Drugs and Magic Remedies (objectionable advertisements) Act compliances besides other regulatory compliances. Medical rationale is prepared for submission to licencing authorities as well as for in-house use.

23. **Manufacturing Site Finalisation**

    Manufacturing licence is applied for the facility where the product is intended to be manufactured.

These are broadly all the steps in manufacturing of Ayurvedic medicines being currently adopted by reasonably good Ayurvedic manufacturing companies in India. Some of the steps have been adopted from the development of pharmaceutical products. Enough care is taken to ensure batch-to-batch consistency and quality of the product provide similar kinds of benefit to the patients batch after batch.

4.9 Summary

Ayurvedic *Bhaishajya Kalpana* made its own progress in the ancient times and adopted all measures to continuously improve upon the dosage forms to make them more effective, stable and palatable. Ayurvedic therapeutic armamentarium has been very dynamic. Starting from basic dosage forms, *Bhaishajya Kalpana* adopted food formats and fermentation products and eventually also accepted *Rasaushadhies*.

Commercialisation of Ayurvedic medicines has added value in terms of adoption of modern dosage forms, modern manufacturing technologies, quality control mechanisms and evaluation of products for safety and efficacy for humanity at large.

References

1. Sharma PV. Charak samhita, vol. 1. Varanasi: Chaukhamba Orientalia; 2014.
2. The Ayurvedic Formulary of India, Part-1. 2nd ed. Government of India, Ministry of Health & Family welfare, Department of Ayurveda, Yoga & Naturopathy, Unani, Siddha, and Homoeopathy, New Delhi, Published by the Controller of Publication, Civil Line, Delhi, 110054; 2003.
3. Ministry of Ayush. Evidence based safety of Ayurvedic medicines, pub. New Delhi: Ministry of AYUSH, Government of India; 2016.
4. Sharma PV. Charak samhita, vol. 2. Varanasi: Chaukhamba Orientalia; 2014.
5. Aeri V, et al. Evaluation of pre-and postfermented aqueous decoction of saraca asoca by high-performance thin layer chromatography. J Planar Chromat. 2015;28. https://doi.org/10.1556/JPC.28.2015.1.0.
6. Singh NK, et al. Estimation of naturally produced water-soluble vitamins in different asava and arishtas using liquid chromatography. J Food Pharm Sci. 2013;1:81–4.
7. Beaudet D, Badilescu S, Kuruvinashetti K, Kashani AS, Jaunky D, Ouellette S, Dieking A, Packirisamy M. Comparative Study on cellular entry of incinerated ancient gold particles (Swarna Bhasma) and chemically synthesized gold particles. Sci Rep. 2017;7:1–12. http://www.nature.com/scientificreports. Accessed 6 Sept 2017.
8. The Ayurvedic Pharmacopoeia of India, Part-I, vol. I, 1st ed. Government of India, Ministry of Health & Family Welfare; Department of Indian Systems of Medicine & Homoeopathy; 1990. p. 15.
9. The Ayurvedic Pharmacopoeia of India, Part-I, vol. VII, 1st ed. Government of India, Ministry of Health & Family Welfare; Department of Ayurveda, Yoga & Naturopathy, Unani, Siddha and Homoeopathy (Ayush), New Delhi; 1990.
10. The Ayurvedic Pharmacopoeia of India, Part-I, vol. VIII, 1st ed. Government of India, Ministry of Health & Family Welfare; Department of Ayurveda, Yoga & Naturopathy, Unani, Siddha and Homoeopathy (Ayush), New Delhi; 2011.
11. The Ayurvedic Pharmacopoeia of India, Part-II, vol. I, 1st ed. Government of India, Ministry of Health & Family Welfare; Department of Ayurveda, Yoga & Naturopathy, Unani, Siddha and Homoeopathy (Ayush), New Delhi; 2007.
12. The Ayurvedic Pharmacopoeia of India, Part-II, vol. II, 1st ed. Government of India, Ministry of Health & Family Welfare; Department of Ayurveda, Yoga & Naturopathy, Unani, Siddha and Homoeopathy (Ayush), New Delhi; 2007.

5 Pharmacological and Pharmaceutical Principles of Ayurvedic Drugs: A Concurrent Appraisal

K. Nishteswar

5.1 Introduction

Pharmacology is the branch of biology concerned with the study of drug action, or in other words, it deals with the effects of drugs on living systems. The drugs employed in the management of various diseases are vegetable, animal, and mineral in origin, and the polyherbal formulations outnumber the mineral and other metallic preparations. In modern pharmacology the drug action is quite often correlated with its chemical structure or active principle. Keeping in mind the era in which Ayurvedic classics were written, it is remarkable that a workable edifice was created by evaluating the effect of drugs and diet, by the only analytical means available then, namely, sensory perceptions. In *Ayurvedic* pharmacology, physiological and biochemical effects of drugs and their mechanism of action in the body are explained with the help of pharmacodynamic principles, namely, *rasa* (taste), *guna* (qualities), *virya* (potency/energy), *vipaka* (biotransformation), and *prabhava* (empirical/inexplicable principle) in terms of bodily components like *tridosha* (three biohumors, *vata*, *pitta*, and *kapha*), *dhatu* (different tissues), *mala* (morbid factors including urine, feces, etc.), *srotas* (channels both macro- and microvessels), and *agni* (enzymes and hormones).

5.2 *Dravya* (Substance/Matter)

The one which is a substratum of the qualities (*guna*) and actions (*karma*) and which is a concomitant cause (*samavayi karana*) is defined as matter (*dravya*) [1]. By this definition, matter happens to be the substratum of qualities and actions, and it is also the concomitant cause of another matter and qualities as well as actions.

K. Nishteswar
Former Professor and HOD, Department of Dravyaguna, Institute for Post Graduate Teaching and Research in Ayurveda, Gujarat Ayurved University, Jamnagar, India

S. Rastogi (ed.), *Translational Ayurveda*, https://doi.org/10.1007/978-981-13-2062-0_5

Table 5.1 Panchamahabhutas with their attributes [6]

No.	*Mahabhuta*	*Guna* (attributes) of *mahabhuta*
1	*Prithvi* (earth/soil)	*Guru* (heaviness), *kathina* (hard), *vishada* (clear), *manda* (slow), *sandra* (dense), *sthula* (thick), *sthira* (stable/immobile), *gandha gunabahulya* (predominance of smell sensation)
2	*Ap* (water)	*Drava* (liquidity), *snigdha* (unctuousness or oiliness), *sheeta* (cold), *guru* (heavy), *manda* (slow), *sandra* (dense), *sara* (flow/mobility), *mridu* (soft), *pichchila* (slimy), *rasagunabahula* (predominance of taste sensation)
3	*Teja/agni* (fire)	*Teekshna* (intense), *ushna* (hot), *ruksha* (dry), *sukshma* (minute/deep penetrating), *laghu* (light), *vishada* (clear), rupagunabahula (predominance of sight sensation)
4	*Vayu* (air)	*Ruksha* (dry), *sukshma* (minute/deep penetrating), *laghu* (light), *visada* (clear), *vikasi* (quick spreading), *vyavayi*, *sheeta* (cold), *sparshagunabahula* (predominance of touch sensation)
5	*Akasha* (space/ether)	*Mridu* (soft), *sukshma* (minute, deep penetrating), *laghu* (light), *vishada* (clear), *shlakshna* (smooth), *vyavayi*, *sheeta* (cold), *khara* (rough), *shabdagunabahula* (predominance of sound sensation)

The capacity to produce something out of its own rests only in the matter. Every substance whether food or medicinal agent is constituted by five proto elements, namely, *prithvi*, *ap*, *teja*, *vayu*, and *akasha* [2]. Soil from which substances like food and drugs are produced is also classified based on *panchamahabhutas*. Substances inherit the qualities of these *mahabhutas* (Table 5.1) from soil and help to maintain bodily physiological functions, as the body is also the product of *panchamahabhutas*. By the theory of *samanya* (generic concomitance)-*vishesha* (variant factor) concept [3], maintenance of health or cure of a disease is monitored by substituting or decreasing the panchabhoutic constituents. Body is constituted by *dosha*, *dhatu*, *upadhatu*, *mala*, *agni*, and *srotas*. These components may be referred as *adhikarana* (target site), and ingested foods or drugs act on them to restore and maintain the healthy state. Ingested substances undergo *paka* (digestive and metabolic phases) with the help of *jataragni* (digestive fire) and its moieties (*dhatwagni* and *bhutagni*) and finally separate into *sara* (essential components) and *kitta* (excretory metabolites) forms [4]. *Sarabhaga* (essential component) replenishes *dhatus* and addresses vitiation of *doshas*, while *kittabhaga* is expelled out through excretory pathways. The phases of ingestion, digestion, metabolism, egestion, and excretion are common for both diet and drugs which are orally administered. According to *Ayurvedic* classics, a substance (diet or drug) has to pass through all these phases by performing the activities with the help of inherent principle, namely, *rasa*, *guna*, *virya*, *vipaka*, and *prabhava* (*rasapanchaka*) [5].

5.3 *Rasa* (Taste)

Rasa refers to the total subjective experience arising on placing any substance in the mouth. Rasa concept described is a pharmacodynamic principle and serves as a tool to explain panchabhoutic constitution of the drug. Rasa is the only quality which is directly perceivable. There are six rasa (*madhura*, sweet; *amla*, sour; *lavana*, salty; *katu*; pungent, *tikta*, bitter; *kashaya*, astringent), and each one is made out of two of the five *panchamahabhutas* [7]. The source material for manifestation of all these tastes is *jalamahabhuta*. The qualities of preceding basic elements (*akasa*, *vayu*, *agni*, *ap*, and *prithvi*) are included in the succeeding ones; so the qualities of *ap* is automatically included in *prithvi*. *Ap* and *prithvi* are the substrata for the manifestation of taste. According to Charaka, out of the six tastes, *madhura rasa* abounds in the qualities of *prithvi* and *jalamahabhuta*, *amla rasa* of *prithvi* and *agni*, *lavana rasa* of *jala* and *agni*, *katu rasa* of *agni* and *vayu*, *tikta rasa* of *vayu* and *akasa*, and *kashaya rasa* of *vayu* and *prithvi*. As a matter of fact, all the *mahabhutas* are present in all the six *rasas*, but the manifestation of the various *rasas* depends on the predominance or otherwise of the qualities of one or more of the *mahabhuta*. Each of the taste has an effect on *dosha*. The *rasa* which is cognized first (by impact with tongue) is considered as *rasa* (primary taste), and the *rasas* which are less apparent or cognizable are called *anurasa* (secondary taste) [8].

According to modern science, human beings can basically recognize five tastes, sweet, sour, salty, bitter, and umami. Distinct cell types located in the taste buds are said to govern the sense of taste, and it can express only one type of specific taste receptor (TR). Four categories of taste bud cells have been recognized as type I, type II, type III, and type IV. Bitter, sweet, and umami taste are recognized by type II cells (or receptor cells). Salt is recognized by type III (or presynaptic cells). There is lack of clarity on salt perception, and type I (glial-like supporting cells similar to astrocytes) or type III cells (presynaptic cells) are said to play a role in its perception. A strong evidence base is unexpectedly gathering on the role of taste upon health and diseases. Recent studies have shown that taste receptors also have several extraoral locations such as the stomach, intestines, liver, pancreas, respiratory system, heart, brain, kidney, urinary bladder, pancreas, adipose tissue, testis, ovary, etc. as being part of a large diffuse chemosensory system. The physiological implications of these taste receptors dispersed in the human body will bring clarity on several concepts used in Ayurvedic pharmacology, such as *rasa*, *guna*, *virya*, and *vipaka*. Ayurveda classifies meat taste as sweet, although modern science classifies it as umami (the Japanese word "umai" means "meaty"); therefore within Ayurvedic framework, umami should be considered as a peculiar sweet submodality. Interestingly, several scientific findings support the Ayurvedic perspective: (1) there are important structural similarities between sweet (T1R2/T1R3) and umami (T1R1/T1R3) taste receptors, both heterodimers having one subunit in common; mice perceive synergistic umami mixtures (glutamate and ribonucleotide) as tasting sweet; and taste cells coexpress the sweet taste and umami taste receptor subunits (all three T1R subunits) [9] (Table 5.2).

Charaka quotes that physician who is well equipped with the knowledge about rasa and dosha can be successful in treating diseases [11]. The enumeration of permutations and combinations of *rasa* and *dosha* helps to prefer the type of drug with a particular panchabhoutic combination/configuration for the therapeutic application of it in the management of diseases. Since the panchabhoutic combination is not directly perceived by *pratyaksha pramana* (direct observation), Acharyas

Table 5.2 Actions (*karma*) of *Shadrasa's* and disorders caused by the excessive usage of substances of dominant *rasa* [10]

Sl. no	Name of rasa	Karma (actions)	Disorders caused by excessive use
1	*Madhura* (sweet)	Bulk promoting, vitalizer, tonic, laxative, diuretic, increases kapha, decreases vata-pitta	Obesity, anorexia, respiratory disorders, lymphadenitis, diabetes, worms, etc.
2	*Amla* (sour)	Appetizer, digestive, carminative, useful in anorexia and harmful for semen, increases kapha-pitta and reduces vata	Blood disorders, swellings, inflammations, burning sensations, skin diseases, anemia, hemorrhage, vertigo, defects of vision
3	*Lavana* (salty)	Moistening, appetizer, digestive breaking, expectorant, harmful for semen, increases kapha-pitta and reduces vata	Impotency, gray hairs, falling of hairs, hemorrhage, gastritis, erysipelas, skin disorders
4	*Katu* (pungent)	Mouth cleansing, appetizer, digestive, bulk reducing, anthelmintic, useful in dyspepsia, increases vata-pitta and decreases kapha	Impotency, unconsciousness, vertigo, debility, burning sensation, thirst
5	*Tikta* (bitter)	Appetizer, digestive, anthelmintic, antipyretic, antipoison, increases vata, decreases pitta and kapha	Emaciation, debility, vertigo, dryness of mouth, nervous diseases
6	*Kashaya* (astringent)	Astringent, absorbent, healing, harmful for semen, increases vata, decreases pitta and kapha	Dryness of mouth, cardiac pain, tympanitis, obstruction in channels, impotency, nervous disorders

preferred *rasa* as a tool which is directly perceivable. Sushruta quotes that dravyas (substances) are also inferred by rasa [12]. He further observes that rasa also helps in identification of panchabhoutic combination, viz., *madhura rasa* containing *dravya*; if possessing *guru* (heaviness) guna, it is presumed that *parthiva* dominance is more in it and similarly *snigdha guna* of *madhura rasa* indicates dominance of *jalamahabhuta*. *Guru* and other gunas (qualities) are present in the *prithvyadi dravyas* (substances of *prithvi* and other *bhuta* predominance), but not in the rasas, and they are ascribed to the tastes, because of intimate coexistence.

5.4 *Vipaka* (Biotransformation)

Rasa indicates the *panchabhoutic* constituents of the *dravya*, and *vipaka* modifies these constituents by transformation into potential forms. *Vipaka* is the transformed state of ingested substance after digestion (may be interpreted as pharmacokinetic principle). This is also called *nishtapaka* (final biotransformation) as opposed to *avasthapaka* or *prapaka* (initial transformation). *Avasthapaka* (gastrointestinal digestion) involves more of a breakdown of complex substances into their simpler components, while *vipaka* takes place in *dhatu* (tissues) initiating biochemical reaction (oxidative and non-oxidative) which ultimately helps in the synthesis of molecule capable of producing different actions [13]. This aspect of the phenomenon depends on *agni*. The terms *dhatwagni* and *kayagni* stand for various cellular enzymes, hormones, and oxygen, which act on the end products of gastrointestinal digestion brought to the tissues by the blood or, in other words, metabolic reactions, viz., catabolic and anabolic. The activity of *nishtapaka* is interpreted in terms of the effects seen on *dosha* (biohumors), *dhatu* (tissues), and *mala* (metabolites). As there are two final effects on the body, *brimhana* (anabolic effect) and *langhana* (catabolic effect), the *vipaka* is said to be of two types—*guru and laghu*. Charaka takes three vipakas as *madhura*, *amla*, and *katu* [14]. Out of these *madhura* is the same as *guru*, while *amla and katu* may be included into *laghu*. Evidently the former classification is according to the effect on *dhatus*, while the latter one is based on *tridoshas*. *Madhura*, *amla*, and *katu* stand for *kapha*, *pitta*, and *vata*, respectively. All these effects (nisthaphala) perceived are explained with help of paired *gunas*, namely, *snigdha-ruksha* and *guru-laghu*. Sushruta opines that in *vipaka*, transformation of *dravya* takes place but not of *rasa*. In the light of this observation, *vipaka* can be redefined as "the process in which drug/dravya metabolizes leading to transformation of *guna* of panchamahabhutas." In other words *vipak*a is the pharmacokinetic principle which explains drug action. Nobody so far confirmed the taste of *amalaki* (*Emblica officinalis*), *guduchi* (*Tinospora cordifolia*), etc. after their completion of metabolism. The drug activity of metabolized active drug molecules may behave like dravyas dominant of *madhura*, *amla*, and *katu rasas*.

5.5 *Guna* (Attribute/Quality)

A principle which remains in *dravya* with inseparable concomitance (*samavaya*), devoid of effort (*nischesta*), and a causative factor (*karana*) in the genesis of similar attribute is defined as *guna* [15]. The *guna*s are of three types: (1) those constituting the distinctive features of the five elements, (2) those common to five elements, and (3) those relating to the soul.

The gunas of the first category are sound (*sabda*), touch (*sparsa*), vision (*rupa*), taste (*rasa*), and smell (*gandha*) constituting the distinctive features of *akasa*, *vayu*, *agni*, *ap*, and pridhvi, respectively. Those of the second category are heaviness (*guru*), lightness (*laghu*), coldness (*sita*), heat (*ushna*), unctuousness (*snigdha*), roughness (*ruksha*), dullness (*manda*), sharpness (*tikshna*), immobility (*sthira*), mobility (*sara*), softness (*mridu*), hardness (*kathina*), non-slimness (*visada)*, sliminess (*picchila*), smoothness (*shlakshna*), coarseness (*khara*), grossness (*sthula*), subtility (*sukshma*), density (*sandra*), and liquidity (*drava*). The gunas of the third category are intellect (*budhi*) including memory (*smriti*), consciousness (*chetana*), patience (*dhriti*), ego (*ahankara*), desire (*iccha*), hatred (*dvesha*), happiness (*sukha*), and misery (*dukha*), etc., and *paradi guna*s (attributes useful for the accomplishment of treatment) include efforts (*prayatna*), predominance (*para*), subordination (*apara)*, propriety (*yukti*), number (*sankhya*), combination (*samyoga*), division (*vibhaga*), separation (*prithaktva*), measurement (*parimana*), transformation (*samskara*), and repetition (*abhyasa*) [16].

Hemadri, the commentator of Ashtangahridaya (an important treatise) while commenting on the evaluation of guna, attributed specific actions to certain gunas, i.e., *guru* being *brimhana* (anabolic), *laghu-langhana* (catabolic), *sheeta-stambhana* (constipative), *ushna-swedana* (sudation/sweating), *snigdha-kledana* (moistening), *ruksha-soshana* (drying), *mridu-slathana* (relaxing), *tikshna-sodhana* (expunging), etc. [17]. *Guna*s attributed to *panchamahabhuta* constituents of dravya are *pridhvi—guru* (heavy), *sthula* (bulky), and *sthira* (stable); predominant in *gandha* (smell), *jala—drava, sita, guru, snigdha, manda,* and *sandra*; predominant in *rasa*, *agni—ruksha, tikshna, ushna, visada,* and *sukshma*; and predominant in *rupa*, *vayu—ruksha, visada,* and *laghu*; predominant in *sparsa* and *akasa-sukshma*, *visada*, and *laghu*; and predominant in *sabda* [7].

The action of drug on *dosha* is explained by Charaka basing on *guna* of the *dravya*. The details are (1) *vata—ruksha, sheeta, laghu, sukshma, chala, visada,* and *khara gunas* which are subdued by dravyas possessing opposite *guna*s, namely, *snigdha, ushna, guru, sthula, sthira, pichchila,* and *shlakshna gunas*. (2) The qualities of *pitta* are *snigdha, ushna, tikshna, drava, amla, sara,* and *katu* which are subdued by *ruksha, sheeta, manda, sandra,* and *sthira gunas. Amla* (sour) and *katu* (pungent) are the rasas, and their opposite gunas, namely, *guru-sheeta-ruksha and guru-sheeta-snigdha*, respectively, are indicated to subdue *pitta*. It appears that *snigdha guna* in a given context aggravates *pitta* and also alleviates it. If the etiological factors of *pitta* vitiation are identified as *katu rasa* dominant, in such cases one has to prescribe drugs possessing *snigdha, guru,* and *sheeta* gunas. (3) The qualities of *kapha* are *guru, sheeta, mridu, snigdha, madhura, sthira,* and *pichchila* which are subdued by *laghu, ushna, kathina, ruksha, sara,* and *vishada* gunas. The gunas of *madhura rasa*, namely, *snigdha, guru,* and *sheeta*, are subdued by *ruksha, laghu,* and *ushna* gunas. In the context of *kapha* possessing *madhura rasa*, it can be alleviated by opposite gunas enumerated by Acharyas.

5.6 *Virya* (Potency/Energy)

The term *virya* means power, potency, and efficacy. In Ayurvedic context the term conveys the idea of energy. Potent *gunas* are considered as *virya* and are identified as two or eight or one among the *gurvadi vimshati guna*s (20 gunas). *Virya* (potential guna) restricts the role of *rasa* and *vipaka* while initiating the drug action. Arunadutta has noted that *rasa* is not stable because it undergoes changes under the influence of *jatharanala* (agni), and it is not the case with gunas, viz., *guru* and the rest. The interrelationship that is stated to exist among *virya, guna,* and *rasa* and, of them, the uniqueness of *virya* have been stressed by Shivadas sen. He observes that *shakti* (energy) is *virya*. "It alone is capable of performing powerful actions. These actions do not suffer from any limitation due to nonattachment of *viryas* to *rasa*." *Virya* is intimately correlated to gunas, viz., *ushna, sheeta,* etc. Since *virya* inheres inseparably (*samavaya* in *dravya*), it is considered to be complementary to rasas. Prof C. Dwarakanath has interpreted *sheeta* and *ushna virya* as potential and kinetic energies, respectively, and categorized 20 gunas into these two groups. Potent gunas are considered as *virya* and are identified as two or eight or one among the *gurvadi vimshati gunas*. The concept of *shadupakramas* (six major therapeutic procedures) gives strength to the version of *gunakarmukata* (guna-induced action) rather than *rasakarmukata* or *vipakakarmukata* [18]. In a nutshell the concept of *virya* reflects the energy or power of potent drug molecules or active principles (secondary metabolites).

5.7 *Prabhava* (Empirical/Inexplicable Principle)

It is also referred as *achintya ashakti* (inexplicable energy). The property of a substance which produces specific actions different from and contrary to those ascribed to *rasa*, *guna*, *virya*, and *vipaka* is known as *prabhava*. For example, both *danti* and *chitraka* are pungent in tastes as well as in *vipaka* and hot in potency (*ushna virya*). But in spite of this similarity, *danti* acts as purgative while *chitraka* does not. The purgative effect of *danti* therefore can be explained only by taking recourse to its *prabhava*—the cause for specific action. Chakrapani quotes that *danti* (*Baliospermum montanum*) root soaked in water loses its purgative principle. The analysis of this observation clearly identifies the principle responsible for purgative property which is water soluble, and the drug administered without that may fail to initiate such activity [19]. Once the drug action is explained basing on active molecule (*utkrishta dravyamsha*), the concept of *prabhava* loses its place from the list of principles of drug action. It is explicit that Acharyas formulated the hypothesis to explain the modus operandi of drugs after observing various activities. In the context of failure of these hypothetical principles to explain the drug action in a rational way, the concept of *prabhava* was formulated which may be interpreted as empirical principle.

Drugs with similar chemical structure will have similar actions. But it is not possible to predict the activity of drug entirely on the basis of chemical structure. Drugs with similar structure having entirely different actions are known as isomers. For example, antazoline and tolazoline appear chemically similar, but the former is an antihistamine and the latter is an adrenergic blocking agent. In the same way, many dissimilar chemical agents are having same action. For example, phenobarbitone, chloral hydrate, and paraldehyde are all depressants of the central nervous system. The concept of *prabhava* may be interpreted with the concept of isomerism.

Charaka states that certain drugs manifest their action by virtue of their tastes, some by virtue of their potency or other qualities, some by *vipaka*, and others by their *prabhava* [20]. Another theory postulated by Charaka, the overpowering or superseding of these principles in case of all of equal strength, i.e., *rasa*, is superseded by *vipaka*, both of them superseded by *virya*, and *prabhava* overcomes all of them. How to assess the state of equal strength among these principles? Let us see the examples furnished by Chakrapani. Honey's *madhura rasa* is overcome by *vipaka* which is *katu*. This example clearly indicates that *vipaka* is *virudha* (opposite) to its rasa and equal strength between *rasa* and *vipaka* is not present in honey. *Anupamamsa* by its *ushna virya* supersedes *rasa* (*madhura*), *vipaka* (*madhura*). In this example also, *balasamyata* is not present. *Prabhava* is such a principle which never considers *balasamyata* (equal strength) or *viruddhagunasamyoga* (combination of incompatible attributes) and exhibits its activity. *Sura* (a type of alcoholic preparation) possesses *amla rasa*, *amla vipaka*, and *ushna virya* and acts as galactogogue which is attributed to *prabhava* principle.

5.7.1 *Vichitrapratyarabdha Dravya*

Usually the *bhutas* or elemental substances which contribute to the constitution of *rasa*, *virya*, *vipaka*, etc. also contribute to the composition of substances which are the substrate for them. These substances are usually classified under the category of *samanapratyarabdhata*. The qualities and actions of such substances are determined and actualized according to their secondary qualities such as the *rasa*, the *virya*, and the rest. There is the special category of substances known as *vichitrapratyarabdha* (born out of peculiar combination of causative factors, i.e., *panchamahabhutas*). In the substances belonging to this category, the collocations of the molecules responsible for the determination of their characteristics, i.e., *rasa*, *guna*, *virya*, and *vipaka*, are of a different order from those of the bhutas or elemental substance which collocate to constitute these molecules. It is because of this structural peculiarity that the effects produced by these substances are at variance with those ascribed to the different secondary qualities mentioned above. For example, both *godhuma* (wheat) and *yava* (barley) possess *swadu* and *guru gunas* (sweet and heavy qualities), yet *godhuma* mitigates *vata* whereas *yava* increases *vata* because of its *katu vipaka* [21].

5.8 Methods of Knowing About Pharmacological Properties of a Drug

The *rasa* (taste) of a *dravya* (substance) is experienced the moment it comes in contact with the tongue (*nipata*). *Vipaka* is inferred post digestion and metabolism looking at the final effects produced in the body (*karma nishta*), while *virya* is identified throughout the stay of the substance in the body (*adhivasa*) and at the beginning through the contact with the tongue [19]. The properties that exist in the causative factors (*panchamahabhutas*) are present in the resultant factors (*karya dravyas*).

A perusal of facts observed and documented by Charaka clearly indicates that *gurvadi gunas* are identified as the only attributes among *rasapanchaka* for initiation of any activity. These *gunas* can be assessed by *nipata* (at tongue level or site of application) or by their concentration in the tissues/cells (*adhivasa*). Assessment of *guna prabhava* can be made by *nipata*, *adhivasa*, and *nishta karma*, and *Acharyas* conveniently used the terms like *rasa*, *vipaka*, and *virya* for identification of *guna at various levels in the body.* Since *gurvadi gunas* are imperceptible and are always inferred by their actions, Acharyas tried to explain their presence in the *dravya* with the help of *rasa* (*nipata*, i.e., contact with the tongue) which is the only perceivable attribute of the drug. Certain *gunas* are perceivable by *nipata* (*tikshna guna* of *Maricha*) also. *Guna* (*virya* a synonym of it) is also assessed by *adhivasa* (contact with bodily tissues and cells) as well as *nishta karma* (i.e., final action), e.g., *snigdha* and *ruksha guna* at the level of the colon, influencing the evacuation of stool and urine.

Rasa is identified at tongue level and it depends on individual's perception. Rasa serves as a tool to infer the Panchabhautika composition of the dravya and facilitates for identification of the spectrum of activity of a particular drug. Acharyas of Ayurveda furnished certain characteristics of individual rasas along with their actions on the body. Since this principle's identification depends solely on the individual's ability to perceive it, a structured proforma is developed to assess the rasa of nonclassical drugs from Ayurvedic perspectives in healthy volunteers [22]. Direct taste perception method was followed in recent studies to determine rasa of folklore medicines like *Curcuma neilgherrensis* Wight [23], *Bulbophyllum neilgherrense* Wight [24], *Leonotis nepetifolia* (L.) R. BR. [25], and *Aspidium cicutarium* SW [26].

Prof. C. Dwarakanath attempted to evolve a method known as "taste threshold" for quantitative determination of intensity of rasa in a given substance [27]. The test is meant for evaluation of the intensity or degree of the taste which finally depends on the tongue only. On these lines, Prof. S.C. Dhyani conducted experiments on 150 well-known Ayurvedic drugs wherein taste of each drug was first assessed by healthy volunteers and then the taste threshold test was conducted to determine the intensity of taste of these drugs [28]. The taste perception and sensibility are complex biophysical and psychological events, and translation of rasa cannot be exactly evaluated without the help of the tongue. When the taste of the drug is explicit, then there shall be no doubt about the perception of taste. But when two or more *Rasas* manifest in the drug with almost equal quantity or intensity, both the tastes may be perceived, and it may be difficult to interpret which is the dominant or *pradhana rasa* (dominant taste). In such cases, taste perception with tongue method may give difference of opinion. Therefore, the taste perception by dilution method helps to solve this problem.

Rasa indicates the panchabhoutic constituents of the *dravya*, and *vipaka* modifies these constituents by transformation into potential forms. *Vipaka* is the transformed state of ingested substance after digestion. *Vipaka* can be assessed based on dosha karma (action on humors), dhatu karma (action on tissues), and mala karma (action on metabolic waste products) [14]. Though assessment of *dosha karma* and dhatu karma is complicated, mala karma can be easily assessed. *Srishtavinmutrata* (easy evacuation of bowels and urine) is the characteristic feature of *madhura* and *amla vipaka* and *badhavinmutrata* (difficulty in evacuation of feces and urine) that of katu vipaka. For assessing the *vipaka* of a *dravya* at *dhatu* level, it requires a minimum of 1 month because *dhatuparinama* from rasa to sukra occurs in duration of 1 month. *Madhura vipaka* is considered as *guru* and *sukrala*. Even though *Srishtavinmutrata* is common for *madhura* and *amla vipaka*, *amla vipaka* is *Sukranasana* (destroys spermatopoeitic tissue). These karmas can be elicited directly in human subjects. *Vipaka* of a dravya can be assessed by *dosha karma* in a single day or by continuous use for several days, i.e., the use of a *katu vipaka* drug increases *vata* whereas a *madhura vipaka* increases *kapha* and acts as *brimhana.*

An attempt has been made to assess *vipaka* of certain drugs by their final action on malas like feces and urine and doshas, namely, *vata*, *pitta*, and *kapha.* Drugs, namely, *bala* and *satavari* (madhura vipaka), *Vrikshamla* and *amalaki* (*amla vipaka* and *madhura vipaka*), *Maricha* and *Pippali* (*katu vipaka* and *madhura vipaka*), kushta and nimba (katu vipaka), and *Lodhra* and *Asoka* (*katu vipaka*) have been taken up for the study. The study was done for a period of 6 days. For the first 2 days, *kapardika bhasma* (250 mg thrice a day) as placebo was given, and from third day onward, the trial drug in decoction form (96 mL twice a day) was given to healthy volunteers for 2 days. The remaining 2 days was taken as follow-up period. The influence of these drugs on doshas and output of urine and feces were assessed by structured proforma. *Madhura* and *amla vipaka* drugs increased the quantity of urine and stool. *Madhura vipaka* drugs increased *kapha dosha* while *amla vipaka* drugs increased *pitta dosha. Katu vipaka* drugs decreased the urine and stool output and increased the *vata dosha* [29].

The *virya* of *dravya* is perceived through two means, viz., *adhivasa* (anumana, inference) and *nipata* (pratyaksha, directly). Here *adhivasa* (anumana) means the *karma* elicited by the *dravya* on bodily components like tissues or cells. *Nipata (pratyaksha)* means direct perception of *virya* through sense organs. When a *dravya* comes in contact with any of the sense organ, it is grouped under *Nipata. Viryas* like *picchila*, *visada*, *snigdha*, *ruksha*, etc. are perceived through *cakshurindriya* (eye); *tikshna virya* may be perceived through *ghranendriya* (nose) and *rasanendriya* (tongue).

Sushruta has enumerated eight types of *virya* and proposed the concept of how these are perceived (Table 5.3).

Out of these eight viryas, *mridu* and *tikshna virya* can be directly perceived through the tongue. *Snigdha* and *ruksha viryas* can be assessed by their effect on mala as *srishtavitmutrata* and *badhavitmutrata*. Charaka has included *guru* and *laghu virya* among *ashtavidha viryas*. These should be assessed like vipaka by their effect on the body such as *brimhana and langhana*. Vaghbata attributed certain karmas to *ushna* and *sita virya*. *Ushna virya* causes *dahana (burning sensation)*,

Table 5.3 Eight types of virya and their means of perception [30]

Sl. no	Virya	Means of perception
1	*Sita*	Sparsanendriyagrahya (touch)
2	*Ushna*	Sparsanendriyagrahya (touch)
3	*Mridu*	Sparsanendriyagrahya (touch)
4	*Picchila*	Both Sparsanendriyagrahya and Caksurindriyagrahya (touch and vison)
5	*Visada*	Both Sparsanendriyagrahya and Caksurindriyagrahya (touch and vison)
6	*Snigdha*	Cakshurindriyagrahya (by observing)
7	*Ruksha*	Cakshurindriyagrahya (by observing)
8	*Tikshna*	Mukha (Ghrana) through the tongue or nose

pachana (digestion), *svedana (sweating)*, etc. *Sita virya dravya* causes *prahladana* and *sthambhana* and acts as *raktapittaprasadana*.

Each substance contains some or the other *guna* out of 20 *guna*s enumerated in the classics. Hemadri's observations draw attention to the final fate of substances (drugs and foods) subjected to *kayagnipaka* or metabolic transformation. In this view the 20 gunas, corresponding to various substances, are reduced into 8 gunas in the first major stage, and in the final metabolic step, the 8 gunas corresponding to metabolites are reduced in to 2 gunas, viz., *ushna* and *sheeta*. These two gunas represent fundamental modes of energy which are effective in performance of actions.

In recent years some efforts have been made to evolve objective parameters to assess *snigdha-ruksha* and *sita-ushna guna*s by animal experimentation. Absolute evaluation of one guna is not possible in living body as infinite factors are related with each and every biological event. In a metabolic study, intestinal secretion and motility test and swimming stress test (swimming-induced hypothermia) were employed to assess the effect of different drugs having *snigdha-ruksha* and *sheeta-ushna* gunas. *Sheeta* and *snigdha guna* drugs have shown an increase in body weight in metabolic experiments compared to *ushna* and *ruksha guna* drugs. *Snigdha guna* drugs decreased the stress-induced hypothermia whereas *ruksha guna* drugs enhanced it [31, 32].

An attempt has been made to assess the effect of *sita* and *ushna virya* drugs (samanapratyarabda dravyas) on basal metabolic rate (BMR). Two *sheeta virya* drugs, namely, *Yashtimadhu (Glycyrrhiza glabra)* and *satavari (Asparagus racemosus),* and two ushna virya drugs, namely, *chitraka (Plumbago zeylanica) and Jatiphala* (*Myristica fragrans*) have been taken for this study. In healthy volunteers initially, BMR was recorded with Mc. Kission metabolizer. Then the drug was administered three times for only 1 day (*chitraka* and *Jatiphala* 2 g each and *Yashtimadhu* and satavari 5 g each). A significant increase ($p < 0.05$) has been observed with yashti, while increase in BMR with *satavari* was not very significant. *Chitraka* and *Jatiphala* brought about a significant decrease in BMR ($p < 0.05$). Therefore *sheeta virya* and *ushna virya* drugs which represent the *saumyatva* and *agneyatva* of a drug or food may be responsible for synthesizing or metabolizing the *dhatus* due to their *santarpaka* or *apatarpaka* actions [33].

According to Ayurveda, *parikshana* (examination) is done by *pratyaksha* (direct observation), *anumana* (inference), and *aptopadesha* (authority of an expert/specialist) [4]. *Rasa* and *virya* present in *dravya* are tested by the tongue through *pratyaksha pramana*. *Virya* and *vipaka* are tested for their action through *anumana pramana*. *Karmaphala* (the effect) is tested on the body by *pratyaksha pramana*, and then *dravyagata karma* (drug activity) is tested by *anumana pramana*. *Sharira krisatva* (leanness of body) is tested by *pratyaksha pramana*, and the *lekhana karma* (anti-obesity activity) of the *dravya* can be inferred with the help of these principles.

5.9 Factors Modifying Drug Activity

Other major factors which influence the pharmacological activities of a drug include soil, collection of the drug (according to season), route of administration, time of administration, dose, dosage form, and use of appropriate *anupana* (vehicle).

5.9.1 Soil

Sushruta indicates selection of soil for drugs having a specific activity, i.e., purgative drugs should be collected from *pridhvi* and *jala* predominant soil and emetic drugs from *agni* and *akasha* predominant soil. Vagbhata advocates to collect medicinal plants from *Jangala* (dry/arid land area) and *Sadharana desha* (land with mixed characteristics, not too dry or marshy). Plants should be collected from *prasathabhumi* (ideal land), and it should be free from big cavities, stones, and anthills. One should not collect medicine from temples, sandy places, cremation ground, etc. The land should be devoid of alkali, with hardly brittle, smooth, soft, stable, black, white, or red soil. The land should be unplowed, near a water source with abundant grasses, and not obstructed by big trees [34]. The effect of ecological conditions on properties of plants was decipherable from the opinion of *Charaka* which states that plants of *Himalayas* are qualitatively better than those of *Vindhyas.* The concept of *Vanya* and *Gramya* varieties of some medicinal plants like *Masha* mentioned in *Nighantus* possesses different medicinal properties, and it reveals a clandestine notion of effect of the ecosphere on plants. *Bhumi* of different types according to the nature of soil are described and advised to collect the plants which are growing on hills for their supremacy in quality. *Sushruta* has explained importance of *Bhumipariksha* only in context of collection of plants products.

5.9.2 Seasonal Collection of Medicinal Plants

The period or season during which drug is collected specifically influences the activity or therapeutic effect. Ayurveda advocates that drugs are required to be collected keeping in view the appropriate habitat (*desha-sampat*), appropriate season (*kala-sampat*), and their effective attributes (guna sampat) [35]. *Charaka* quotes the importance of *ritu* in germination and growth of medicinal plants. Proper season has been qualified as the season during which the plant intended for collection should have *rasa* in abundance (at level of one *rasa*), *virya*, and *Gandha*. *Charaka* has discussed the effect of stars, planets, moon, sun, and air and fire on the manifestation of *rasa*, *virya*, *vipaka*, and *prabhava* of drugs. He highlighted the role of *Kala* in the formation of drug properties and mentioned specific seasons for the collection of different parts. He also describes the direct effect of seasonal disturbances on the *Aharadravya Sangraha.* He categorically pointed out that the drugs growing seasonally are only to be collected. *Acharya Chakrapani* further clarified that root of medicinal plant with *ushna virya* should be collected in *greeshma ritu* and *sheeta virya* drugs should be collected in *Shishira ritu* (Table 5.4).

Susrutha not agreeing with popular concepts of collection of medicinal plants opined that drugs of cold potency should be collected during cold seasons (*Varsha*, *Shishira*, *Hemanta*) and those of hot potency during hot season *(Sharad*, *Vasanta*, *Greeshma).* Susrutha suggests to collect the drug basing on *virya* instead of part used of the plant.

Table 5.4 Time of collection of plants according to the part used

Useful part	*Sushruta Samhita*	*Charaka Samhita*	*Rajanighantu*
Mula	*Pravrit*	*Grishma/shishira*	*Shishira*
Patra	*Varsha*	*Varsha/vasanta*	*Shishira*
Shaka	–	*Varsha/vasanta*	–
Pushpa	–	*Yathartu*	*Vasanta*
Phala	*Grishma*	*Yathartu*	*Vasanta*
Sara	*Vasanta*	*Hemanta*	–
Twak	*Sharat*	*Sharat*	–
Kanda	–	*Sharat*	*Hemanta*
Ksheera	*Hemanta*	*Sharat*	–
Panchanga	–	–	*Sharat*

Shishira, February–March; *Vasanta*, March–April; *Grishma*, May–July; *Varsha*, August–September; *Sharat*, October–November; *Hemanta*, December–January

Modern researches reveal that the chemical processes of plant metabolism and some of the physical processes are regulated by temperature. Each species has its own optimum temperature requirement in which it grows optimally. In addition, some of the other environmental factors like humidity, duration of light, soil, soil structure, water, air, flora, and fauna can also affect plant growth directly or indirectly. Thus, collection should be by considering all these factors. Thus, with changing trend, it can be rationally postulated that cultivated field is an extended type of *Bhumidesha* that should be taken into consideration while ascertaining drug qualities. Drug should be collected in the right phonological stage in the right season. There is a vivid description about collecting the *Aahara (food)* and *Aushadhi dravyas* (drugs), and they are collected in fully grown stage.

The WHO while recommending good agricultural and collection practices (GACP) has also advocated that medicinal plants should be harvested during the optimal season to ensure the production of medicinal plant materials and finished herbal products of the best possible quality [36]. The time of harvest depends on the plant part to be used. Modern scientific validations also reveal that seasons have impact on availability of active principles in medicinal plants. The active principles and other constituents of plants vary quantitatively at different seasons of the year, and plant materials are usually best collected during the particular seasons.

5.9.3 Some Scientific Validation on Collection Practices

5.9.3.1 *Tinospora cordifolia* (Thunb.) Miers

Guduchi (*Tinospora cordifolia* (Thunb.) Miers, Menispermaceae), a dioecious creeper, has the highest concentration of total phenolics and total sugar in summer season and starch and tannin content in winter season. However, tinosporaside and berberine were seen in highest concentration in monsoon season. Studies also revealed highest antioxidant potential in winter season as well as in late summer season. Female plant was observed to be having better therapeutic phytoconstituents, and the best harvesting seasons were found to be winter or late summer for antioxidant potential and immunomodulator activities and monsoon for antidiabetic activity of *T. cordifolia* [37].

5.9.3.2 *Glycyrrhiza glabra* Linn

Studies have revealed influence of seasonal variation on antioxidant and gastroprotective activities of licorice extracts. Chemical profile of licorice quantitatively varied at different harvest times, and these fluctuations determined changes in its bioactivities. The specimens of the plant collected from May to November showed the most favorable free radical scavenging and antioxidant effects, whereas the best gastroprotective effect was in May. The major therapeutic constituents, liquiritin and glycyrrhizin, were found to be higher in February and May contributing to the superoxide radical scavenging and gastroprotective effects. Similarly, glabridin and glabrene were highest in November enhancing antioxidant and DPPH scavenging activities of licorice [38].

5.9.3.3 *Ocimum basilicum* Linn

Best antioxidant activity is observed in *Ocimum basilicum* in winter season with IC50 value 4.8 μg/mL [39].

5.9.3.4 *Alstonia scholaris* R. Br

Seasonal variation on antineoplastic activity of *Alstonia scholaris* R. Br. in HeLa cell has been observed on studying samples of the drug collected during monsoon, summer, and winter. The exposure of HeLa cells to different extracts prepared from the stem bark collected in monsoon, winter, and summer seasons resulted in a dose-dependent increase in the cell-killing effect, and the highest cell-killing effect was observed for the extract prepared from the summer collections [40].

5.9.3.5 *Momordica charantia* Linn

Seasonal variation was found to influence the antidiabetic activity of *Momordica charantia* fruits. The highest value of antidiabetic activity was found in spring season, followed by summer, autumn, and winter season. This variation may be attributed to the difference in quantity or quality of the active compounds in the fruits, as different seasons of the year could directly or indirectly affect the availability of some precursors that the plant needs for the biosynthesis of the active ingredients [41].

5.9.3.6 *Desmodium gangeticum* (L) DC

Desmodium gangeticum plant has shown quantitative variation in chemical constituents in different seasons. The variation was found coinciding with the growth period of the plant, i.e., lowest percentage was seen in the immature stage and highest percentage on fully flowering. It was also seen that in the fully ripened fruiting plants the percentage of lupeol decreases. Plants growing in higher altitude regions showed a higher concentration of marker compounds suggesting the influence of the geographical region on bioconstituents [42].

5.9.3.7 *Calotropis procera* (Ait) R. Br

Different plant parts such as apical bud, mature leaves, stem, whole plant, and flowers of *Calotropis procera* have different concentrations of phytoconstituents in different seasons. Protein and carbohydrates were highest in summer in all the plant parts. Concentration of protein was more pronounced in flowers. Tannin content is pronounced in the apical buds and stem in monsoon and summer, respectively. Apical bud showed highest concentration of phenols in winter [43].

5.9.3.8 *Plumbago zeylanica* Linn

Plumbagin content of *Plumbago zeylanica* roots collected from 13 phytogeographical regions of India has shown genotypic variations on high-performance liquid chromatography. Highest amount was detected in plants from Coimbatore, Tamil Nadu, and lowest was found in plants from Kolli Hills, Tamil Nadu. Seasonal variation was also observed in the synthesis of plumbagin in *Plumbago* plants. Expression analysis of polyketide synthase gene in roots was studied using quantitative real-time polymerase chain reaction to get better insight into its role in plumbagin synthesis. Results showed that expression of polyketide synthase gene is correlated with the level of plumbagin content in the roots of the plants [44].

5.9.3.9 *Achyranthes aspera* Linn

The seasonal variations in antibacterial activity of different parts of *Achyranthes aspera* have shown highest activity for hexane extracts of the plant collected during January against all the tested bacteria [45].

5.10 Diurnal Variations

Daily changes are observed in medicinal plants apart from seasonal variations. Circadian rhythms are known to control stomatal opening, gene expression, transcription, and timing of photoperiodism and to drive growth and development, although the control mechanisms remain unknown. Daily fluctuations were seen in the essential oil of wild basil herb, or *Ocimum gratissimum* (Lamiaceae), where levels of eugenol in the essential oil were observed to drop from 98% at 12 a.m. to 11% at 5 p.m. [46].

5.11 Effect of Lunar Cycles

Lunar cycles also influence the growth and phytochemical production in plants. Ayurvedic classics specified the collection of drug according to season and auspicious period when the moon is in the constellation of *Pushya*, *Aswinior Mrigashira.* Percentage oil of *Acorus calamus* Linn. within the rhizome varies with intensity of lunar phases. The total constituents, osmotic pressure in sap (root), and plant growth are relatively high during full moon phase when compared to new moon phases. Growth of plants recorded in ten replicates with one control was set in during experimentation. The maximum growth was seen during the month of October, and chemical constituents were found to be high in percentage during this month [47]. Garlic cloves were found to contain maximum percentage of oil during full moon day. *Adhatoda vasica* was found to contain maximum quantity of chemical constituents for developing maximum osmotic pressure in sap root in the day preceding, during, and immediately after full moon day [48]. In a recent study to evaluate the effect of lunar cycles on phytoconstituents, *ashwagandha* root (*Withania somnifera*) was found to contain maximum withanolide concentration in the samples collected in *greeshma ashadha poornima* (full moon day of *greeshma ashadha*) [49]. Thus the moon rays have a profound effect on the cell sap within the plants which in turn affects the transpiration, root pressure, and presence of active principles.

Harvesting of medicinal plants should be done considering all these factors. The best harvesting time for some of the commonly used medicinal plants are given below [50].

Kalmegh (*Andrographis paniculata*): The best harvesting time was observed at 120 days after sowing to get higher biomass containing maximum andrographolide content.

Tulasi (*Ocimum sanctum*): Harvesting done on bright sunny days yield oil of good quality and higher quantity. The oil and eugenol content is maximum at the flower initiation and seed-setting stages.

Usheera (*Vetiveria zizanioides*): The plants planted in July should be harvested after 18 months to get the maximum oil yield. The yields of root and oil percentage vary with changes in environmental conditions.

Sarpagandha (*Rauvolfia serpentina* (Linn.) Benth. ex Kurz): It is reported that roots dug out in winter (December), when plants have shed their leaves, are richer in total content of alkaloids than the roots harvested in August.

Markandika (*Cassia angustifolia*): Young senna leaves and pods contain a high sennoside content. It is also found that senna plants produce foliage containing higher sennosides between 50 and 90 days of sowing.

Vidanga (*Embelia ribes*): Studies have clearly identified the importance of attainment of maturity prior to collection. The fruits of *Embelia* are harvested on a large scale much before it attaining maturity. A comparison on the unripe and mature fruits showed huge variation in embelin, 1.67% in unripe fruits collected in October whereas mature fruits collected in December on an average contained 4.64% embelin which clearly points out that the fruits should be harvested after attaining maturity to get better quality produce.

Dhattura (*Datura metel*): The plant attains optimum vegetative growth as well as the highest percentage of alkaloids by July (5 months after sowing), when the first harvest is taken. It is recommended to harvest the leaves in the early morning or late afternoon. In studies in India, it was found that mature leaves of about the middle of the stem of *D. metel* had the maximum alkaloid content and that very young fruits possessed a higher content of alkaloid than older fruits. In *Datura metel* grown experimentally in Iran, the highest scopolamine content was found in the stem (0.3%) and young leaves (0.25%) of 6-week-old plant and in the roots (0.2%) of 16-week-old plant.

Medicinal plants should be collected in the right season in the right phenological stage. As a general rule, leaves are collected from the plants during the flowering period, as plant is very active at this time. The sap movement and photosynthetic activity are maximum, and leaves contain maximum percentage of active constituents. As the moisture decreases their constituents, they are collected in dry weather. Bark is collected in spring or early summer as the cambium is very active and due to thin cell wall bark gets easily separated. In some other cases, bark is collected in other season. Wild cherry bark is collected in autumn as it contains maximum percentage of active constituents at this season, while *Cinchona* bark is collected in rainy season as it gets easily separated. The usual time for collection of leaves is when flowers are beginning to expand. At this time it is rational to assume that the leaves are in the healthiest state and contain optimum quantity of the product of plant metabolism to produce desirable therapeutic action. Collection of flower must always be done in dry weather because the petals which are damp when gathered become badly discolored during drying. Fruit and seed drug should be collected when the fruit or seed is fully matured. Roots and rhizome are usually collected when their tissues are fully stored with reserve food being assumed that the phytoconstituents will be high during this season. In temperate region autumn is therefore the season of collection. Resin and gums should be extracted in summer. Due care should be given in the primary processing and storage of medicinal plants to protect them from mycotoxin-producing fungi. Degradation of alkaloids and medicinally valuable components of stored plant drugs due to fungal infestations has been reported [51].

5.12 Routes of Drug Administration

Routes of drug administration play an important role in the elucidation of drug action. A drug may exert different effects when given by different routes. Thus, oral magnesium sulfate acts as saline purgative. When injected, it is a depressant of the central nervous system and acts as an anticonvulsant. On the other hand, hypertonic magnesium sulfate, given as a retention enema, can be used to reduce intracranial tension. *Madanaphala* when given orally acts as emetic and if administered with *Vasti Dravays* (ingredients of enema) facilitates for its quicker transportation in the colon by its *Urdwabhagahara* (removal of malas distributed in upper portion of body) property and acts as a synergistic for toning up the nervous system or relieving intracranial tension [52].

5.13 *Anupana* (Vehicle)

The route of administration largely determines the latent period between administration and onset of action. Poor absorption of the drug, inactivation in the gut, or degradation of the drug during the first passage through the liver can be prevented by administration of *anupanas* like honey, pepper, betel leaf juice, etc. Suitable *anupana* should be used to augment the action of the drug. Just as the oil spreads quickly when put into water, so also the quick absorption and spread of the medicine are facilitated due to the addition of *anupana* [53]. The concept of *anupana* matches with the modern concept of bioavailability enhancers. A "bioenhancer" is an agent capable of enhancing bioavailability and bioefficacy of a particular drug with which it is combined, without any typical pharmacological activity of its own at the dose used. These are also termed as "absorption enhancers" which are functional excipients included in formulations to improve the absorption of a pharmacologically active drug. The term "bioavailability enhancer" was first coined by Indian scientists at the Regional Research Laboratory, Jammu, who discovered and scientifically validated piperine as the world's first bioavailability enhancer in 1979 [54]. The particle size of the drug also affects the absorption. Fine powders of the herb quickly get absorbed than coarse particle Churna. Metals in Bhasma (incinerated fine powder or nanometallic particles) absorb quickly than coarse powder of metals or minerals. Acid drugs (*amalaki*, *Nimbu*, *Amlavetasa*, etc.) are rapidly absorbed from the stomach. Basic drugs (containing Ksharas) are not absorbed until they reach alkaline environment of the small intestine (e.g., *Apamarga*, *Aswagandha*, *Sourjakshara*, *Shanka Bhasma*, etc.). The alkaline environment, in which the major component of the drug exists in an unionized form, facilitates its absorption.

5.14 Time of Administration of Drug

For better efficacy, *bhaishajya kala* (time of administration) also should be considered while administering the medicine. Time of administration depends upon the extent and rate of digestion, absorption, biotransformation, and excretion of the ingested/administered drug. Vagbhata has delineated 11 oushadhakalas considering vitiated doshas, roga (disease), and rogi bala (strength of the patient) [55]. They are:

1. *Abhakta* (without food) for *kapha* dominant and strong persons
2. *Pragbhaktam* (before food) for diseases caused by vitiated *apanavata* (a subtype of vata) and diseases of lower extremities and obesity
3. *Madhyabhaktam* (during meal) for diseases of vitiated *samana vata* and *pitta dosha* and diseases of alimentary tract
4. *Adhobhaktam* (after meal) for diseases of vitiated *vyana* and *udanavat*a and diseases of upper part of the body and emaciation
5. *Sabhaktam* (mixed with food) for children and persons with aversion toward medicine and diseases affecting all parts of the body
6. *Antarabhaktam* (in between meal) for vitiated vyana vata disorders
7. *Samudgam* (at the commencement and at the end of meals) for hiccup, kampavata, and convulsions
8. *Muhurmuhu* (frequent administration) for *swasa*, *kasa*, hiccup, *trishna, chardi*, and *visha*
9. *Sagrasam* (mixed along with one morsel)
10. *Grasantaram* (in between the morsels) for disorders of vitiated pranavata,
11. *Nisi* (bed time) for *urdhajatrugata roga* (diseases of head and neck)

5.15 *Matra* (Dosage/Posology)

Dose is defined as the amount of drug in weight and volume that is necessary to provide a desired effect. In clinical practice it is called as therapeutic dose, while for experimental purposes (in animals) it is called as an effective dose (ED). The frequency of drug administration is mainly determined by its biological half-life. Chakrapani in his book *Chakradatta* mentions that there is no fixity of a dose of drugs [56]. It should be decided according to doshas, digestive fire (*agni*) strength (*bala*), age, disease, drugs, and bowels (*koshtha*). Sarngadhara details about the dose (matra) of drugs to be used in pediatric to geriatric patients [57]. During the first month of life of the baby, the dose of medicine to be administered should be one Raktika (125 mg) given with milk, honey sugar, or ghee. With each succeeding month, the dose should be increased by one ratti, till the first year when the dose will be one masha (0.97 g). Further increase will be one masha for each successive year till the age of 16 years. From 16 to 70 years, the dose should be same. After 70 years it has to be gradually decreased as in the case of children.

5.16 Contraindications of Drugs

Ayurvedic literature gives details of drug-drug and drug-diet incompatibilities (*virudha*). Sodhana procedures described for drugs and the use of suitable anupana along with the administered drugs help to minimize the adverse drug reactions. Acharyas mentioned contraindications for the usage of certain drugs in particular conditions. For example, *Haritaki* (*Terminalia chebula*) is contraindicated in emaciated and weak persons, pregnant ladies and those who were subjected to bloodletting therapy. It is advised to avoid *Surana* (*Amorphophallus campanulatus*) in skin diseases (*dadru, kushta*) and bleeding disorders. *Vatada* (*Prunus amygdalus* Baill. var. *dulci*) is also contraindicated in bleeding disorders (Raktapitta) [58]. There have been reports of a possible interaction between garlic (*Lashuna*) and warfarin that could increase the risk of bleeding in people taking blood-thinning medication. Similarly *Ardraka* (*Zingiber officinale*) also increases the risk of bleeding when used along with anticoagulants. To avoid the adverse drug reactions, medicines should be administered considering the constitution of the patient (*prakriti*), age (*vaya*), disease (*vikruti*), tolerance (*satmya*), psychological state (*satwa*), digestive capacity (*aharashakti*), capacity for exercise (*vyayama shakti*), quality of tissues (*sara*), physical proportions of the body (*samhanana*), and strength (*bala*) [59].

5.17 Dosage Forms and Shelf Life

Panchavidhakashayakalpanas (five different dosage forms) are described in therapeutic system of Ayurveda, which is further subclassified as upakalpanas. These include different dosage forms like *Swarasa* (juice), *Kwatha* (decoction), *Kalka* (paste), *Churna* (powder), *Vati* (tablet), *Taila* (oils), *Lepa-malahara* (ointment), *Asava* and *Arista* (self-generated alcoholic preparations), *Avaleha* (linctus), *Bhasma* (incinerated powder), *Pisti* (paste), etc. Among them some have very short shelf life period such as *Swarasa* which has to be utilized immediately on preparation, and other dosage forms have longer shelf life such as Asava, *Arishta*, *Bhasma*, etc. The use of modern packaging technology and preservatives have tremendously impacted the shelf life period of Ayurvedic medicines.

5.18 Value Addition/Potentiation of Drug Activity

Charaka suggested the method for increasing the therapeutic efficacy of the drug. A drug triturated with its juice increases its potency. If a drug is added with ingredient having identical potency, then effect of recipe will enhance even if taken in small quantity. He further states that "By virtue of appropriate *Samyoga* (addition of ingredients), *Vishlesha* (elimination of ingredients), *Kala* (appropriate time of administration) and *Samskara* (processing) even a small quantity of a drug may produce more powerful effects and otherwise even a recipe in large quantity may produce very mild effect." In a way this concept reflects the theory of synergism.

5.18.1 Methods of Differentiating a Good and Bad Drug

Acharya Sushruta mentioned the qualities of ideal drug (*prasastha bheshaja*) as one grown in ideal geographical region; procured on a good day; administered in proper dose; pleasing to the mind; possessing pleasant odor, color and taste; and balancing the vitiated doshas without causing any discomfort. To maintain quality standards for the manufactured medicinal products, care should be taken right from cultivation and collection of plant materials [60]. While harvesting plant materials, care should be taken to collect only healthy ones. Plants which are infested with fungi, pests, bacteria, etc. should be avoided. The World health Organization (WHO) guidelines on good agricultural and collection practices (GACP) for medicinal plants are primarily intended to provide general technical guidance to obtain medicinal plant materials of good quality for the sustainable production of herbal products classified as medicines. Based on these, the government of India has set forth guidelines for good agricultural practices and good field collection practices for medicinal plants to ensure and enhance the quality of ASU (Ayurveda, Siddha, and Unani) medicines. The Ayurveda Pharmacopoeia of India (API) provides general standards for the plant drugs which are used in medicine. Evaluation of a drug means confirmation of its identity and determination of its quality and purity. It is necessary because there may be biochemical variations in the same drug, deterioration due to treatment and storage, and chances of substitution and adulteration [61]. Drugs may be identified on the basis of their morphological, histological, chemical, physical, and biological studies. Morphological evaluation refers to evaluation of drugs by color, odor, taste, size, shape, and special features like touch texture, etc. By microscopic and histological methods, one can confirm the structural details of plant origin. Special diagnostic characters like palisade ratio, vein islet number, and stomatal index help to confirm leaf identity. Chemical evaluation (qualitative and quantitative chemical evaluation) is very useful in detecting adulteration. Further the purity of crude drug is ascertained by quantitative estimation of active chemical constituents present in them. Various chromatographic techniques (TLC, HPTLC, HPLC, etc.) help to ascertain the quality of drugs. Assessment of biological efficacy is also important in differentiating a good drug from a bad one.

Conclusion

Every substance or matter (*dravya*) is constituted by combination of certain mahabhutas. The causative factors for initiation of drug action are enumerated under *rasapanchaka*, i.e., *rasa*, *guna*, *virya*, *vipaka*, and *prabhava. Rasa* (taste) is a useful tool to understand the probable activity of drug as well as its panchabhoutic constitution. Gunas (attributes) of dravya capable to exert the activity are referred by the name "*virya*." *Vipaka* helps to synthesize these *gunas/virya*. *Rasa* and *guna (virya)* are considered as pharmacodynamic principles, and *vipaka* is interpreted as pharmacokinetic principle. The unknown principle which contributes for specific action of a drug is referred as *prabhava.* Any activity of a drug can be explained rationally with the chemical composition or secondary metabolites. Soil in which drug grows and period of harvesting also influence chemical constituents of plants. The other factors like dose, dosage form, time, and route of drug administration modify the drug activity.

References

1. Sharma RK, Dash B, editors. Charakasamhita, Vol I. Reprint Chowkhambha Sanskrit Series. Varanasi; 2014. p. 21.
2. Sharma RK, Dash B, editors. Charakasamhita, Vol I. Reprint Chowkhambha Sanskrit Series. Varanasi; 2014. p. 451.
3. Sharma RK, Dash B, editors. Charakasamhita, Vol I. Reprint Chowkhambha Sanskrit Series. Varanasi; 2014. p. 26.
4. Acharya YT, editor. Charakasamhita vimanasthana. Varanasi: Choukhambha Prakasan; 2013. p. 70.
5. Sharma RK, Dash B, editors. Charakasamhita, Vol III. Rep Chowkhambha Sanskrit Series. Varanasi; 2009. p. 15.
6. Pandey GS, editor. Bhava prakasha, Chap. 4. Varanasi: Choukhambha Bharati Academy; 2015.
7. Sharma RK, Dash B, editors. Charakasamhita, Vol I. Reprint Chowkhambha Sanskrit Series. Varanasi; 2014. p. 452.
8. Sharma RK, Dash B, editors. Charakasamhita, Vol I. Reprint Chowkhambha Sanskrit Series. Varanasi; 2014. p. 463.
9. Gilca M, Dragos D. Extraoral taste receptor discovery, a new light on pharmacology, Evid Based Complement Altern Med. 2017;Article ID 5435831, 30p.
10. Sharma RK, Dash B, editors. Charakasamhita, Vol I. Reprint Chowkhambha Sanskrit Series. Varanasi; 2014. p. 465–9.
11. Sharma RK, Dash B, editors. Charakasamhita, Vol I. Reprint Chowkhambha Sanskrit Series. Varanasi; 2014. p. 458.
12. Acharya YT, editor. Susruta sammhita. Reprint Chaukhamba Sanskrit Sansthan. Varanasi; 2013. p. 174.
13. Dwarkanath C. Digestion and metabolism in *Ayurveda*. Varanasi: Chaukhambha Krishnadas Academy; 2003. p. 11, 71, 5, 9.

14. Sharma RK, Dash B, editors. Charakasamhita, Vol I. Reprint Chowkhambha Sanskrit Series. Varanasi; 2014. p. 473.
15. Sharma RK, Dash B, editors. Charakasamhita, Vol I. Reprint Chowkhambha Sanskrit Series. Varanasi; 2014. p 37.
16. Sharma RK, Dash B, editors. Charakasamhita, Vol I. Reprint Chowkhambha Sanskrit Series. Varanasi; 2014. p. 35, 459.
17. Harisadasiva S (editor). Ashtangahridaya, Chaukhamba Sanskrit Sansthan Varanasi; 2012. p 12, 13.
18. Dwarkanath C. Digestion and metabolism in *Ayurveda*. Varanasi: Chaukhambha Krishnadas Academy; 2003. p. 270, 2–3, 5, 8.
19. Sharma RK, Dash B, editors. Charakasamhita, Vol I. Reprint Chowkhambha Sanskrit Series. Varanasi; 2014. p. 477.
20. Sharma RK, Dash B, editors. Charakasamhita, Vol I. Reprint Chowkhambha Sanskrit Series. Varanasi; 2014. p. 478.
21. Nishteswar K. Text book of Dravyaguna. Varanasi: Choukhambha Surabharathi Prakashan; 2007. p. 71.
22. Nishteswar K. Assessment of rasa (taste) of non-classical drugs- a pharmacodynamic principle. Ann Ayurvedic Med. 2014;3(1–2):29–35.
23. Shyam Prasad M, Ramachandran A, Nishteswar K, Chandola HM. A preface study on exploring the pharmacodynamics of Curcuma neilgherrensis Wight.-A folklore medicine. Indian J Tradit Knowl. 2013;12(2):288–94.
24. Kumari H, Nishteswar K. A pilot study on Rasa (taste quality) determination of an extra ayurvedic pharmacopoeial drug Bulbophyllum neilgherrense Wight. Ann Ayurvedic Med. 2013;2(3):72–9.
25. Pushpan R. Experimental and clinical evaluation of Leonotis nepetifolia (L.) R.Br. w.s.r to its anti-arthritic activity-A tribal claim, Ph.D. thesis work of Dravya guna Department, IPGT & RA, Gujarat Ayurved University, Jamnagar; 2014.
26. Hardik M. An experimental evaluation of Antihyperlipidemic activity of Kukkutn khi (Aspidium cicutarium SW) A folklore Herbs., M.D. thesis work of Dravyaguna Department, IPGT&RA, Gujarat Ayurved University, Jamnagar; 2014.
27. Mitchell PH. Text book of general physiology. Michigan: Mcgraw-Hill; 1956. p. 220.
28. Dhyani SC. Rasapanchaka. 3rd ed. Varanasi: Chowkhamba Sanskrit Series; 2008. p. 66–87.
29. Dave NH. Vipaka karmanishtaya. Thesis, Jamnagar: IPGT&RA, Gujarat Ayurved University; 1988
30. Acharya YT, editor. Susruta Sammhita. Reprint Chaukhamba Sanskrit Sansthan. Varanasi; 2013. p 175, 183.
31. Balerao SS. A comprehensive study of gunas and evolution of some objective parameters in the context of Snigdha and Ruksha Gunas. Thesis, Jamnagar: IPGT&RA, Gujarat Ayurved University; 1998.
32. Santosh M. Evolution and evaluation of some objective parameters for ushna and sita gunas based on panchabhoutik theory and experiments. Thesis, Jamnagar: IPGT&RA, Gujarat Ayurved University; 2008.
33. Nishteswar K. Basic concepts of Ayurvedic pharmacology. Varanasi: Choukhambha Sanskrit Series Office; 2009. p. 109–14.
34. Harisadasiva S, editor. Ashtangahridaya. Varanasi: Chaukhamba Sanskrit Sansthan; 2012. p. 770.
35. Acharya YT, editor. Charakasamhita vimanasthana. Varanasi: Choukhambha Prakasan; 2013. p. 276.
36. Anonymous. Good Agriculture and collection practices for medicinal plants. Geneva: WHO; 2003. p. 11.
37. Choudhry N, Singh S, Siddiqui MB, Khatoon S. Impact of seasons and dioecy on therapeutic phytoconstituents of Tinospora cordifolia, a rasayana drug, BioMed Res Int. 2014:11p.
38. José C, Tůmová L, Areche C, et al. Variations in the chemical profile and biological activities of licorice (Glycyrrhiza glabra L.), as influenced by harvest times. Acta Physiol Plant. 2013;35(4):1337–49.

39. Hussain AI, Anwar F, Sherazi STH, Przybylski R. Chemical composition, antioxidant and antimicrobial activities of basil (Ocimum basilicum) essential oils depends on seasonal variations. J Food Chem. 2008;108(3):986–95.
40. Jagetia GC, Baliga MS. The effect of seasonal variation on the antineoplastic activity of Alstonia scholaris R. Br. in HeLa cells. J Ethanopharmacol. 2005;6(1-2):37–42.
41. Kolawole OT, Ayankunle AA. Seasonal variation in the anti-diabetic and hypolipidemic effects of Momordica charantia fruit extract in rats. Eur J Med Plants. 2012;2(2):177.
42. Jayanthy A, Prakash Kumar U, Remashree AB. Seasonal and geographical variations in cellular characters and chemical contents in Desmodium gangeticum (L.) DC. An Ayurvedic medicinal plant. Int J Herbal Med. 2013;1(1):34–7.
43. Falguni S. Range of phytochemical variations in calotropis procera. Int J Med Arom Plants. 2011;1(2):180–3.
44. Panda S, Kamble A. Genotypic and seasonal variation of plumbagin content from different populations of Plumbago zeylanica L. in India. Proc Natl Acad Sci India Sect B Biol Sci. 2016;86:165–9.
45. Suniland R, Yadav JP. Seasonal variation in antibacterial activity of different parts of Achyranthes aspera against some bacteria. Int J Med Arom Plants. 2012;2(3):369–75.
46. de Vasconcelos Silva MG, Craveiro AA, Matos FJA, Machado MIL, Alencar JW. Chemical variation during daytime of constituents of the essential oil of Ocimum gratissimum leaves. Fitoterapia. 1999;70:32–4.
47. Karnick CR Effect of phases of moon on the growth and active principles of Acorus calamus(Bach). Nagarjuna J. 1977. June issue.
48. Karnick CR Effect of lunar phase-days on the growth and active constituents of medicinal plants- Series I: adhatoda vasica nees. Nagarjuna. 1997. June issue.
49. Tavhare SD, Nishteswar K, Shukla VJ. Effect of seasonal variations on the phytoconstituents of Aswagandha (Withania somnifera(L) Dunal) w.r.t to lunar cycles. Anc Sci Life. 2016;35(3):150–8.
50. Farooqi AA. Cultivation of medicinal and aromatic crops. Bangalore: Universities Press Limited; 2011.
51. Anonymous. Good field collection practices for Indian Medicinal Plants, NMPsB, Dept. Of AYUSH. WHO: New Delhi; 2009.
52. Nishteswar K. Basic concepts of Ayurvedic pharmacology. Varanasi: Choukhambha Sanskrit Series office; 2009. p. vii.
53. Srivastava S, editor. Sarngadharasamhita. Varanasi: Choukhambha Orientalia; 2013. p. 174.
54. Navin A, Bedi KL. Bioenhancers, revolutionary concept to market. J Ayurveda Integr Med. 2010;1(2):96–9.
55. Harisadasiva S, editor. Ashtangahridaya. Varanasi: Chaukhamba Sanskrit Sansthan; 2012. p. 219.
56. Prabhakara Rao G, editor. Chakradatta. Varanasi: Choukhambha Orientalia; 2014. p. 8.
57. Srivastava S, editor. Sarngadharasamhita. Varanasi: Choukhambha Orientalia; 2013. p. 53.
58. Pandey GS, editor. Bhava prakasha nigantu. Varanasi: Choukhambha Bharati Academy; 2015. p. 6, 679, 576.
59. Acharya YT, editor. Charakasamhita vimanasthana. Varanasi: Choukhambha Prakasan; 2013. p. 652.
60. Acharya YT, editor. Susruta sammhita. Reprint Chaukhamba Sanskrit Sansthan. Varanasi; 2013. p. 148.
61. Kokate CK, Purohit AP, Gokhale SB. Pharmacognosy, vol. I & II. Pune: Nirali Prakashan; 2010.

6 Ayurvedic *Rasayana* Therapy: A Rational Understanding Necessary for Mass Benefits

Sanjeev Rastogi, Subhash C. Lakhotia, and Ram H. Singh

6.1 Introduction

Conquering death has been an eternal desire of the mankind. Numerous myths are associated with the fountain of youth or the elixir which can provide immortality. *Amrita* (nectar for immortality) is an imaginary substance from Indian mythology which is cherished for such properties. Since eternity appears unachievable, the quest for not growing old and maintaining the energy and vigor of youth continues. Although growing old and eventually dying is an eternal truth, efforts have been directed to defy it as long as possible. Every culture around the globe had something or the other with similar objectives. The preservation of the dead bodies of their Pharaohs in the pyramids by Egyptians was the epitome of the belief that someday man will conquer the death and so all the dead can eventually be alive again. The story of sage *Chyavan* having regained his youthfulness after using a *Rasayana* called *Chyavanprash* (named after him who consumed it initially) in Indian mythology has a similar notion of defying aging and regaining the lost youthfulness. In this scenario, the Ayurvedic *Rasayana* therapy emerged to provide unmatched benefits in delaying aging by inhibiting the functional decline in various body tissues that are associated with aging. *Rasayana* in its essence is about methods that promote "healthy aging" through the use of specific drugs, formulations, and dietary and lifestyle plans. Conventionally such drugs and formulations are also called

S. Rastogi (✉)
Department of Kaya Chikitsa, State Ayurvedic College and Hospital, Lucknow University, Lucknow, India

S. C. Lakhotia
Cytogenetics Laboratory, Department of Zoology, Banaras Hindu University, Varanasi, India

R. H. Singh
Department of Kaya Chikitsa, Faculty of Ayurveda, Institute of Medical Sciences, Banaras Hindu University, Varanasi, India

S. Rastogi (ed.), *Translational Ayurveda*, https://doi.org/10.1007/978-981-13-2062-0_6

Rasayana. In contemporary sense a comprehensive plan of using *Rasayana* formulations for the intended effects is called *Rasayana* therapy, and their effects in the clinical and biological sense are called *Rasayana* effects.

Rasayana was the culmination of earliest systematic study and application in the area of restorative medicine based upon the principles of Ayurveda. Unfortunately, with the passage of time, further refinements in its practice have not been made, and as a result it got gradually shrouded in myths and mystery resulting in frequent mis- or improper usage.

Advances in recent decades in understanding of aging have revived interest in antiaging factors and thus also in the *Rasayana* therapy. This has been also catalyzed by a global resurgence of interest toward natural/traditional medicine systems, in which Ayurveda remains a prominent player because of its documented antiquity. In current times, the *Rasayana* therapy is possibly the most sought after, notwithstanding the fact its basis remains poorly understood. Antiaging and super nutrition are high interest areas in biological research [1]. Consequently, the claims about the super nutritious values of *Rasayana* that can bring about qualitative changes in cells and tissues leading to their improved functioning and thus delay the decay leading to aging have helped keep the debate alive, even though the claims of such dramatic effects have rarely been seen in practice.

Despite the extraordinary praise received by *Rasayana* all through the history of Ayurveda, its applications in real practice in current times are limited. For a common man, *Rasayana* often means preparations consisting of some precious ingredients (like gold, silver, ashes of gems) that provide additional sexual vigor, although in standard Ayurvedic practices such formulations actually represent another class called *Bajikarana*. However, due to lack of clarity, they have got linked with *Rasayana*. Such lay belief has often been exploited in the consumer market in India, and elsewhere, through promotion of formulations in the name of *Rasayana*, claiming improved manliness for the consumers. Unfortunately, many Ayurvedic physicians also do not find the preventive and health maintenance properties of *Rasayana* attractive enough in the face of cure dominant contemporary medical practices. Moreover, the complex and cumbersome regimes associated with traditional *Rasayana* therapy also render them hard to be practiced. Unavailability of any immediate and tangible short-term benefit through the use of *Rasayana* in state of health or disease has further limited its use in clinical practice.

Rasayana is one important branch of study of Ayurveda among its eight divisions. Its textual praise in preventive and restorative health care is attractive enough to enquire about its utility in realistic terms. To substantiate these, there is need for finding the rationality and translational value of *Rasayana* principles and defining their practical, comprehensible, and deliverable usages.

The exploration of this kind is not only meant to validate the concept of *Rasayana* described in Ayurvedic texts by looking at them in a scientific perspective and enriching it with cutting-edge evidences but also to find the areas of the clinical applicability with a clear understanding of methods of application, primary and secondary goals of therapy, and its temporal relationship. If this kind of translation of *Rasayana* concept of Ayurveda can be done with the help of biological and material sciences, it would possibly be one of the biggest help to the mankind in this century. This chapter on Ayurvedic *Rasayana* therapy is focused on this theme.

6.2 What Is *Rasayana* and What Is It About?

Conventionally *Rasayana* is the formulation having some special therapeutic effects. These effects are related to improved functional performance, cognition, strength, and delayed aging observable through delaying the obvious telltales of aging. Vivid descriptions about *Rasayana* are available in three great texts of Ayurveda (*Brihattrayi*, namely, Charaka Samhita, Sushruta Samhita, and Ashtanga Hridaya). Besides these, *Rasayana* is discussed in most of the later texts of Ayurveda, evidencing its sustained presence throughout the history of Ayurveda. With the introduction of alchemy in Ayurveda (*Rasashastra*), the whole *Rasayana* concept took a giant leap by proposing mercury and other mineral-metal-based fast-acting formulations having superior properties compared to the herb alone *Rasayana* proposed in the early Vedic period [2].

Charaka Samhita (~500 BC), one of the most revered texts of Ayurveda, begins its treatment section (*Chikitsa Sthana*) with a highly illustrative description of *Rasayana* and *Bajikarana*. This reflects the importance of *Rasayana* as a preventive, restorative, and curative measure before recommendation of the therapeutic interventions for a disease. *Rasayana* are the means and methods of bringing qualitative improvements at cellular levels,[1] and this can either be drug based, food based, or nondrug based. On the basis of their actions, *Rasayana* are further defined as the one which arrests disease and the other symptoms of aging.[2] Further to Charaka, Sushruta described *Rasayana* in a more advanced and illustrated manner. Whereas Charaka primarily focused upon bringing qualitative and subsequently functional changes at the cell and tissue levels with the help of *Rasayana*, Sushruta recommended use of *Rasayana* for many morbid conditions as well. This disease-specific *Rasayana* approach of Sushruta is visible from the name of its chapter dealing with *Rasayana* (*Sarvopghat Shamaniya Rasayana*, i.e., *Rasayana* which conquers all the assaultive events). Later texts of Ayurveda followed almost similar trend of describing *Rasayana* till eighth century when Nagarjuna, the founder of *Rasashastra*, started experimenting with mercury and other metals as ultimate *Rasayana* to bring immortality [2]. In whatever way the *Rasayana* are described in Ayurveda, there is a consensus about methods of their use. Ayurveda recommends a specific regime of using *Rasayana*, and irrespective of type of *Rasayana* to be used, the preparatory phase is essentially the same. Similarly there is a consensus about special attributes associated with various *Rasayana* in relation to the dose and duration of their use and their effects upon particular body tissue or function of the body. Ayurveda proposes a highly meticulous plan of use of each *Rasayana* together with special precautions to be observed during the use of *Rasayana*, if the suggested benefits are to be obtained.

1 दीर्घमायु: स्मृति मेधाम आरोग्यम तरुणम वय:। प्रभा वर्ण स्वरौदार्य देहेन्द्रिय बलं परम॥

वाक्सिद्धि प्रणति कान्ति लभते ना रसायनात। लाभोपायो हि शस्तानाम रसादीनाम रसायनम ॥ च.चि. १/७-८.

Long life, memory, intellect, health, young age, improved glow, voice and strength of the body, flexibility and shine are the benefits of rasayana. Methods of procuring improved quality of body tissues are called rasayana (Charaka Samhita Chikitsa Sthana, Rasayana Paad 1/7–8).

2 रसायनम च तज्ज्ञेयम यज्जराव्याधि विनाशनम।

Rasayana is the one which eliminates aging and its related diseases.

6.3 Methods of Using *Rasayana*: Optimal Age of Beginning the Use

Use of *Rasayana* should be initiated early. Ayurveda recommends it to be started in early or middle age. This philosophy of Ayurveda is in tune to the current scientific understanding of beginning of aging and degenerative processes in human beings [3]. We are aware that aging is a gradual process occurring over time and is marked with multiple programmed and orchestrated events at cellular level. Considering the continuously ongoing events of cellular injuries as a result of metabolic processes, it is also believed that aging actually begins at birth [4]. Aging has also been linked with number of cell divisions a cell may undergo. Following Hayflick's limit [5], a cell may normally divide for a limited number of times in its life span, and this number is usually correlated with a partial loss of telomeres with each cell division. Telomeres are the chromosomal caps responsible for complete replication of the genetic material in a cell, a precondition of normal mitotic cell division. The gradual loss of telomeres at each cell division marks the senescence of cell [6].Using *Rasayana* early in the age with its intention to reduce aging may, therefore, be an approach to prepare cells to stabilize their genomic architecture. This may suggest that it would be good to begin the *Rasayana* in early childhood itself, but possibly because of complexities associated with preparing a person to become more receptive to *Rasayana* effects, this is postponed till *purve vayasi* (early age, may be the early adulthood) or *madhya* (middle) age.

6.3.1 Methods of Using *Rasayana*: Getting Ready for the Intended *Rasayana* Use

The preparations required for *Rasayana* intake in Ayurveda find a corollary in cleaning a cloth before coloring it in order to get the best results. Ayurveda proposes a thorough *Samshodhana* (bio-cleansing) protocol to be followed before a *Rasayana* intervention to ensure best possible results. There are multiple reasons for recommending a preparatory phase before the actual *Rasayana* intake. The most important of such explanation revolves around the theme that *Samshodhana* leads to a cleaning of the *srotus* (minute conduits in body) which would allow the drug to reach the target tissue for maximum effects. *Samshodhana* is also supposed to increase *Samshodhana* (metabolic fire) and hence may increase any biotransformation required to manifest the ultimate *Rasayana* effect at target site. Many unresolved questions, however, still remain. *Samshodhana* is a generic process of bio-cleansing, and its various components like *Vamana, Virechana*, and *Vasti* have generalized effects besides having their specific roles upon a particular *dosha* because of their predominant action/s on a particular system. It is, therefore, imperative to know if a particular *Samshodhana* is to be recommended for a particular *Rasayana* directed to affect a specific system. For example, if we intend to invigorate nervous system, shall we go for *Vasti* (for its *vata* correcting potential) before we initiate a neuro-regenerative *Rasayana* to get optimal results? Similarly, *Vamana* and *Virechana*, which are specific for *kapha* and *pitta* disorders, are more specific to cardiovascular,

Table 6.1 Composition of *Haritakyadi Churna*, a preferred *Samshodhana* drug before *Rasayana* intake

Component	English name
Haritaki	*Terminalia chebula*
Saindhava	Rock salt
Amalak	*Emblica officinalis*
Guda	Jaggery
Vaca	*Acorus calamus*
Vidanga	*Embelia ribes*
Rajani	*Curcuma longa*
Pippali	*Piper longum*
Vishvabheshaja	*Zingiber officinale*

respiratory, and hepatobiliary digestive systems. It would also be imperative to understand what the biological correlate of the *srotoshuddhi* is. Does it imply the improved drug absorption because of cleaner micro conduits, or does it improve biotransformation by making the cellular environment more sensitive to a particular direction of reaction? Does it result in better absorption as the ultimate benefit, and, therefore, would *Samshodhana* lead to a reduction of required dose for the desired therapeutic action? For satisfactory answers to these issues, appropriate pharmacokinetic studies on drug absorption and elimination cycles in the body are needed. In this context, it would be useful to understand if *Srotoshodhana* affects cell-cell contacts, like the tight junctions, which permit passive transport of solute or macromolecules in a dynamic manner between cells [7].

As a practical measure for *Samshodhana*, Charaka recommends only one preparation, namely, *Haritakyadi Churna*, for *Shodhana* of the body (C. S. Ch.Sth.1/25-28). This combination of nine drugs in equal proportion (Table 6.1) is to be used with hot water in a dose of about 10 g per person after appropriate *Snehana* and *Swedana*, before *Rasayana* intake. The *Samsarjana* (convalescent food practice) protocol after this *Shodhana*, preceding the *Rasayana* intake, is also substantially different than conventional *Samsarjana* practice. Contrary to the usual *Panchakarma* recommendation of gradual introduction of rice, lentils, meat, and wheat in a predefined meal course pattern based upon the intensity of *Shodhana*, in context of *Rasayana*, an oat gruel (*Yavaka Yavagu*) processed with *ghrita* alone is recommended for 3–7 days as per the intensity of *Shuddhi*[3] (purification). This is done in order to completely eliminate the traces of routine food and nutrients from the intestinal tract and adjacent tissue. The drug recommended for *Shodhana* contains *Haritaki* (*Terminalia chebula*) which suggests that the purpose of the drug here is to induce *Virechana* (therapeutic purgation). This textual reference of Charaka gives an inference that possibly the primary *Samshodhana* required prior to *Rasayana* is

3 त्रिरात्रम यावकं दद्यात पंचाहं वाअपि सर्पिषा। सप्ताहं वा पुराणस्य यावत्छुद्देस्तु वर्चस:॥

शुद्ध कोष्ठम तु तं ज्ञात्वा रसायनमुपचारेत। वय: प्रकृति सात्म्यज्ञो यौगिकम यस्य यद भवेत॥ च.चि. १/ २७-२८.

For three to seven days yava along with ghee should be given till the cleaning of the body from old excreta. Upon complete cleaning, Rasayana should be used on the basis of age, Prakriti and suitability (Charaka Samhita Chikitsa Sthana Rasayana Paad 1/27–28).

Virechana alone and not other kinds of *Samshodhana* procedures like *Vamana* and *Vasti.* It is believed that consumption of oat meal for 3–7 days as the sole food prior to *Rasayana* might promote effects of *Rasayana* through *Malashuddhi* (clearing of the old excreta) and *Koshtha Shuddhi* (clearing of the gastrointestinal tract) so that the subsequent *Rasayana* intake evokes better response.

Oat is a known source of dietary fiber having numerous gastrointestinal effects. It is found to delay gastric emptying and small intestine motility. Due to prolonged satiety after the oat meal, it may suffice at its own as a full meal when recommended pre *Rasayana.* In the large intestine, its soluble fiber increases the fermentation activity and produces butyric acid which enhances growth of probiotic bacterial strains. It increases production of microbial mass and thereby aids the removal of nitrogen via feces. It also increases wet weight of stools, thereby alleviating constipation. Short-chain fatty acids such as butyric acid enhance cell proliferation of the colonic mucosa [8]. Removal of extra nitrogen through feces, enhanced cell proliferation in colonic mucosa, and enhanced growth of probiotic bacterial strains might be some contributors to *Mala Shuddhi* and *Koshtha Shuddhi* believed to follow the oat consumption before *Rasayana* intake.

6.3.2 Choosing the Appropriate *Rasayana*? What Is My *Rasayana*?

The choice of *Rasayana* is entirely dependent upon age, *Prakriti* (innate constitution), and *Satmya* (individual susceptibility) of the intended user (see Footnote 3). This notion recognizes the fact that there can be differential choices as per age, *Prakriti*, and *Satmya.* This description of Ayurveda proposes the use of *Rasayana* in a highly individualized and dynamic manner rather than as a generic recommendation.

Ayurveda prescribes a highly precise way of selecting the right *Rasayana* for intended use on the basis of matching individual's needs and tolerances. Age reflects the specific functional decline in various tissue and organ systems, and, therefore, the choice of *Rasayana* in relation to age may be related to support the specific functions that decline with age. *Prakriti*-based choice of *Rasayana* means choosing the *Rasayana* that have properties slightly opposite to that *Prakriti* to maintain a balance in net *dosha.* A *Pitta Prakriti* individual may not be recommended *Bhallataka* (marking nut)-based *Rasayana* although the same may be a good choice for a *Kapha Prakriti* individual. Individual susceptibility also has a similar implication that all *Rasayana* may not be equally suitable to every individual. Milk is one specific example in the case. Despite its huge praise as a *Rasayana*, it is not tolerated by everyone and hence may not be recommended as a generic *Rasayana* to all.

6.3.3 Methods of *Rasayana* Intake: Indoor and Outdoor Ways

Rasayana can be used through *Kuti Praveshik* (in door) or *Vatatapik* (outdoor) methods. Among the two, *Kuti Praveshik* method is found superior to *Vatatapik* method on account of providing a controlled intervention and hence facilitating the outcome. It is, however, noteworthy that because of the complexities associated with *Kuti Praveshik* mode, it is not the commonly used method of *Rasayana* therapy.

6.3.3.1 Designing a Kuti for Kuti Praveshik Mode of Rasayana Intake

A meticulous architectural plan for making a *Kuti* (room or indoor ward for *Rasayana* patients) is recommended in classical Ayurvedic texts [9]. A *Kuti* is suggested to be built in northeast direction, covering enough space at an auspicious place having abundance of raw materials. A three-walled *Kuti* is recommended to be built with small window in the wall in order to make the *Kuti* clean, sanitized, and pleasing in every season. This might be a way of providing an all-weather natural air conditioning to keep the room warm or cool as per the need of the weather [10].

6.3.3.2 Entering into the Kuti

A highly ritualistic plan of entering into the *kuti* is recommended marked by the entry on an auspicious day and time with a clear state of mind. A prior *Samshodhana* of the body is essential before entering into *Kuti*. It is also important that the entry should not be immediately after the *Samshodhana* but after a gap so that the person regains his/her normal vital status after having undergone the *Samshodhana*. The gap can be of 3–7 days as required for restoration of the *Samshodhana* through *Samsarjana* after the *Samshodhana*.

Ayurveda proposes that immediately after the *Samshodhana*, there is a diminution of *Samshodhana* which is proportional to the intensity of the *Shuddhi* (major, moderate, or minor cleansing). In normal course of *Samshodhana*, this diminished *Samshodhana* is required to be rekindled with a specific dietary plan beginning from simple starch to complex protein and fat diet over a scheduled period which is again judged by the degree of detoxification. More intensive *Samshodhana*, therefore, requires a longer observance of *Samsarjana* to restore the diminished *Samshodhana*. A basis for the diminished *Samshodhana* following *Samshodhana* seems to lie in the greater shedding of enzyme-producing cells in the gut lumen upon a forced expulsion because of *Vaman* (vomiting) or *Virechana* (purgation) [11]. Intestinal cells are known to be regularly shed in the lumen and to be replaced by new cells regenerated at the base of the crypts of Lieberkuhn [12]. A complete renewal of the functional villous epithelium by the stem cells of the crypts of Lieberkühn takes place every 2–6 days [12, 13]. It is likely that a forced expulsion during the *Samshodhana* process may enhance the epithelial shedding, resulting in a transient deficiency of the enzyme-secreting cells in proportion to the intensity of *Samshodhana*. Therefore, the period required for recovery may also vary accordingly.

6.3.4 Methods of *Rasayana* Intake: How Long Should It Be Used?

Although described in explicit details, some key information regarding usages of *Rasayana* are missing in Ayurvedic texts. One such information is about the total duration of *Rasayana* use. There is no general plan for determining the net length of *Rasayana* use although in some individual cases it is specified. In general, this period is suggested to be between 1 and 3 years unless specified otherwise. It is also important to note that this is the minimum period required to perceive the benefits of *Rasayana*. However, the classical texts do not state if the *Rasayana* intake should be stopped after the minimal period or may be continued to get long-term or additional benefits.

6.3.5 Safety of *Rasayana*

Ayurvedic texts note that adverse effects of *Rasayana* may happen if the standard principles of using the *Rasayana* are not meticulously adhered to. Such adverse effects are more often mode-dependent rather than being preparation dependent and, accordingly, are more pronounced in *Kuti Praveshik* mode of *Rasayana* application. It is noted that if a disease occurs because of improper intake of *Rasayana* or appears during the *Rasayana* intake, the same should be immediately stopped and a proper management for the disease should be rapidly planned.[4] Ayurvedic texts, however, do not discuss in detail the possible complications following use of any *Rasayana*. Consequently, information on this aspect remains incomplete for use in real practice and needs further studies on the mechanisms of actions and pharmacokinetic effects of *Rasayana*.

6.4 Benefits of *Rasayana*

Besides its possible specific applications for certain diseases, *Rasayana*, in general, are believed to have multiple functions that improve the quality of life. Such benefits are primarily related to a few functional and anatomical attributes of the body, as described in Ayurvedic texts (see Footnote 1) (Table 6.2). Besides these generic benefits shared by *Rasayana* in general, specific *Rasayana* preparations for specific benefits are also described, which are dependent upon their composition and methods of use.

Table 6.2 Physical, physiological, and mental attributes of *Rasayana* use

Physical attributes	Physiological attributes	Mental attribute	Overall impact
Taruna vaya (young-looking appearance)	*Prabha* (glow)	*Smriti* (memory)	*Deerghayu* (longevity)
Pranati (flexibility)	*Varna* (color)	*Medha* (intellect)	*Aarogya* (healthy state)
Deha bala (physical strength)	*Swarodarya* (pleasing voice)		*Vaaksiddhi* (ability to perform what is said)
	Indriya bala (strong senses)		
	Kanti (luster)		

4 रसायन विधिभ्रंशाज्जायेरन व्याधयो यदि। यथास्वमौषधं तेषां कार्यं मुक्त्वा रसायनम॥ च.चि.१/२९.

If any complications occur due to improper intake of Rasayana, it should be stopped immediately and the disease should be treated properly (Charaka Samhita Chikitsa Sthana Rasayana Paad 1/29).

6.4.1 Physical and Physiological Attributes of *Rasayana*

Taruna vaya (young age), *Pranati* (flexibility), and *Deha Bala* (body strength) are possibly the most common features that are promoted by *Rasayana*. *Taruna vaya* is directly related to the lower biological rather than the chronological age. *Taruna vaya* essentially implies being young in appearance as well as in functions. This means that whatever it takes to attain this youngness, it needs to be omnipresent in the body through actions upon every cell so that their functions and appearances match those at younger age. Many studies have revealed the physical, physiological, and mental changes occurring in the body with aging [14, 15]. It is also known that aging occurs at different rates in different body tissues [16, 17]. In this context, *Rasayana* may have generic age-stabilizing effects, besides tissue-specific actions. Interestingly, Ayurveda describes usage of generic as well as the tissue-specific *Rasayana*. For example *Amalaki* (*Emblica officinalis*) is proposed as the best age stabilizer (*Vaya Sthapana*), while a number of tissue-specific *Rasayana* or *Kamya Rasayana* are also proposed for various tissue-related functions in the body [18].

Multiple theories for human aging exist, although none of them has been established as the sole mechanism of aging. Such theories, however, help in understanding the possible sequence of events that eventually culminate in cellular senescence and finally the death. Among the prominent theories in this context are extrinsic (stochastic) and intrinsic (developmental-genetic) cause theories. The former suggests the cumulative cellular damage from free radicals and radiation, errors in protein synthesis, and protein cross-linking as the causal mechanisms for cell aging, whereas the latter hypothesize intrinsic, preprogrammed, genetic control of cellular aging. In either case, *Rasayana* is proposed to affect factors that lead to cellular senescence. Ayurveda recognizes both the extrinsic and intrinsic causes of senescence. It is believed that exposure to *Vata* predominant food and lifestyle leads to an early aging, possibly due to damage to cells because of free radicals, oxidative and radiation stresses, and poor nutrition [19]. At the same time, Ayurveda also considers a genetically programmed mechanism of aging by believing in a decadal reduction of functional efficiency of tissues. As presented in Table 6.3, *Sharangadhara Samhita* (twelfth century AD) presents a precise account of this decadal decline of biological functionality of various body tissues by presuming 100 years as the average life span [20].

The differential rates of aging of different tissues are now well known so that at a given point of time in life of an individual, some tissue may correspond to the chronological age, while others may be biologically older because of faster aging [17]. The current average Indian life span is about 68 years [21]. It would be interesting to examine if the decadal decline of function, as enunciated in the above referred text, should be considered in reference of 100 years or should be normalized to the contemporary 68-year life span. It is also important to note that this decline refers to a healthy aging. In cases of rapid aging, due to pathogenesis or faulty lifestyle, the decline in functions can be quicker besides a selective premature loss of some specific functions. A number of *Rasayana* have been proposed to delay such common functional declines.

Table 6.3 Decadal decline of tissue functioning during aging

Age	Declining functional domain	Modern corollary
10 years onward	*Balyam*	Childhood
20 years onward	*Vriddhi*	Growth
30 years onward	*Chavi*	Skin glow
40 years onward	*Medha*	Cognitive capacity
50 years onward	*Tvaka*	Skin luster
60 years onward	*Drishti*	Visual acuity
70 years onward	*Shukra*	Virility
80 years onward	*Vikram*	Courage
90 years onward	*Buddhi*	Intellect
100 years onward	*Karmendriya*	Physical mobility

While recommending *Rasayana*, Ayurveda comprehensively outlines the various reasons of premature aging leading to years lost in disability (YLD) and years of life lost (YLL) and proposes that avoidance of such causes along with appropriate *Rasayana* intake may allow one to live the full span of life in a good functional state.[5] *Rasayana* therapy, therefore, can be considered as a remarkable intervention to reduce the disease adjusted life years (DALY) [22].

Varna, Prabha, and *Kanti* are three visible skin attributes associated with *Rasayana* use. *Varna* refers to color of the skin, whereas *Prabha* and *Kanti* refer to glow and luster of the skin, respectively. Skin color is the net outcome of a complex interplay of melanin, carotene, oxygenated hemoglobin, and deoxygenated hemoglobin. Out of these, particle size, shape, and location of melanin play crucial role in determining the skin color. The nearer the melanin particles are to the surface, the darker the skin appears [23]. *Prabha* and *Kanti*, on the other hand, are more reflective of radiance of skin which represents status of skin perfusion and oxyhemoglobin levels. The skin, which has good perfusion with good oxyhemoglobin level in the blood, radiates more vibrantly hence displays improved *Kanti*.

Aging affects the skin in multiple ways, and there are more age-related changes in the skin than those reflected through its *Varna*, *Prabha*, and *Kanti* alone. As a result of aging, the skin becomes darker, less elastic, thinner, fragile, and rough with reduced epidermal turnover so that a wound in later ages takes more time to heal. The characteristic wrinkling of the skin in old age is due to loss of subcutaneous fat and reduced bonding between epidermis and dermis. Epidermal thickness decreases about 6.4% per decade on average, with an associated reduction in epidermal cell numbers. The overall volume of subcutaneous fat typically diminishes with age,

[5] सर्वे शरीर दोषा भवन्ति ग्राम्याहारादम्ल लवणकटुक्षारशुष्कशाकमांस तिल पलल पिष्टान्न भोजिनां विरूढ नव शूक शमी धान्य विरुद्धासात्म्य रुक्ष क्षाराभिष्यन्दि भोजिनां क्लिन्न गुरु पूति पयुर्षित भोजिनां विषमाध्यशन प्रायाणां दिवास्वप्न स्त्री मद्य नित्यानां विषमातिमात्रव्यायाम संक्षोभित शरीराणांम भय क्रोध शोक लोभ मोहायास बहुलानाम; अतोनिमित्तम हि शिथिलीभवन्ति मांसानि, विमुच्यन्ते सन्धय:,विदह्यते रक्तम, विष्यन्दते चानल्पं मेद:, न संधीयते अस्थिषु मज्जा, शुक्रं न प्रवर्तते, क्षयमुपैत्योज:, स एवम भूतो ग्लायति, सीदति, निद्रा तन्द्रा आलस्य समन्वितो निरुत्साह: श्वसिति,असमर्थश्चेष्टानां शारीरमानसीनां, नष्ट स्मृति बुद्धिच्छायो रोगाणाम अधिष्ठान भूतो न सर्वमायुरवाप्नोति।तस्माद एतान दोषान अन्वेक्षमाण:सर्वान यथोक्तान अहितानपास्य आहार विहारान रसायनानि प्रयोक्तुम....। च.चि. १ रसायनाध्याय द्वितीय पाद/ ३.

although the proportion of total body fat increases with aging [24]. Reactive oxygen species (ROS) plays a key role in skin aging by causing damage to the cellular structures including the membranes and DNA. Contrary to the internal tissue aging, the skin is also exposed to external environment which causes an extensive damage to skin tissue. There are also changes in its neurosensory perception, permeability, response to injury, repair capacity, and increased incidence of some skin diseases.

In view of such wide range of effects of aging on the skin, *Rasayana* intending to act on skin aging should have an ability to address such diverse age-related changes in the skin. In view of the obvious visibility, changes in the skin are often the first telltale signs of aging, and again, because of their obvious visible impacts, they attract greater attention for reducing the changes. A large number of local applications are being tried to address the visible signs of skin aging, although such local applications appear to miss the point that aging is a cellular process and any intervention to reduce this has to act at cellular level.

Besides conventional *Rasayana* drugs, Ayurveda also proposes highly beneficial effects of *Abhyanga* (oil massage) on skin aging. Although not considered directly within the purview of *Rasayana*, *Abhyanga* has good reasons to be considered as *Rasayana* because of its *Alpajara* (delayed aging) effects. Beneficial effects of massage are multidimensional. Besides improving blood circulation, it also stimulates parasympathetic nervous system, giving the person calm and relaxed feeling [25]. This improves the serotonin levels, induces good sleep, and reverses the catastrophic effects of stress hormones. It reduces the transepidermal water loss (TEWL) and hence maintains the tissue turgidity to help keeping it soft and supple. Sesame (*Sesamum indicum*) oil, commonly recommended as massage oil in Ayurveda, has its own antiaging benefits for being rich in tocopherol and linoleic acid. An increased wound healing was reported following local use of ozonated sesame oil [26]. Oil massage is a regular health-keeping practice in India and is reported to cause increased body weight in infants who receive regular massage [27]. A better skin integrity is also observed among the babies who are massaged with sunflower oil [28]. Ayurveda proposes that a regular *Tailabhyanga* renders the skin with properties like *Sutwaka* (beautiful skin), *Susparsha* (better touch perception), *Priya Darshana* (good looking), and *Alpa Jara* (less affected by aging) (Charaka Samhita Su. 5/85-89). All of these properties are comparable to those of *Rasayana,* and hence, *Tailabhyanga* may be considered as *Rasayana*.

6.4.2 *Medhya Rasayana* for Improving Mental/Brain Activity

Smriti (memory) and *Medha* (intellect) are two important cognitive attributes offered by *Rasayana*. Besides being associated with all *Rasayana*, Ayurveda proposes a special *Medhya Rasayana* category which is specialized in cognitive care. *Mandukparni* (*Centella asiatica*), *Yashtimadhu* (*Glycyrrhiza glabra*), *Guduci* (*Tinospora cordifolia*), and *Shankhpushpi* (*Convolvulus pluricaulis*) are four such *Rasayana* providing special *Medhya* effects. These plants have special intake methods and special parts to be used for *Medhya* purpose [29]. Among these, *Shankhpushpi* is considered as the best and is recommended to be consumed as a *Kalka* (paste) of whole plant [30]. Besides these recommendations from Charaka under the category of *Medhya Rasayana*, a few more herbs are in practice for similar purposes. These are *Aindri* (*Bacopa monnieri*), *Jyothishmati* (*Celastrus paniculatus*), *Kushmanda* (*Benincasa hispida*), *Vacha* (*Acorus calamus*), and *Jatamamsi* (*Nardostachys jatamansi*).

6.4.3 Impact of *Rasayana* in Totality

Deerghayu (long life) and *Arogya* (disease-free status) are proposed to be the eventual effects of all *Rasayana*. Almost all the *Rasayana* recommended in Ayurveda act primarily on increasing the life span to the maximum possible extent in reference to human life. References are suggestive of 100 years as the optimal age of human being, and so most *Rasayana* target to achieve this age span, and doing so they essentially target eliminating the diseases which may act as a limiting factor in availing this objective.

How much time is required for a *Rasayana* to give rise to this effect? Is it a lifetime intervention or an intervention having lifetime effects? For specific *Rasayana* formulations, Ayurveda has a recommendation of consuming for a period of 1–3 years. At the same time, food- and lifestyle-based nondrug *Rasayana* are recommended to be used consistently throughout the life (*Nitya Rasayana*). There are many *Rasayana* which are primarily active on certain systems, tissues, and functions and hence also act on diseases pertinent to those systems or tissues. *Chyavanprash*, for example, is considered as *Rasayana* acting on respiratory system and hence is effective in conditions like *Kasa* (cough) and *Shvasa* (dyspnea). *Chyavanprash* also has anabolic properties (*Angavardhana*) and hence is employed to counter the emaciation consequential to respiratory diseases. *Brahma Rasayana* in particular is able to create calmness and purity of mind (*Aarsh Satva*) and hence can be employed as a *Rasayana* in all psychological and psychiatric illnesses. *Bhallataka* (*Semecarpus anacardium*) is highly recommended in *Kapha* disorders and is also recognized to promote intellect and appetite (*Medhagni Vardhana*). *Pippali* (*Piper longum*) *Rasayana* is recommended for various respiratory conditions.

What should be the dose of one *Rasayana*? Ayurveda recommends the *Rasayana* dosage in reference to individual *Agnibala* (digestive capability). In most cases it is recommended to be an amount that does not reduce the normal food intake. Food is recommended to be taken only after the initial dose of *Rasayana* is digested and one feels hungry. In some cases a second dose in the evening is also recommended. In most conditions, a special course of meal is recommended during the *Rasayana* intake. These include milk, *Mung yush* (*Mung* broth), *Yava* (barley), etc. in specific cases.

6.5 Herbometalic and Mercurial Compounds as Fast-Acting *Rasayana*

With the emergence of *Rasashastra* (Ayurvedic Alchemy), mercury and other metals (like gold, silver, iron, copper, zinc, etc.) and mineral-based formulations were prepared through various specialized methods, which rendered them nontoxic and at the same time highly active. This was a turning point in the history of Ayurvedic clinical practices. Alchemy in India was started in post-Vedic period (400–800 AD), initially with the primary intent of preparing an elixir of life for imparting immortality and later for the transmutation of base metals into gold [31]. *Rasashastra* describes number of preparations composed of mercury and sulfur and other metals and herbs, having special properties of countering the effects of aging and subsequently increasing the life span. These herbo-metallic compounds are sensu stricto not considered and used as *Rasayana*, despite their being mentioned as *Rasayana* in *Rasashastra* classics like *Rasaratna Samuccaya*. These formulations are also not as commonly used as *Rasayana* because of a general apprehension of toxicity associated with mercury and other heavy metals. However, many studies have not only endorsed their being nontoxic but also their consideration under *Ayurveda* to deliver benefits that are typically associated with traditional *Rasayana*. This is also noteworthy that such preparations, on account of their faster actions and high penetrability, were not required to be taken in a strict *Kutipraveshik* manner and were able to give their therapeutic effects in relatively shorter periods with small doses. Several experimental studies on mercury- and sulfur-based compound *Ras Sindoor* in recent years have examined biological effects of this formulation in different animal model systems and also its physicochemical nature and potential metal toxicity. Besides improving the general well-being and certain cell stress responses in the *Drosophila* model [32], *Ras Sindoor* ameliorated neurodegeneration in fly models of Huntington's and fly and rat models of Alzheimer's diseases [33, 34]. In all cases, there was no evidence of cellular or organismic toxicity due to the heavy metal. Biophysical studies on *Ras Sindoor* revealed that the Ayurvedic method of preparation of *Ras Sindoor* results in the final product being completely nontoxic nanoparticles [35, 36].

6.6 Nondrug *Rasayana*: Food, Lifestyle, Behavior, and Values Giving Rise to *Rasayana* Effects

Besides drug-based *Rasayana*, various dietary substances, lifestyle measures, behavior, and values are also recommended to have *Rasayana* effects of their own. These may collectively be called as nondrug *Rasayana*. *Ghrita* and milk are best examples in food category.[6] A regular use of milk and *ghrita* is considered as *Rasayana* in Ayurveda. *Amalaki* itself is proclaimed as best *Vayasthapana* (age stabilizer), and, therefore, use of its fruit itself also gives *Rasayana* effects. Substantial work has recently been carried out to examine the effects of *Amalaki Rasayana* (a formulation derived primarily from *Amalaki* fruits) on aging and other biological parameters using fruit fly models [32, 37]. This *Rasayana* was found to improve the thermal, starvation, and oxidative stress tolerances in *Drosophila* which may explain its antiaging effects [37]. *Amalaki Rasayana* administration in rats also reduced the age-associated DNA damage in brain cells [38] and improved the telomerase activity in rat blood cells [39]. Such beneficial effects of *Amalaki Rasayana* also contribute to its antiaging effects. More significantly, this formulation was also found in fly and rat models to substantially alleviate the neurodegeneration associated with diseases like Huntington's and Alzheimer's [33, 40]. *Amalaki Rasayana* was also found having beneficial effects upon myocardial energetics, muscle contractile function, and exercise tolerance capacity [41].

A comprehensive value-based lifestyle (*Achara Rasayana)* is also proclaimed in Ayurveda to have effects similar to those of *Rasayana* intake.[7] Principal recommendations in *Achara Rasayana* are related to interpersonal behavior, mental attitude, values and moral, spirituality, dietary habits, etc. (Table 6.4). Most of these recommendations are helpful in reducing internal and external conflicts and thus help in avoiding stress. These recommendations of Ayurveda are very much in tune with what is called *eudaemonic* well-being (a collective assembly of positive behaviors inclusive of self-acceptance, positive relations with others, autonomy, environmental mastery, purpose in life, personal growth, etc.) [42]. A *eudaemonic* lifestyle is found to reduce the broad-based morbidity and mortality and thus helps in achieving the objectives of good health and long life as envisaged for *Rasayana*. Ayurveda in a highly appreciable manner identifies four possible modes of leading the life, namely, *Hitayu* (life helpful to others), *Ahitayu* (life unhelpful to others), *Sukhayu* (life pleasurable to self), and *Dukhayu* (life

---

6 क्षीर घृताभ्यासो रसायनानां । च.सू.२५/४०.

A practice of consuming milk and ghrita on daily basis is like Rasayana (Charaka Samhita Sutra Sthana 25/40).

7 सत्यवादिनम अक्रोधमं निवृत्तं मद्यमैथुनात । अहिंसकमनायासं प्रशान्तम प्रियवादिनम।
जप शौच परं धीरं दान नित्यं तपस्विनम। देवगोब्राह्मणाचार्य गुरु वृद्धार्चने रतम॥
आनृशंस्यपरं नित्यं नित्यं करुणवेदिनम । समजागरणस्वप्नं नित्यं क्षीरघृताशिनम॥
देशकालप्रमाणज्ञं युक्तिज्ञम अनहंगकृतम। शस्ताचारम असंकीर्णम अध्यात्म प्रवणेन्द्रियम॥
उपासितारं वृद्धानामास्तिकानां जितात्मनाम। धर्मशास्त्र परं विद्यान्नरं नित्यरसायनम॥
गुणैरेतैः समुदितैः प्रयुंगक्ते यो रसायनम। रसायन गुणान सर्वान यथोक्तान स समश्नुते॥ च. चि. १-४/ ३०-३५.

The one who adheres to truth, does not get angry, has abandoned alcohol and sexual indulgence, nonviolent, calm and pleasing in speech, has spiritual interests, clean, donor, respectful to elders, teachers, Brahmins and deities, empathetic, has a balanced sleep and awake cycle, consumes milk and ghrita routinely, does carefully as per the need of season, and place, careful in behavior, has a control on sensual desires, interested in reading spiritual texts gets all the benefits of Rasayana even if he does not consume any Rasayana (Charak Samhita Chikitsa Sthaan 1 Rasayan Paad 4 / 30–35).

Table 6.4 Acts enumerated under *Achara Rasayana*

Class of attributes	Description	Current understanding
Mental attributes	*Satyavadinam*	Adherent to truth
	Akrodham	Non-anger
	Ahimsakam	Nonviolent
	Prashantam	Cool
	Priya vadinam	Speaking pleasantly
	Japa	Spiritually inclined
	Shauch	Inclined toward cleanliness
	Dheer	Patience
	Daan	Donations
	Tapasvinam	Dedicated
	Deva go brahmanaacharya guru vruddha archana	Respectful to God, Brahmin, scholars, teacher, elderly
	Aanrishansaya	Non-harsh
	Karunavedinam	Empathetic
	Shastaacaaram	Appropriate behavior
	Asamkeernam	Open-minded
	Adhyatma pravan	Spiritually oriented
	Upasita vriddhanam astikanaam	Praising the elderly and devotees
	Jitaatmananam	Having self-control
Habits	*Nivrattam madya maithunat*	Having abandoned alcohol and sexual indulgence
	Sam jaagaran swapnam	Balanced sleep and wake cycle
Physical attributes	*Anayasam*	Not doing excessive physical activity
Food habits	*Nityam ksheer ghritashinam*	Daily intake of milk and *ghrita*
Cognitive attributes	*Deshkaal pramaanagya*	Knowing of behaving as per time and place
	Yuktigyam	Knowing of taking action as per appropriate need
	Dharmashaastra param vidyaanaram	Inclined toward studies and spiritual books

miserable to self). Out of these, Ayurveda recommends *Hitayu* as the most gratifying and thus promotes all the values and measures which promote *Hitayu* [43].

6.7 *Rasayana* Principles and Contemporary Practices: Identifying the Gaps and Structuring the Bridges

Ayurveda presents a vivid account of measures and approaches helpful to make the foundation of delayed aging, a desire of mankind since antiquity. Such measures are highly diverse and include various drug and nondrug approaches. Ayurveda's drug-based measures include herbs, minerals, and metals in isolation or in combination. Non-drug measures are composed of various dietary and lifestyle habits. Such methods have been so highly praised in Ayurvedic literature that metaphorically they provide a connotation of enabling a person with sustainable superhuman strengths and a maximally expanded life span. Ayurvedic account of *Rasayana* seems to be the earliest written account of conceptualizing betterment of human race through postnatal applications aiming at improving the post-birth quality and appearance. The idea of "euphenics" was also proposed by Lederberg in 1960 [44].

6.7.1 Gaps in Understanding the Mechanisms of Biological Actions of Different Rasayana

Considering the importance of herbal preparations in Ayurveda and all traditional health-care systems [45–47], numerous studies have been undertaken during the past several decades to identify the "active principle/s" in different herbal preparations that have the most potent effect for a given health condition. In fact, genesis of most of the modern medicines can be traced back to this kind of research. However, this reductionist approach to identify the "active principle" in the herbal formulations is not in consonance with the holistic approach of Ayurveda. Almost all the *Rasayana* are complex formulations of herbal or herbo-mineral mixtures, most of which, as discussed above, are used in conjunction with other lifestyle practices. Despite the traditional medicines being at the roots of modern medicine, some degree of mutual suspicion and contempt has emerged between practitioners of modern and traditional medical systems due to differences in their underlying approaches. This is aggravated especially because the mechanistic details of the modes of actions of Ayurvedic *Rasayana* and other practices are not understood in terms of contemporary understanding of biological and material systems. This calls for unbiased scientific inquiries to understand the modes of actions of the diverse *Rasayana* at molecular, cellular, and organismal levels using good experimental planning and models. The true spirit of Ayurveda would be revived, and mankind would gain from its advantages only through in-depth studies of the ancient texts together with rationally designed experimental studies directed to understand the biological effects of various Ayurvedic formulations and practices. It is indeed necessary that the experience-based practices be supplemented by experiment-based evidences and understanding [46–50].

The emergence of Ayurvedic biology [46, 51] during the past decade is a very significant development in this context from the viewpoint of rejuvenation of the age-old Ayurveda. Such in-depth and unbiased basic researches on the underlying principles and their modes of actions on different constituents of the body, including at cellular and subcellular levels, are providing better understanding of the mechanisms and efficacies of various principles, practices, and formulations that are fundamental in Ayurveda. It is highly desired that well-coordinated basic science studies are undertaken to understand the mechanisms of actions of each of the *Rasayana* described in classical texts so that we can understand their modes of actions at molecular, cellular, and tissue levels in the context of contemporary biological and material sciences. It would also be useful to examine the physiological and other changes at organism level that follow the administration of a given *Rasayana*. Basic science studies would also help in sorting out myths that would have inevitably crept in during the thousands of years of Ayurveda's history. More importantly, such basic studies would also unravel novel therapeutic applications of even the most commonly used Ayurvedic formulations. For example, basic studies in *Drosophila* and rat models have shown [33, 34, 40] that *Amalaki Rasayana* and *Ras Sindoor* can be very effective in suppressing the increasingly common neurodegenerative ailments like Alzheimer's and Huntington's diseases.

Another major issue that hampers widespread usages of Ayurvedic *Rasayana* formulations is the quality control. Being complex mixes of multiple herbal extracts and products, it is nearly impossible to develop efficient physicochemical quality control measures for the diverse *Rasayana*. A detailed understanding of biological actions of the given *Rasayana*, prepared in the prescribed manner, in a suitable model system can provide good-quality control parameters.

It is not out of context here to see what Ayurveda proposes as a possible mechanistic explanation to *Rasayana*. Charaka proposes the *Rasayana* as a means of producing better quality cells and tissues through optimal nutrition in order to achieve their best functional status (*labho paayo hi shastanaam rasadeenam rasaayanam*) (see Footnote 1). This opens up the possibility that *Rasayana* act through improved nutrition dynamics so that some essential nutrients reach the target tissue and optimize the cellular functions. It is likely that the protocol mode associated with *Rasayana* consumption (*Samshodhana* etc.) also further facilitates the essential nutrients to reach the target tissue. Obviously, massive and organized efforts are essential to initiate appropriate experimental studies on modes of actions of the diverse *Rasayana* and other formulations described in *Ayurveda*. Then only we would understand the underlying mechanisms and let the masses take full advantage of this age-old health-care knowledge base.

6.7.2 Contemporary Rasayana Practices: Minding the Ethical Gaps

The context of *Rasayana* looks highly inspiring when read from a preventive and promotive perspective, but it can also be depressive when one looks at some of the prevailing practices. Contemporary practice of *Rasayana* seems to have often missed the essence of practicing *Rasayana* and *Bajikarana* in their own contexts. Whereas *Rasayana* is primarily meant for improving functional abilities and longevity so that its practitioner can utilize them in a higher societal pursuit, *Bajikarana* essentially focuses upon improving functional abilities from a pleasure-seeking personal perspective. Failing to appreciate this distinction, we see that many *Rasayana* drugs are promoted commercially for their value as an aphrodisiac. *Shilajatu* is an apt example in this context which, despite being a highly praised *Rasayana*, is primarily promoted as an aphrodisiac. *Triphala* is another example in the series. Despite the high praise of *Triphala* as *Rasayana,* in practice it is being recommended mostly as a purgative. Lay and popular media have contributed to such misinformation by putting word *Rasa* in *Rasayana* in the context of pleasure-seeking aphrodisiac activity.

In the context of *Rasayana's larger aim being directed to* societal purposes, Ayurveda clearly defines criteria for the people eligible to undergo *Rasayana* therepy.[8] These criteria primarily call for a mental and physical integrity and cleanliness of the prospective recipient in order to assure the use of additional abilities for the right causes. These criteria, however, are relaxed when the recipient is sick and if the *Rasayana* is intended primarily for curative purposes. Such ethics-bound selectivity in choosing the right recipient is often missing in contemporary *Rasayana* practices. Such concerns have been expressed in the context of eugenics, euthenics, and euphenics practices [52] and cannot be overlooked in relation to contemporary practices of *Rasayana* therapy.

6.7.3 Gaps in Awareness: Rasayana Market and Consumers

Getting beyond the ethical concerns of practicing *Rasayana*, the other concerns are based on ground realities of gaps between the knowledge available in the classical texts of Ayurveda and the one required for making a decision about its use. The primary concerns are about finding the relevance of using *Rasayana* in the contexts they have initially been promoted. Many *Rasayana* preparations are available as the over-the-counter products in the market, and a large population is using them regularly on their own as health supplements. Unfortunately so far, there is no definitive evidence that the "*Rasayana* effect" has been achieved in terms of "healthy aging" and endowment of better functional abilities following the use of such *Rasayana*. *Chyavanprash*, a highly praised and consumed *Rasayana*, is a good example. An amount equal to 2.5 crore kg of *Chyavanprash*, worth Rs. 500 crores, is being sold every year in India and elsewhere [53]. Its intended use is variable as per the personal choice. Some prefer it using in winter as a protection against respiratory tract diseases, whereas others use it throughout the year. Considering a 2.5 kg/person consumption on average, we can presume a gigantic 1 crore population as an all-time regular consumer of *Chyavanprash* at any given point of time. This looks to be an amazingly large massive application of *Rasayana* at community level. However, are we really able to make any noticeable difference in health status among the consumers and nonconsumers of *Chyavanprash*? Besides this, there is another flipside story associated with *Chyavanprash*. The consumption of this highly

8 यथास्थूलमनिर्बाह्य दोषान्छारीरमानसान। रसायनगुणैर्जन्तुर्युज्यते न कदाचन॥

योगा ह्यायु:प्रकर्षार्था जरा रोग निबहर्णा:। मन:शरीर शुद्धानाम सिध्यन्ति प्रयतात्मनाम ॥

तदेतन्न भवेद्वाच्यम सर्वमेव हतात्मसु। अरुजेभ्यो अद्विजातिभ्य : शुश्रूसा येषु नास्ति च॥ च.चि.१-४/ ३६-३८.

Until a person is clean externally as well as internally, physically as well as mentally, Rasayana never gives its desired effects. Those who have a control on their desires, and those who have a clean mind and body, if use Rasayana for curing a disease or for delaying aging, get all the benefits of Rasayana. Those who do not have a self-control, are not sick, not respectful to elders should not be given a course of Rasayana (Charaka Samhita Chikitsa Sthana 1, Rasayana paad 4/ 36–38).

acclaimed *Rasayana* was banned in 2008 for athletes by Indian Olympic Committee on the pretext that about 20% brands of *Chyavanprash* contain or produce compound-mimicking epiandrosterone, an anabolic steroid banned by International Olympic Committee [54]. Allegations of adulterating Ayurvedic drugs with synthetic medicines, steroids, and analgesics for their enhanced effects are not new. A recent addition in the list is of sildenafil, tadalafil, and/or vardenafil adulteration to Ayurvedic *Rasayana* drugs and aphrodisiacs [55]. The *Chyavanprash* story, however, has also to be looked at from a different viewpoint since it is having anabolic properties of its own, leading to an increase in body weight (*anga vardhan*). Obviously, it is crucial to actually identify the mechanisms and basis for the anabolic effects of *Chyavanprash* in order to recommend its usage in a specific and controlled manner.

Indian Ayurvedic drug industry currently is worth about Rs. 4000 crore [56]. *Chyavanprash* alone accounts for about 12.5% share of this market, making it one of the largest-selling Ayurvedic products in the global market. It is indeed disappointing that despite this being the most acclaimed, marketed, and sold Ayurvedic product, very little is done to prove and maintain its credentials. Very few scientific studies have actually examined the claimed health benefits of *Chyavanprash*, and even these studies are of limited value because of their small sample size, short study duration, and other methodological limitations [57]. One study by Yadav et al. is worth highlighting here as being the sole study speaking about classical *Rasayana* effect of *Chyavanprash* in terms of genoprotection preventing the smoking-induced mutations [58]. We do not however find a single study being conducted to ascertain the appropriate period of intervention as recommended in Ayurveda.

6.7.4 Gaps in the Practice: Concern of Lack of Trust Reflecting the Knowledge Gap

Ayurvedic practitioners themselves often do not trust the claims endorsed for various *Rasayana*, and hence they do not practice it. The consumers, because of the unawareness, also do not get the proclaimed benefits of *Rasayana* since their intentions are mostly limited to gain some petty health benefits to make them disease free during changing weathers or sometimes for aphrodisiac benefits. Ayurvedic pharmaceutical companies have no interest in undertaking R&D in *Rasayana* because they are able to get their share from the market without investing in such researches. Researchers in Ayurveda are not interested to work on this for the perceived complexity and intangibility associated with the subject. Due to such disinterest, what is found is that there is a gross mismatch between principles and practice of *Rasayana*, almost to the point where good practices are becoming nonexistent. In view of these, *Rasayana* has largely become an endangered wisdom. Its retrieval to its past glory, proactive steps to preserve and to promote this wisdom are urgently required.

Besides saving this science as an ancient wisdom from becoming extinct, there are stronger reasons to look back at *Rasayana* for its healthy aging propositions. The life expectancy in India has increased to 68.78 years. The ratio of elderly population in India is rapidly increasing with its share reaching about 8% of the current total population. This is expected to reach 12.5% by 2030 and 19% by 2050 as per UN Population Fund India report 2017 [59]. This means that by 2050 about one-fifth of Indian population will be above 60 years hence requiring extra care related to aging. Any current proposition which can offer a healthy aging to this upcoming "going to be old" population is most fascinating and desired proposition. The best proactive mode for this could be the introduction of *Rasayana* to school-going children, on a similar note as is thought for managing malnutrition, anemia, and worm infestations in the children through various national health programs.

There are wide gaps in what is known about usages of *Rasayana* and what is required to be known to ensure its evidence-based practice. Ayurvedic texts at places do not clearly elaborate about standard operating guidelines of using *Rasayana* in every individual context. As discussed above, many questions, in the context of use of *Rasayana* in reference to drug and general, do not have clear answers.

Bringing clarity for its deliverables, rational protocols of its use including the dose and duration determinations, standardization of the preparations, and defining the usage in healthy and sick population are some areas which need clear evidences for using and recommending *Rasayana* in specific conditions. Ayurvedic hospitals and institutions may need to come forward to generate long-term observation-based data to find prospective benefits of using various *Rasayana* in different segments of populations. There is a strong need for determining the differences between outpatient-based and inpatient-based *Rasayana* intake in order to establish any superiority of the latter over the former. Need of *Samshodhana* prior to *Rasayana* is also required to be reexamined on the basis of scientific evidences. Long cohort studies may be required to differentiate between disease occurrences in a control unexposed and exposed populations consuming *Rasayana*. Finally, a number of scientific evidences may be required to put forward the genome-based mechanism involved behind the *Rasayana* effects. The recently initiated Ayurvedic biology studies have started giving clues about the cellular mechanisms underlying the actual *Rasayana* effects of various *Rasayana* preparations. Much more, however, is still required to be carried out on clinical grounds from the Ayurvedic community itself in order to generate real-life data for substantiation of what is observed in clinic and what is being found in research laboratories so that the gap between what is known and what needs to be known gets progressively reduced.

Conclusion

Ayurvedic *Rasayana* therapy looks promising when viewed from its textual point. There are elaborated and explicit details in Ayurveda regarding use of various *Rasayana* in conditions of health and disease. Whereas in relation to disease, it focuses on offering a cure for a particular ailment, in the context of general health, it offers qualitative improvements in the quality of life. This qualitative change is proposed to be in the form of subjective functional improvements and also in the form of objective visible changes in signs of aging. Although *Rasayana* is one of the most important disciplines of *Ashtanga* Ayurveda, its understanding and consequently its practice continue to be on decline in recent times.

The gaps between the textual references and the practical needs and the lack of clear answers to situations in routine clinical practice underlie the general disinterest of practitioners toward its practice. Complexities associated with its use, intangibility of effects, and need of long-term usage are further limiting factors. However, despite these limitations, potential of *Rasayana* in the current context of increasing life span and consequent increase in requirement of care of the elderly population needs a revisit. Ayurvedic proposal of starting *Rasayana* at early age is highly attractive in this regard if it is shown to lead to a disease-free state at later ages.

It is believed that to attain such objectives, more clear theoretical and practical understanding of its principles is essential to provide dependable, action-oriented, and reproducible evidence-based applications which would help reduce the high burden associated with diseases and disabilities of the aging population.

References

1. Wenzel U. Nutrition, sirtuins and aging. Genes Nutr. 2006;1(2):85–93. https://doi.org/10.1007/BF02829950.
2. Savrikar SS, Ravishankar B. Introduction to "Rasashaastra" the iatrochemistry of Ayurveda. Afr J Tradit Complement Altern Med. 2011;8(5 Suppl):66–82. https://doi.org/10.4314/ajtcam.v8i5S.1.
3. Aunan JR, Watson MM, Hagland HR, Søreide K. Molecular and biological hallmarks of ageing. Br J Surg. 2016;103:e29–46.
4. Mendoza-Núñez VM. What is the onset age of human aging and old age? Int J Gerontol. 2016;10:56. https://doi.org/10.1016/j.ijge.2015.06.0042015.
5. Hayflick L, Moorhead PS. The serial cultivation of human diploid cell strains. Exp Cell Res. 1961;25:585–621.
6. Childs BG, Gluscevic M, Baker DJ, Laberge R-M, Marquess D, Dananberg J, van Deursen JM. Senescent cells: an emerging target for diseases of ageing. Nat Rev Drug Discov. 2017;16:718–35.
7. Weber CR. Dynamic properties of the tight junction barrier. Ann N Y Acad Sci. 2012;1257:77–84. https://doi.org/10.1111/j.1749-6632.2012.06528.
8. Mälkki Y, Virtanen E. Gastrointestinal effects of oat bran and oat gum: a review. LWT Food Sci Technol. 2001;34(6):337–47.
9. Gaur BL, Commentary on Charaka Samhita. New Delhi: Rasthriya Ayurveda Vidyapeeth; 2011.
10. How homes kept cool before the age of AC. http://blog.solarcity.com/how-homes-kept-cool-before-the-age-of-ac/. Last accessed on 29 Oct 2017.
11. Rastogi S, Chaudhari P. Convalescent food practices in Ayurveda. In: Rastogi S, editor. Ayurvedic science of food and nutrition. New York: Springer; 2014. p. 67–80.
12. Williams JM, Duckworth CA, Burkitt MD, Watson AJM, Campbell BJ, Pritchard DM. Epithelial cell shedding and barrier function: a matter of life and death at the small intestinal villus tip. Vet Pathol. 2015;52(3):445–55. https://doi.org/10.1177/0300985814559404.
13. Mayhew TM, Myklebust R, Whybrow A, et al. Epithelial integrity, cell death and cell loss in mammalian small intestine. Histol Histopathol. 1999;14(1):257–67. [PubMed].
14. Boss GR, Seegmiller JE. Age-related physiological changes and their clinical significance. West J Med. 1981;135(6):434–40.
15. Nigam Y, Knight J, Bhattacharya S, Bayer A. Physiological changes associated with aging and immobility. J Aging Res. 2012;1:Article ID 468469, 2 pages. https://doi.org/10.1155/2012/468469.

16. Wheeler HE, Kim SK. Genetics and genomics of human ageing. Philos Trans Roy Soc B Biol Sci. 2011;366(1561):43–50. https://doi.org/10.1098/rstb.2010.0259.
17. Horvath S. DNA methylation age of human tissues and cell types. Genome Biol. 2013;14(10):R115.
18. Singh RH, Rastogi S. *Rasayana* therapy and rejuvenation. In: Rastogi S, editor. Evidence-based practice in complementary and alternative medicine. Berlin: Springer; 2012.
19. Ornish D, Lin J, Chan JM, et al. Effect of comprehensive lifestyle changes on telomerase activity and telomere length in men with biopsy-proven low-risk prostate cancer: 5-year follow-up of a descriptive pilot study. Lancet Oncol. 2013;14(11):1112–20. https://doi.org/10.1016/S1470-2045(13)70366-8.
20. Shrivastava S. Commentary on Sharangadhara Samhita. Varanasi: Chaukhambha Orientalia; 1999.
21. Life expectancy at birth, total (years). https://data.worldbank.org/indicator/SP.DYN.LE00.IN. Last accessed on 22 Oct 2017.
22. Metrics: disability-adjusted life year (DALY). http://www.who.int/healthinfo/global_burden_disease/metrics_daly/en/. Last accessed on 30 Oct 2017.
23. Everett JS, Budescu M, Sommers MS. Making sense of skin color in clinical care. Clin Nurs Res. 2012;21(4):495–516. https://doi.org/10.1177/1054773812446510.
24. Farage MA, Miller KW, Elsner P, Maibach HI. Characteristics of the aging skin. Adv Wound Care. 2013;2(1):5–10. https://doi.org/10.1089/wound.2011.0356.
25. Diego MA, Field T. Moderate pressure massage elicits a parasympathetic nervous system response. Int J Neurosci. 2009;119(5):630–8. https://doi.org/10.1080/00207450802329605.
26. Valacchi G, Lim Y, Belmonte G, Miracco C, Zanardi I, Bocci V, Travagli V. Ozonated sesame oil enhances cutaneous wound healing in SKH1 mice. Wound Repair Regen. 2011;19:107–15. https://doi.org/10.1111/j.1524-475X.2010.00649.x.
27. Dhar S, Banerjee R, Malakar R. Oil massage in babies: Indian perspectives. Indian J Paediatr Dermatol. 2013;14:1–3.
28. Mirmohammadali M, Hosseini-Baharanchi FS, Dehkordi ZR, Bekhradi R, Delaram M. The effect of massage with oils on the growth of term infants: a randomized controlled trial. Open J Pediatr. 2015;5(3):223–31. https://doi.org/10.4236/ojped.2015.53034.
29. Kulkarni R, Girish KJ, Kumar A. Nootropic herbs (*Medhya Rasayana*) in Ayurveda: an update. Pharmacogn Rev. 2012;6(12):147–53. https://doi.org/10.4103/0973-7847.99949.
30. Shastri KN, Chaturvedi GN. Charaka Samhita. Varanasi: Chaukhambha Bharati Academy; 1986.
31. Ali M. A brief history of Indian alchemy covering pre-Vedic to Vedic and Ayurvedic period (circa 400 B.C.-800 A.D.). Bull Indian Inst Hist Med Hyderabad. 1993;23(2):151–66.
32. Dwivedi V, Anandan EM, Mony RS, Muraleedharan TS, Valiathan MS, Mutsuddi M, Lakhotia SC. In vivo effects of traditional ayurvedic formulations in Drosophila melanogaster model relate with therapeutic applications. PLoS One. 2012;7:e37113.
33. Dwivedi V, et al. Ayurvedic Amalaki Rasayana and Rasa-Sindoor suppress neurodegeneration in fly models of Huntington's and Alzheimer's diseases. Curr Sci. 2013;105:1711–23.
34. Saba K, et al. Energetics of excitatory and inhibitory neurotransmission in aluminum chloride model of Alzheimer's disease: reversal of behavioral and metabolic deficits by Rasa Sindoor. Front Mol Neurosci. 2017;10:323. https://doi.org/10.3389/fnmol.2017.00323. eCollection2017.
35. Ramanan N, Lahiri D, Rajput P, et al. Investigating structural aspects to understand the putative/claimed non toxicity of the Hg based ayurvedic drug Rasasindura using XAFS. J Synchrotron Rad. 2015;22:1233–41. https://doi.org/10.1107/S1600577515012473.
36. Mukhi P, Mohapatra S, Bhattacharjee M, et al. Mercury based drug in ancient India: the red sulfide of mercury in nanoscale. J Ayurveda Integr Med. 2017;8(2):93–8. https://doi.org/10.1016/j.jaim.2017.01.009.
37. Dwivedi V, Lakhotia SC. Ayurvedic Amalaki Rasayana promotes improved stress tolerance and thus has anti-aging effects in Drosophila melanogaster. J Biosci. 2016;41(4):697–711.

38. Swain U, Sindhu KK, Boda U, et al. Studies on the molecular correlates of genomic stability in rat brain cells following Amalaki rasayana therapy. Mech Aging Dev. 2012;133:112–7.
39. Guruprasad KP, Dash S, Shivakumar MB, et al. Influence of Amalaki Rasayana on telomerase activity and telomere length in human blood mononuclear cells. J Ayurveda Integr Med. 2017;8(2):105–12. https://doi.org/10.1016/j.jaim.2017.01.007. Epub 2017 Jun 9.
40. Tiwari V, Saba K, Veeraiah P, Jose J, Lakhotia SC, Patel AB. Amalaki Rasayana improved memory and neuronal metabolic activity in AbPP-PS1 mouse model of Alzheimer's disease. J Biosci. 2017;42:363–71. https://doi.org/10.1007/s12038-017-9692-7.
41. Kumar V, Aneesh KA, Kshemada K, et al. *Amalaki Rasayana,* a traditional Indian drug enhances cardiac mitochondrial and contractile functions and improves cardiac function in rats with hypertrophy. Sci Rep. 2017;7:8588. https://doi.org/10.1038/s41598-017-09225-x.
42. Ong AD, Patterson A. Eudaimonia, aging, and health: a review of underlying mechanisms. In: Vittersø J, editor. Handbook of Eudaimonic Well-being. International handbooks of quality-of-life. Cham: Springer; 2016.
43. Rastogi S, Chaudhari P. Ethics as a modality affecting health and healthcare practice: revealing the real strengths of traditional healthcare. Asian Bioethics Rev. 2015;7(4):371–9. https://doi.org/10.1353/asb.2015.0030.
44. Lederberg J. Molecular biology, eugenics and euphenics. Nature. 1963;198:428–9.
45. Patwardhan B, Mutalik G, Tillu G. Integrative approaches for health: biomedical research, ayurveda and yoga. London: Academic Press; 2016.
46. Valiathan MS. Ayurvedic biology: the first decade. Proc Indian Natl Sci Acad. 2016;82(1):13–9.
47. Lakhotia SC. Ayurvedic biology—an unbiased approach to understand traditional health-care system. Proc Indian Natl Sci Acad. 2016;82(1):1–3.
48. Valiathan MS. Ayurveda and modern science. Aryavaidyan. 2017;XXX(3):5–9.
49. Patwardhan B. Bridging Ayurveda with evidence-based scientific approaches in medicine. EPMA J. 2014;5(1):19.
50. Lakhotia SC. Validation of Ayurvedic formulations in animal models requires stringent scientific rigor. J Ayurveda Integr Med. 2010;3:171–2.
51. Valiathan MS. Ayurvedic Biology: a decadal vision document. Bengaluru: Indian Academy of Science; 2006.
52. Wolbring G. Eugenics, euthenics, euphenics: the underlying issue is that someone decides, based on values, which characteristics should be part of society and which are not. GeneWatch. 1999;12(3):8–10.
53. Chyawanprash market in India. http://www.mbarendezvous.com/general-awareness/chyawanprash-market-in-india/. Last accessed 5 Nov 2017.
54. Pump iron, don't eat Chyawanprash. http://www.hindustantimes.com/india/pump-iron-don-t-eat-chyawanprash/story-WUSwByiwxc6JjlIgMJK6SM.html. Last accessed on 5 Nov 2017.
55. Savaliya AA, Shah RP, Prasad B, Singh SJ. Screening of Indian aphrodisiac ayurvedic/herbal healthcare products for adulteration with sildenafil, tadalafil and/or vardenafil using LC/PDA and extracted ion LC–MS/TOF. J Pharm Biomed Anal. 2010;52(3):406–9.
56. Industry Scenario. http://vibrantAyurveda.in/?page_id=2083. Last accessed on 5 Nov 2017.
57. AnanthaNarayana DB, Durg S, RamManohar P, Mahapatra A, Aramya AR. Chyawanprash: a review of therapeutic benefits as in authoritative texts and documented clinical literature. J Ethnopharmacol. 2017;197:52–60. https://doi.org/10.1016/j.jep.2016.07.078.
58. Yadav JS, Thakur S, Chadha P. Chyawanprash Awaleha: a genoprotective agent for bidi smokers. Int J Hum Genet. 2003;3(1):33–8.
59. Caring for our elders: early response India Ageing Report 2017. http://india.unfpa.org/sites/default/files/pub-pdf/India%20Ageing%20Report%20-%202017%20%28Final%20Version%29.pdf. Last accessed on 5 Nov 2017.

Part II

Translational Ayurveda: Clinical Practice

Understanding Cancer: Expanding the Horizon Through Applying the Collective Wisdom of Ayurveda and Conventional Medicine

7

Sanjeev Rastogi, Sen Pathak, and Ram Harsh Singh

7.1 Introduction

Cancer is the world's second largest cause of death. A disease of unknown etiopathogenesis, it affects everyone irrespective of cast, creed, gender, or geography. Cancer generally is associated with high morbidity and mortality. About 8.2 million deaths occurred worldwide in 2012 were reported due to cancer. This number is expected to be nearly doubled (13 million) in the next two decades [1]. The incidence of cancer is continuously growing over the past many years. Fourteen million new cancer cases were reported worldwide in 2012. A 70% rise of such cases (22 million) is expected to occur in the next two decades and hence raises an alarm.

Cancer is marked with a silent course of occurrence, relentless progress, multiple system affliction, enigmatic etiopathogenesis, and fewer options of cure. All these features collectively entail the cancer to be a disease of high priority in medical fraternity in terms of finding ways for its early diagnosis and possible managements. This priority eventually warrants for a clarion call to look out seriously in the realm of cancer through initial visualization and subsequent effective utilization of all kinds of knowledge available as a help to understand and eventually to manage it more effectively. Such resources and tools upon their thorough screening may help initiating the newer domains of research and subsequently prove to be of value in proposing better management of the disease.

S. Rastogi (✉)
Department of Kaya Chikitsa, State Ayurvedic College and Hospital, Lucknow University, Lucknow, India

S. Pathak
Department of Genetics/Cancer Biology, The University of Texas M.D. Anderson Cancer Center, Houston, TX, USA

R. H. Singh
Department of Kaya Chikitsa, Faculty of Ayurveda, Institute of Medical Sciences, Banaras Hindu University, Varanasi, India

S. Rastogi (ed.), *Translational Ayurveda*, https://doi.org/10.1007/978-981-13-2062-0_7

From our experiences of the past, we have learned that a research should always be novel in terms of "moving forward" without missing to accommodate the learning from the past. This "move forward but don't forget to have an eye on your back" approach seems most appropriate for the conditions like cancer where a lot is still beyond the understanding of science despite its sharp progress in the past few decades. Sometimes referred as "reverse innovation," this method can be employed in cancer [2] through serious review of unorganized and unexplored knowledge available at various scattered sources in the form of ancient scriptures, texts, practices, and beliefs. A serious lookout at what is practiced at the ethno-cultural community levels referring as traditional understanding and treatment to cancer may be of immense help. There may be a number of such practices prevailing globally to represent the culture-based understanding of the disease and its management. Our concern here is however limited to the domain of Ayurveda, a traditional health-care wisdom of the Orient with a focus upon its proposals about cancer in order to see how these can help the current world knowing this disease better in terms of finding some help in designing more effective preventive and curative solutions for the same in the future.

Besides agony and unpredictability associated with it, cancer has huge economic implications too. The global direct cost incurring upon prevention and treatment of the disease and the indirect cost incurring in the form of lives lost, disability caused, and losses to the families are estimated to be of the extent of $2.5 trillion in a year [3]. Seeing the huge economic burden of cancer, this is obvious to think that a large sum should be invested for researching in areas like prevention, early diagnosis, palliation, and cure of cancer. Unfortunately, a gross mismatch between the burden of cancer and investments made toward its eventual reduction is also evident in particular to the areas like geographical locations, types of disease, treatment modalities, and socioeconomic status [4]. A large scope of systematic investment therefore still remains due to an equity-based understanding of cancer in the multiple areas of its concern which eventually may matter in designing a better preventive or curative strategy aiming at ultimate reduction of cancer burden.

Now that about 250 years of an organized research had been carried so far in the area of cancer, we need to evaluate where we have reached ultimately. Commencing from linking chimney soot to the incidence of scrotal squamous cell carcinoma in 1775 by Percivall Pott, it took great strides while passing through chemotherapy till reaching to the making of The Cancer Genome Atlas (TCGA) [5]. Although the progress made in this period has been impressive in many areas, we see that a large part of information crucial to cancer-related care is still missing.

What causes, prevents, or cures cancer? These are the fundamental questions still unanswered despite them being most vital from the perspectives of a patient suffering with cancer, the caregivers, or a treating physician. This situation warrants for a more serious review of the way we have conventionally been looking at cancer so far.

7.2 Paradigm Shift in Health Understanding: Reverse Innovation, Grassroots Innovation, and Glocalization and Their Relevance in Health and Disease Research

While looking at the possibility of a paradigm shift within cancer understanding, it is obvious to note that this may require a thought convergence of all possible cancer doctrines into a common visible end point. Three independently emerging (although overlapping some time) concepts, namely, reverse innovation, grassroots innovation, and glocalization, need a worthy discussion here. Reverse innovation as a word and concept has a large credit to Govindarajan and Trimble [6] who have originally described this to explain the possibility of innovative indigenous ideas and technologies originating in the developing world and subsequently finding a place in the developed world. Contrary to the usual sight of downstreaming of the high-end technologies from the developed to developing countries, this concept proposed the reverse and hence appropriately termed "reverse innovation." Although primarily pleading on the backdrop of business conglomerations, looking at opportunities far from the places of their origin, interestingly Govindarajan and Trimble begin their argument of reverse innovation quoting a good example of how an Ayurvedic recipe (containing coconut water, carrot juice, rice water, carob flour, and dehydrated bananas) traditionally used in Bangladesh for managing acute dehydration was able to find a place in Lancet [7, 8]. Upon subsequent explorations, it bloomed as a breakthrough which disproved the conventional scientific belief of the developed world about the role of sugar in infective diarrhea. (Sugar was believed to promote pathogens in gut in case of infective diarrhea. Later it was found to enhance salt and water absorption. This has subsequently made the foundation for revealing sodium-glucose cotransport mechanism which was considered one of the most important medical advances of the century.) The intervention subsequently found a number of applications besides the one for which it was originally described. An excerpt from "Reverse Innovation: Create far from Home win everywhere" (Govindarajan and Trimble [6]) says:

> "Earlier in the 1960s, there were epidemic outbreaks of cholera in Bangladesh and elsewhere in South Asia. The key to keeping cholera patients alive was simple: Keep them hydrated. According to Dr. Mehmood Khan, Chief Scientific Officer of PepsiCo (which now owns Gatorade), Western doctors who went to help stem the epidemic were surprised to discover a centuries-old local treatment for the severe diarrhea caused by cholera. The concoction included ingredients such as coconut water, carrot juice, rice water, carob flour, and dehydrated bananas. At the time, Western medical opinion held that putting carbohydrates in the stomachs of patients suffering from diarrhea would cause cholera bacteria to multiply and the disease to worsen". "Yet for thousands of years, this was the normal treatment used in Ayurvedic medicine," says Khan.
>
> "By giving carbohydrate and sugar in the solution with salt, uptake was quicker, and patients rehydrated faster". The success of the treatment was covered in the British medical journal Lancet, and it made its way to a doctor at the University of Florida. The doctor saw a common problem in the need for rapid re-hydration. If such a treatment worked well for cholera patients, it would surely work for healthy football players.

This example makes it a point of considering ancient wisdom in health care everywhere to find help for better understanding about a disease and eventually about its better management. This is particularly important for conditions where satisfactory answers are still far from the immediate sight of modern medicine. Cancer, for obvious reasons, tops the priority list here. A “reverse innovation” in medicine may be considered far ahead of “reverse pharmacology” which is an extremely narrow application of the whole traditional health-care wisdom, limited to the search of leads from Ayurveda (or from other traditional health-care sources) in order to develop new molecules and drugs, an avenue which otherwise has been an extremely time-consuming and expensive affair in current pharmaceutical industry [9].

Better understanding about a disease seems to have higher advantage which may be gained through applying reverse innovation in the area. It argues to utilize the old wisdom to expand the dimension of current understanding in various domains of health care inclusive of (but not limited to) prevention, etiopathogenesis, disease categorization, individual susceptibility, and the personalized care. Reverse innovation to a large extent also seems to be a cross application of different knowledge systems for common goals.

“Grassroots innovations,” on the contrary of reverse innovation, looks more lateral in its applications [10]. It refers to modest and innovative solutions of day-to-day problems faced by an indigenous population. It is referred as “my problem–my solution” approach which is very apt to an ethno-cultural setting defined by a specific geographical area and socioeconomic category. A self-sustainable model of living has given such populations an opportunity to deal with their problems with their own resources. We know by the precedence of history that such approaches have remained successful most of the time. Folklore medicine is one such approach where the health-care problems are understood in context of the culture and are dealt with the resources available within the surrounding ecosystem. Plenty of such approaches are also prevalent in the folklore management of cancer [11].

Such folklore practices are neither the high-tech approaches nor have many referrals in ideal textual contexts. Their power however lies in the fact that they are practiced and believed and show relief in many cases. This grassroots innovation also makes sense to be explored in terms of cancer management.

“Glocalization” or adaptation of global strategies to suit the local needs [12] is another promising thought, making a sense in looking at cancer with applying global technology narrowed down to meet the local needs. Corporate world has acknowledged this strategy well by suitably modifying their technologies as per the local needs in many areas. There are strong reasons to believe that this can have a thorough application in the area of health care too. General Electric (GE), a big player in health-care technology, has adopted this strategy to radically modify its high-end sophisticated ECG machine to suit to the affordability, running cost, portability, and capacity to deal with dust and power fluctuation common to Indian background. All these factors were otherwise limiting the expansion of affordable cardiac health care in remote areas of India. MAC 400, a newer portable version of ECG machine by GE, has changed the cardiac diagnostic scenario at primary care setting in India by making a global technology available at the doorstep in a highly customized format [6].

Although done by the multinational giants primarily with the commercial motives, it has shown the world a way that this customization of global technology is the future key of evolving effective health care for the most needy who do not fit into the context of advanced high-tech solutions owing to their high capital and running cost and also not being able to address the local problems. Glocalization, in this context, can be extensively helpful in finding easy diagnostic and therapeutic solutions by means of assuring affordable technologies available to everyone in need.

A lot in the world is still required to be explored, and while doing so, this is of utmost importance to understand where our predecessors have already reached. A keen interest in observing at ancient wisdom and practices of health care may help us find clues to turn previous observations into scientific reality and vice versa. This may save much time and money needed to reinvent the wheel every time and may add a push to see further and farther by "standing upon the shoulders of giants" as acknowledged by Isaac Newton in 1676 in his letter to Robert Hook:

> "If I have seen a little further, it is by standing on the shoulders of Giants."

This phrase is as meaningful today as it was four centuries back, and similarly it is as meaningful to health-care science as it is to any other domains of science. Recognizing the power of previous knowledge, Stephen Hawking in his book *On The Shoulders of Giants: The Great Works of Physics and Astronomy* stated:

> "Each generation stands on the shoulders of those who have gone before them, just as I did as a young PhD student in Cambridge, inspired by the work of Isaac Newton, James Clerk Maxwell and Albert Einstein." [13]

It is for that matter Charaka, Sushruta, and Vagbhata, the all-time great legends of Ayurveda, and many more on the league are no less than such giants whose shoulders have given us a strong foundation of health-care science to stand upon and to look beyond what can ordinarily be seen and understood at our own.

7.3 Cancer: What Makes It So Special?

Besides the high burden of cancer in terms of its morbidity, mortality, and economic impact, for a biologist, there are many more reasons of high concern about cancer. Cancer, originating from a single organ-specific cell, is a silent illness manifesting only when it reaches at advanced stages. Nearly 46% of cancers are diagnosed only when they reach their later stages [14]. A late diagnosis of cancer limits the outcomes due to the limited therapeutic options available at late stages. Cancer in its most forms presents with a relentless and rapid progress limiting the life opportunities once its diagnosis is made. Cancer metastasis is an exclusive phenomenon which perpetuates its impact from a local to a systemic disorder. Its enigmatic etiopathogenesis is yet another cause of concern. Because of its obscure etiology in many cases, a definitive preventive strategy to cancer cannot be adopted. Limited treatment opportunities and a ubiquitous presentation have made cancer a much sought after pathology at research forums. In this kind of state, the current strategy to deal with cancer is to prevent it wherever it is possible, diagnose it at the earliest when the primary prevention fails, and treat it on a war footing once it is diagnosed.

Cancer prevention is made possible in certain conditions where a clear association between causative factors and ensuing pathogenesis is established [15]. For many other cancer types, however, prevention is not yet possible owing to the complex interplay between environmental and individual factors leading to the ultimate pathology. Prevention is also not possible in many other instances where a multifactorial etiopathogenesis is expected to play a role in the causation of cancer. Prevention of cancer is also practically not possible where the causes despite them being known to have associations with certain type of cancer cannot be practically removed [16].

Diagnostic delay is another cause of concern in cancer. This delay in most instances is because of the absence of warranting signs and symptoms related with the disease. Unlike other diseases, cancer does not have its own set of warning signs and symptoms to sense its early presence. In most conditions, cancer features are actually the secondary features manifesting as a result of functional compromising at local, organ, or system level. Due to high resilience of human physiology, such symptoms however often arise very late and hence cause a late diagnosis [17]. Besides this patient-sided delay in the diagnosis, there are reasons of delay due to the lack of appropriate attention and resources at primary and secondary care points. There are issues like cost, availability, and accessibility of screening methods involved in the diagnosis of cancer adding to the diagnostic delay. Sometimes, the delay is also due to the absence of an appropriate technology to make an early and quick diagnosis of cancer within the affordable and accessible reach of the common people.

7.4 Cellular Events in Cancer

Molecular mechanism involved in the cancer pathogenesis is thoroughly studied in the past few decades. It is now known that in cancer, a few cells become rebellious to follow the rules of a civilized normal cell society. These rules are related to cell division, differentiation, and cell death. Through an intricate molecular mechanism of intercellular communication and operating through cell division, differentiation, and death, the body keeps a strict check upon the actual number and type of cells available in the organ at one point of time. The mechanism involved in such case operates through molecular, biochemical, and cellular signals eventually affecting the cell behavior. A mutation subsequently affects the cellular genome resulting in rearrangement, subsequently leading to activation/upregulation of telomerase activity. Unfortunately, despite this clarity of the molecular mechanism of the cancer pathogenesis, it is not yet completely known how a particular cell behaves erratically and what are the protective factors that save other cells from behaving erratically despite being exposed to similar causative factors.

7.5 Ayurvedic Wisdom of Health and Disease: What Leads to Disease, and What Prevents It?

This is well observed that everyone does not essentially fall sick. In a cross section of population, some live a healthy and long life, whereas others are unhealthy and short-lived. Cancer demographics in Western countries show that more than one in every three individuals has a possibility of suffering with cancer [18]. Now this is a pressing question finding what makes the one destined to suffer from cancer and prevents the others to have the same fate. Ayurveda proposes a few generic rules for remaining healthy.[1] These rules in general are related to eating and lifestyle habits, personal values, and behavior. A contravention of these rules eventually invites illness and renders one unhealthy. Besides the breach of these generic health rules, there are clearly defined risk factors also which play crucially in the net development of a disease. Although in cancer, such risk factors are not so explicitly detailed, these are highly specific in many other diseases. In context of diabetes, greediness about sweet food and avoidance of physical activity are identified as two most important risk factors which determine the incidence and prognosis of the disease on individual basis.[2,3]

7.6 Genetic Susceptibility of Diseases

Elaborating further upon the causes of diseases, Ayurveda identifies genetic associations as one important determining factor for being affected or unaffected with a disease upon being exposed to a set of causative factors. By virtue of a *dosha*-specific tuning of the body for particular setting of physiological functioning, various body types, namely, *vata*, *pitta*, or *kapha* or their various combinations, have a greater chance of being affected with disorders coming under the functional domain of predominant *dosha*. It is for this reason a *vata* predominance makes the person more susceptible to

---

1 नरो हिताहार विहार सेवी समीक्ष्यकारी विषयेषु अवसक्त।दाता समः सत्य परः क्षमावान आप्तोपसेवी च भवति अरोगा॥ चरक संहिता.

One who is selective in choosing his food and life style, analytical, not deeply involved in sensual pleasures, giver, remains equal in all situations, truthful, forgiver and respectful to elders remains away from diseases (Charaka Samhita).

2 गृध्नुमभ्यवहार्येषु स्नान चंक्रमण द्विषम। प्रमेह क्षिप्रमभ्येति नीडद्रुममिवाण्डजः॥ च.नि.४/५०

Diabetes comes to them quickly and repeatedly who are greedy (for food), unclean and do not walk.

3 मन्दोत्साहम अतिस्थूलम अतिस्निग्धम महाशनम । मृत्युःप्रमेह रूपेण क्षिप्रमादाय गच्छति॥ च.नि.४/५१

The one who is lazy, obese, eats fatty meal in large quantity is soon approached by death in the form of diabetes.

suffer with neurodegenerative disorders comparing to the people with other *dosha*-specific dominance. The same is true for *pitta* and *kapha* which cause an increased possibility of being affected with hepatobiliary, acid peptic and blood-related disorders, and respiratory and cardiac diseases, respectively, among people having a dominance of such *dosha*. As a precaution, Ayurveda therefore specifically proposes that the people should be highly selective for their food and routine activities in order to keep a tight balance of their governing *dosha* preventing the same to become exuberant. This is now well established that Ayurvedic *dosha* specifications and subsequent physiological functioning are having genetic basis and depend upon up- or downregulation of a particular set of genes responsible for specific functions [19, 20]. By proposing a watch upon food and routine activities, Ayurveda offers handy tools to keep such up- and downregulated gene activity regularly monitored and kept under check and balance.

7.7 Epigenetic Causes of Diseases

Besides genetic susceptibility about the disease, Ayurveda proposes multiple other endogenous and exogenous factors playing specific roles in pathogenesis. An excessive, inappropriate, or inadequate application of factors like *kala* (timings/season), *buddhi* (intellect), and *indriyartha* (substances of interaction with five senses) is perceived as the possible cause of all diseases.[4]

Such factors can be elaborated further as are illustrated in Table 7.1.

Table 7.1 Epigenetic causes of diseases

	Atiyoga (excessive presence)	*Ayoga/hina yoga* (inadequacy or absence)	*Mithya-yoga* (in appropriate presence)
Kala (timing/season)	• Excessive presence of light or dark in the surroundings causing misappropriation of biological clock in response to light dark cycle • Excessive seasonal manifestations like extreme hot and cold weather or prolonged seasons	Inadequacy or absence of any such components	Inappropriate presence of such components in the surroundings. Examples are inappropriate dark and light exposures during day and night and inappropriate hot and cold exposures during winter and summer
Buddhi (intellect)	Excessive thinking	Inadequate or absent thinking	Faulty or inappropriate thinking
Indriyartha (substrate of perception)	Excessive contact with substrates of perceptions	Inadequate or absent contact with substrates of perception	Faulty or inappropriate contact with substrates of perception

4 काल बुद्धीन्द्रियार्थानाम योगो मिथ्यान च अतिच। च.सू.१/५४.

A faulty application of time, intellect and sensual perception (in the form of inappropriate, inadequate or excessive application of any one among these or their combination) leads to diseases.

Such exogenous factors, upon their regular and sustained exposure, cause a sustained change in the body physiology through down- or upregulations of various proteomic and metabolomic pathways. The metabolic and genetic changes instigated by the stress pathways (often the by-product of a *kala, buddhi*, and *indriyartha* misappropriation) are involved in the pathogenesis of cancer through a cascade involving genomics, transcriptomics, proteomics, and finally metabolomics [21].

7.8 Determinant of Health: Ayurvedic Postulates

Ayurveda proposes the health as a perfect blend of multiple percepts functioning harmoniously. Such percepts are mostly indicative of physiological functioning of the body such as *dosha* (physiology regulators), *agni* (metabolic regulator), and *dhatu mala kriya* (the process of metabolic transformation leading to synthesis and eventually waste production). Besides such physiological percepts of health, an eventual happy state of *atman* (the pure, unbiased, and absolute self), *indriya* (perceptive organs), and *manas* (the mind) also forms an essential composite of health.[5] A balanced physiology along with a balanced cognition therefore forms two essential components of health in an independent and a mutually dependent manner.

7.9 Ayurvedic Postulation of Oncogenesis

Ayurvedic biology proposes a functional distinction of three *doshas* on the basis of their functional expertise [22]. In reference to the cancer biology where unhindered cell division, exuberant cell growth, and subsequent cell proliferation are important steps besides an impedance to cell death, this is important to understand how this may be deciphered in terms of Ayurvedic biology. Categorically referring to the cell biology, cell division is an attribute of *vata*, metabolism of *pitta*, and growth of *kapha*. *Vata* has a functional attribute of early senescence, whereas *kapha* has a tendency to delay the senescence. If we categorize the hallmarks of cancer in terms of Ayurveda, some interesting parallels may be drawn (Table 7.2). During normal course, the three *doshas* are found to be regulated through a counter-regulatory mechanism. Excess of one *dosha* therefore leads to the deficit of another *dosha* having the opposite properties. Excessive *vata* therefore also produces signals like deficient *kapha*. Deficiency signals are easiest to be trapped by the body, and a correction of excess *dosha* is often made by replenishing the *dosha* with opposite property. It is for this reason that common pathologies usually present with involvement of one *dosha* alone and are easy to treat. In complex pathogenesis, however, this counter-regulation of *dosha* is lost resulting in multiple *dosha* involvement and at the same time resulting in *bidoshik* or *tridoshik* pathologies which are more complex and

---

5 समदोष: समाग्निश्च: समधातु मल क्रिय:। प्रसन्नात्मेन्द्रिय मन: स्वस्थ इत्यभिधीयते। सुश्रुत संहिता.

Table 7.2 Six hallmarks of cancer and their link with Ayurvedic biology

Hallmark	Features	*Dosha* involved
1. Immortality	Produce telomere proteins to enable indefinite cell divisions	*Pitta* and *kapha*
2. Produce go signals	Produce its own chemical message to start division	*Vata*
3. Override stop signals	Escape the signals to stop division	*Vata*
4. Resistance to cell death	Override the senescence signals	*Kapha*
5. Angiogenesis	New blood vessel formation to ensure nutrition	*Pitta* and *kapha*
6. Metastasis	Spreading at far away places	*Vata*

difficult to treat. Table 7.2 gives us a clear view that all three *dosha*s are involved in cancer pathogenesis, hence making it a *tridoshaja* pathology which at an advanced stage is either difficult to treat or is untreatable.

7.10 Hallmarks of *Tridoshaja* Diseases

Unlike *monodoshik* pathogenesis, *tridoshik* diseases are characterized by many unique features in terms of their course, clinical presentation, and treatability. It often erupts as a subsequent *dosha* involvement in existing *monodoshik* pathology met without adequate reparative measures. Such conditions are often long-standing having a chronic onset and long course of presentation. Once the pathology is set in, the consequences may rather be faster than the process of pathogenesis. Clinical presentation of a *tridoshik* disease may be highly diverse due to the involvement of all three *doshas*. This may eventually have a multisystem involvement leading to a multisystem failure by virtue of derangement of all three governing *doshas*. *Tridoshik* pathogenesis is also difficult to treat or untreatable due to the involvement of multisystem and the failure of counter-regulatory mechanism. *Tridoshaja* pathology therefore looks to be the one affecting the whole *milieu interior* of the body to the extent that it leads to a sustained repression to the effective cellular functioning in the body.

Besides arising as the complication produced out of *monodoshik* pathogenesis, there are many genetic factors which may lead to *tridoshaja* pathology. Such genetic factors are more important in reference to the pathologies like cancer where a clear and sharply defined etiopathogenesis could not be established but where the etiology is pervasive and constantly available. *Viruddha Ahara* (incompatible diet and food combinations) is one such factor leading to *tridoshaja* pathologies. By means of incompatibility of food, Ayurveda proposes a comprehensive and exhaustive outlook of the factors which may render the food unwholesome and as a subtle cause of disease. Such factors are related to food in reference to its consumption timings, space, quantity, quality, processing, and various combinations of food preparations. This is noteworthy to understand that a wholesome food may turn into unwholesome if not being consumed as per the principles of Ayurvedic dietetics [23]. Any derangement of *agni* (metabolic fire) and subsequently produced *ama* (product of faulty digestion or metabolism) can be another sustained factor presenting with a large possibility of producing a systemic disorder upon its prolonged presence. Deranged *agni* may be transient resulting due to the faulty routines or may be sustained due to competently erratic routines. What is most important is that a deranged *agni* produces faulty metabolites which may not be able to nourish the tissue as they are desired to and may also have antinutritive and anti-transportive properties which hinder the tissue nutrition. Such products may also result in reduced cellular absorption and transportation, hence causing a sustained nutritional stress.

Suppression of natural urges is yet another subtle and sustained cause of *tridosha* pathogenesis. In normal routine, many involuntary and natural urges are voluntarily suppressed. Such suppression hypothetically may result in partial reabsorption of the waste which the body wished to eliminate. Habitual suppression of such natural urges if practiced for a long time may eventually result in complex *tridoshaja* pathogenesis.

For all of such factors which eventually lead to *tridosha* pathology, the characteristics shared by all of them are their pervasive presence and their mild yet sustained impacts upon their initial exposures. It is however their sustained presence for substantial time which actually develop *tridosha* pathology in a person.

7.11 Sustained Repression Model of Oncogenesis: A *Tridoshaja* Pathology

Biological systems respond to new environmental signals by making appropriate reprogramming of their cellular and metabolic functions in order to ensure the survival under new situations. Such responses may range between apoptosis if the signals are too intense and sharp and cell proliferation if such signals are modest but constantly present [24, 25]. Threats exceeding the cellular threshold may lead to cell death, whereas a sustained suboptimal threat for a long period may lead to cellular proliferation. From Ayurvedic perspectives of pathogenesis, this may be hypothesized that a long-standing *dosik* imbalance in the body may work as a sustained environmental signal compelling a reprogramming of cellular and metabolic functions aiming to optimize the chances of cell survival. Upon such exposures, cells may opt to behave as a community to resist the changes threatening to their survival. In a biological system, cells have an intricate intercellular communication system through which the stress message may be communicated among all having a potential of being affected by the situation [26]. As a result, some cells may be recruited to resist the situation by reprogramming their cell system to ensure survival in extreme situations. This may eventually make a cell resistant to death despite of unfavorable situations around. This might be a trigger of the initiation of cancer (Fig. 7.1).

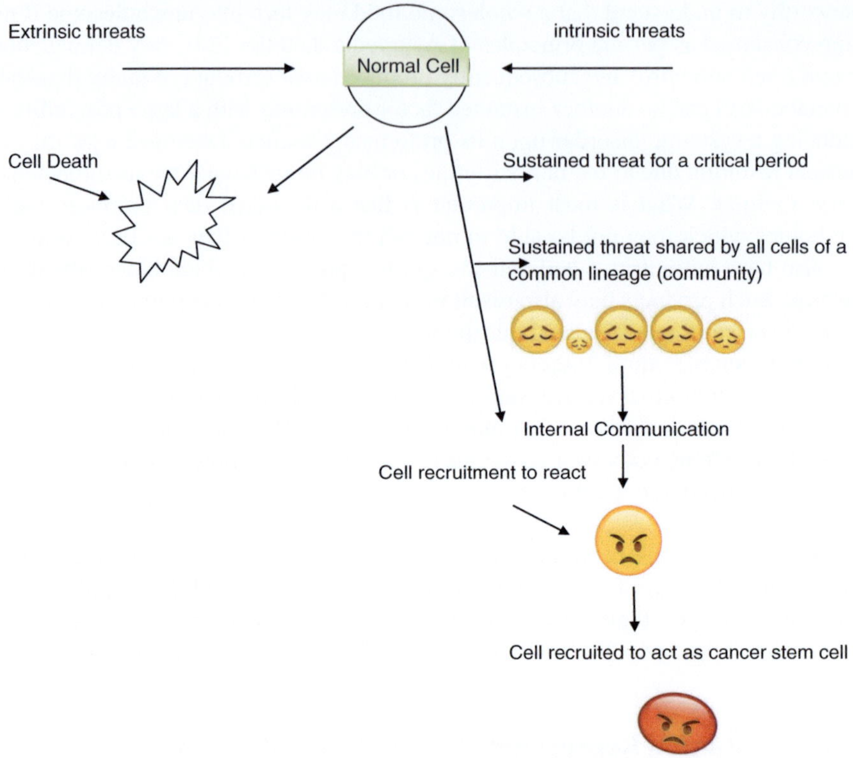

Fig. 7.1 Sustained repression model of oncogenesis: a *tridoshaja* pathology

7.12 Cancer in Ayurveda: Exploring the Ancient Wisdom

Textual description of cancer in Ayurveda is largely limited to the obvious localized swellings visible through the naked eyes (*utsedhasaamanya*[6]). *Granthi* (isolated nodular swellings), *apachi* (multiple nodular swellings), *galaganda* (a solitary swelling limited to the front of the neck), and *arbud* (small elevated swelling like a hill) together comprise the clinical entities where an elevated swelling (*utsedha*) remains the principal presenting feature. A highly illustrative description about such swellings follows subsequently to differentiate one condition from the other on the basis of root cause. Ayurveda largely follows an "analogous approach of disease categorization" where the diseases are categorized on the basis of common presenting features rather than on the basis of diverse sources of their origin. This broad classification based upon the primary symptoms and signs usually follows a more convincing way of looking into the pathogenesis through a detailed clinical examination differentiating between all possible pathogenesis based on the respective

6 रोगाश्चोत्सेध सामान्यात अधिमांस अर्बुदादयः। (चरक संहिता सूत्र स्थान १८/३३)

Diseases marked by visible localized swelling are like localized muscle growth and tumors.

dosha and *dushya* involvements (identifying the possible causative factors and the site of the tissue where the pathogenesis is taking place). It is for this reason that the description of *utsedha* in Ayurveda is not ipso facto parallel to what is understood as cancer in biology, but it essentially encompasses cancer as one among several possible pathologies causing an isolated elevated swelling at some body part. The cancerous status in most of such entities is defined clinically through a few obvious telltales of cancer like *aruja* (painless) and *achala* (fixed, adhered to the supporting tissue)[7] well recognized in cancer biology [27]. Subsequent to this presentation, these are also categorized as difficult to be treated (*krucchasadhya*) and untreatable (*asadhya*). The later condition is warned as *vivarjita* (not to be handled) for its poor prognosis. *Sadhya* (treatable), *krucchasadhya* (difficult to be treated), and *asadhya* (untreatable), therefore, seem to be the earliest attempt of differentiating between various stages of a cancerous condition on the basis of their treatability. Such stages are described distinctly in reference to various solitary lumps. In the case of swelling in the neck (*galaganda*) resembling to thyroid pathologies, the signs of cancerous pathology are much pronounced. A chronic standing (*samvatsara ateet*, existing for more than 1 year), associated breathing difficulty (*krucchacchvasantam*), loss of weight (*ksheena*), change in voice quality (*bhinnaswara*), loss of appetite (*arochaka*), and soft skin all through the body (*mridusarvagaatram*) is considered untreatable and hence recommended to be avoided.[8] Such features of an untreatable stage of *galaganda* are now well-recognized features of thyroid malignancy [28]. What has been considered untreatable referring to various localized swellings in Ayurveda can now be inferred as warning signs of ensuing malignant pathology, hence warranting an earliest attention and intervention.

7.12.1 Granthi

These are the encapsulated swellings containing some liquid material inside. The inside material may be a transparent secretion (*vatikgranthi*), hot secretion (*paittikgranthi*), white thick secretion (*kaphajagranthi*), or cheesy secretion (*medogranthi*). Based upon the nature of secretions, these clinical entities look similar to cystic swelling, infective swelling, abscess, or sebaceous cyst. Additionally, an aneurismic, engorged swelling of the vein is described as *siraj granthi*. *Granthi* are always painful; however, it varies in nature and intensity on the basis of primary pathology.

---

7 ग्रन्थि: सिराज: स तु कृच्छसाध्यो भवेद्यादि स्यात सरुजश्चलश्च। अरुक स एवाप्यचलो महांश्च मर्मोत्थितश्चापि विवर्जनीय ॥ (सुश्रुत संहिता निदान स्थान ११/८-९)

A nodular swelling of veins is considered difficult to be treated if it is painful and movable. However, it is untreatable if is without pain, fixed, big and arising at a vital place.

8 कृच्छ्राच्छ्वसंतम मृदु सर्वगात्रम संवत्सरातीतम अरोचकार्तम ।क्षीणं च वैद्यो गलगण्डिनं तं भिन्न स्वरं चैव विवर्जयेत्तु॥(सुश्रुत संहिता निदान स्थान ११/३०).

A patient of galaganda having difficulty in breathing, soft body parts, older than a year, loss of appetite, weight loss, and change in voice should be discarded by physician for being untreatable.

7.12.2 Apachi

These are rounded, immobile, smooth, non-tender, multiple, nodular, skin-colored swellings commonly found at axillary (*kaksha*), clavicular (*akshakasthi*), and submandibular (*hanvasthi*) region. This description resembles to that of lymphadenopathies of various etiologies.

7.12.3 Arbuda

Arbuda are described as rounded (*vrutta*), fixed and immovable (*sthira*), expanded (*mahantam*), deep-rooted (*analp mulam*), slowly progressive (*chirvruddhaya*), and nonsuppurative swellings arising due to vitiated *dosha* influencing the connective tissue (*mamsa*). *Arbuda* is of six subtypes, namely, *vata, pitta, kapha* on the basis of inflicting *dosha*, *rakta* (blood), *mamsa* (muscles), and *medas* (fat-rich connective tissue). Features of *arbuda* are similar to those already described for *granthi*.[9]

7.13 Cancer as a Clinical Specialty in Ayurveda

Possibly, first time in reference to a clinical division of Ayurveda, a specialty is described referring to the study of tumors. A person skilled with the knowledge of tumors is referred as *arbudagya*. A person who knows about the metastasis of the primary tumor (*adhyarbuda*) and also knows about its prognosis (as is the case of *dwirbuda*) is called as *arbudagya*.[10] Such terminology is found nowhere in Ayurveda in reference to any other clinical specialty apart from a gross clinical subdivision between medical and surgical specialties. An *arbudagya* may therefore be considered as an Ayurvedic oncologist in contemporary sense.

Expanding the clinical understanding about localized swellings, a vivid clinical description is available in Ayurveda. Such description is available to describe various features like association of pain, feeling on touch, size and shape, discharge, mobility, color, number, place of origin, and progression of the swelling as listed in Table 7.3. Upon looking at this highly illustrated clinical description of the swellings as is available in Ayurveda, an expansion to the contemporary knowledge of subtyping of various tumors may easily be approached.

9 गात्र प्रदेशे क्वचिदेव दोषा: सम्मूर्च्छिता मांसमभिप्रदूष्य।वृत्तं स्थिरं मन्दरुजं महान्तम अनल्पमूलं चिर वृद्धयपाकम ॥ कुर्वन्ति मांसोपचयम्तो शोफं तदर्बुदं शास्त्रविदो वदन्ति।वातेन पित्तेन कफेन चापि रक्तेन मांसेन च मेदसा च॥ तज्जायते तस्य च लक्षणानि ग्रन्थे: समानानि सदा भवन्ति ॥ (सु.नि.११/ १३-१४)

10 यज्जायते अन्यत खलु पूर्व जाते ज्ञेयं तद अध्यर्बुदम अर्बुदज्ञै:। यद द्वन्दजातं युगपत क्रमाद्वा द्विरबुदं तच्च भवेद असाध्यम ॥ सु. नि. १२/२१

Table 7.3 Differentiating clinical features of tumorous swellings (*utsedha*) in Ayurveda

Signs/symptoms	Differentiating features
1. Pain	*Toda* (piercing pain) *Bheda* (cutting pain) *Daha* (burning) *Chosh* (burning) *Prajjvalit* (like burning in fire) *Alpa vedana/ruja* (mild pain) Manda rujam (mild pain)
2. Shape and size	*Vrutta* (rounded) *Unnat* (elevated) *Vigrathita* (nodular) *Mahan* (big)
3. Feeling on touch	*Amridu* (hard) *Ushna* (hot) *Sheet* (cold) *Pashanavata* (stony hard) *Snigdha* (oily)
4. Discharge	*Accha* (clean) *Ushna* (hot) *Shukla ghanam cha puyam* (whitish thick like pus) *Pinyaaksarpiprtimam* (cheesy, like the sesame paste)
5. Mobility	*Achalai* (fixed) *Sthira* (immobile) *Chala* (mobile)
6. Color	*Krishna* (black) *Raktasapeeto* (reddish yellow) *Avivarna* (normal colored) *Ananyavarna* (skin colored)
7. Number	*Dwirbuda* (two tumors at the same time) *Adhyarbud* (another tumor at the side of primary tumor)
8. Place of origin	*Hanvasthi* (submandibular) *Kaksha* (axilla) *Akshakasthi* (supraclavicular) *Bahu* (arm) *Manya* (cervical region) *Gala* (neck) *Rakta* (blood) *Mamsa* (muscles) *Mahasrotus* (GI tract)
9. Progression	*Chirabhivriddhi* (slow progress) *Varshgananubandhi* (remains for many years)
10. Other features	*Atikandu* (severe itching)

7.14 Cancer Management Opportunities in Ayurveda

Cancer is largely a result of lost balance between cell division and cell death. As a result, the cells fail to respond to conventional signals of stopping the cell division and eventually die. The mechanism of cellular immortality appears at molecular level and is marked by a genomic, biochemical, and subsequent physiological changes in order to ensure the cell survival. Ayurvedic perception of *tridosha* pathophysiology immediately warrants for stoppage of all such practices which may lead to a suboptimal intrinsic change in the microenvironment around the cell. There can be preventive strategies for cancer based upon Ayurvedic principles of healthy living. These preventive measures are usually generic but may also have some specific roles to play in cancer prevention if Ayurvedic postulates of oncogenesis are given a chance and consideration.

Cancer management of Ayurveda may be categorized on the basis of its preventive, promotive, and curative strategies. Prevention of cancer can be obtained by carefully avoiding the factors having a potential to lead *tridosha* pathogenesis. Avoiding *adhayasna* (eating food without the digestion of earlier intake), *visamasana* (irregular eating habits), *apathya* (unhealthy food not suitable to the individual), and *viruddhahara* (incompatible food and dietary combination) types of food practices may be a help in this regard. Avoiding natural urge retention (*vegavarodha*) may also be a crucial preventive point.

Promotion of health may be practiced by consuming pathya (food which is compatible on individual basis). There are certain foods which are categorically considered healthy and hence can have an unrestricted use. Such edibles are mung (*Phaseolus mungo*), milk, honey, rock salt, and hot water. Besides this, Ayurveda also proposes a category of conditionally healthy food which are having a recommendation of consumption in limited quality and frequency [29]. On the other hand, there is also a category of completely unhealthy food which is required to be absolutely avoided.

Ayurveda recommends a routine seasonal detoxification for healthy people to eliminate the accumulated waste in the body regularly produced through various biological processes. Like all biological processes, Ayurvedic biology proposes a seasonal accumulation-collection-suppression/dissemination (*sanchaya-prakopa-prashama/prasara*) cycle of *dosha*. All *dosha*s have a season-specific accumulation and tendency to either go into natural suppression or into flaring up and dissemination, the later becoming the prelude to various *dosha*-specific pathologies. As a preventive strategy, Ayurveda proposes a routine cleansing of such accumulated *dosha* by specifically designed cleaning process specific to *dosha* type. For *vata*, *pitta*, and *kaphavasti*, *virechana* and *vaman* are recommended as specific methods of eliminating them and, therefore, bringing back a normal physiological balance of *dosha*. Such practices, if observed regularly, may reduce the chances of any *dosha*-specific pathology to initiate and therefore may reduce the chances of cancer occurrence also.

Besides food, *rasayana* is another health promotive key strategy of Ayurveda. *Rasayana* is classically defined as the means of promoting healthy biological system through providing essential nutrients and growth factors and also through scavenging the metabolic toxins having a system damaging potential.[11] It is for this

[11] लाभोपायो हि शस्तानाम रसादीनाम रसायनम ॥ च.चि. १/७-८.

Methods of procuring improved quality of body tissues are called rasayana (Charaka Samhita ChikitsaSthana, RasayanaPaad 1/7–8).

reason that *rasayana* is proposed to have antiaging effects. Cancer incidence is known to increase with age [30]. This is largely believed that through adoption of suitable strategies to prevent age-related cellular damages, such age and cancer incidence relationship may suitably be modified [31]. Ayurveda proposes *rasayana* as important intervention to prevent or to delay aging-related physiological or pathological consequences[12] which may have an association with cancer too. A few general health restoratives like amalaki (*Embelica officinalis*) which is pronounced as *vayasthapananamshrestha* (best age stabilizer), haritaki (*Terminalia chebula*) as *pathyanam shreshtha* (best suitable substance), and *ksheer ghritaabhyaas*[13] (practice of consuming milk and *ghrita*) can have their pronounced effects upon general health of an individual and can help in reducing the incidence of cancer as well.

Achara rasayana (ethics-based general principles of conduct) is one significant recommendation of Ayurveda for proposing its benefits at par with actual *rasayana*.[14] This means a practice of code of conduct and behavior may be as helpful in restoration of youthfulness and health as *rasayana* themselves.

For people who had been on unhealthy lifestyles and are willing to be shifted to healthier ones, Ayurveda proposes a scientific plan to make gradual and effective changes by giving the system an opportunity to adapt. Such protocol is referred as *padamshika* protocol where the changes are executed in parts and not instantly or suddenly. *Sarvarasabhyasa* (practicing the consumption of all tastes) is also one highly recommended strategy of Ayurveda to remain healthy. Ayurveda finds taste as a representation of five essential elements available in a substance, and hence taste discrimination may lead to disturbance in elemental composition of body as well. Consuming substances representing all tastes will nullify this possibility of food-based *doshik* imbalance to appear.

Besides such preventive and promotive approaches, there are local and systemic approaches to treat cancer. *Kshara* (chemical cauterization) and *Agnikarma*

---

12 रसायनम च तज्ज्ञेयम यज्जराव्याधि विनाशनम।

Rasayana is the one which eliminates aging and related diseases.

13 क्षीर घृताभ्यासो रसायनानां । च.सू.२५/४०

A practice of consuming milk and ghrita on daily basis is like Rasayana (Charaka Samhita Sutra Sthana 25/40).

14 सत्यवादिनम अक्रोधमं निवृत्तं मद्यमैथुनात । अहिंसकमनायासं प्रशान्तम प्रियवादिनम।
जप शौच परं धीरं दान नित्यं तपस्विनम। देवगोब्राह्मणाचार्य गुरु वृद्धार्चने रतम॥
आनृशंस्यपरं नित्यं नित्यं करुणवेदिनम । समजागरणस्वप्नं नित्यं क्षीरघृताशिनम॥
देशकालप्रमाणज्ञं युक्तिज्ञम अनहंगकृतम। शस्ताचारम असंकीर्णमअध्यात्म प्रवणेन्द्रियम॥
उपासितारं वृद्धानामास्तिकानां जितात्मनाम। धर्मशास्त्र परं विद्यान्नरं नित्यरसायनम॥
गुणैरेते: समुदिते: प्रयुंगक्ते यो रसायनम। रसायन गुणान सर्वान यथोक्तान स समश्नुते॥ च. चि. १-४/ ३०-३५.

The one who adheres to truth, does not get angry, has abandoned alcohol and sexual indulgence, nonviolent, calm and pleasing in speech, has spiritual interests, clean, donor, respectful to elders, teachers, Brahmins and deities, empathetic, has a balanced sleep and awake cycle, consumes milk and ghrita routinely, does carefully as per the need of season, and place, careful in behavior, has a control on sensual desires, interested in reading spiritual texts gets all the benefits of Rasayana even if he does not consume any Rasayana (Charak Samhita ChikitsaSthaan 1 RasayanPaad 4 / 30–35).

(thermal ablation) are two such highly practiced procedures of Ayurveda recommended for complete uprooting of local superficial nonmalignant tumors. A highly precised technique is recommended in Ayurveda to practice such methods. Conventional *samshodhana* (elimination) and *samshamana* (palliation) are also recommended for various types of cancers on the basis of *doshik* prevalence and the strength of the sick and of sickness (*rogi* and *rogabala*).

7.15 Cancer in Ayurveda: Questions Yet to Be Answered

Despite this highly commendable inference about cancer pathobiology and its management obtained by reviewing Ayurvedic literature, we find a number of questions still unanswered. There are large and visible gaps between the classical text and real clinical practice which hinder the translational possibility of the knowledge spread through Ayurvedic texts. Unless these gaps are bridged, there may not be a smooth transition from book to bedside referring to cancer. The classical description of *arbud* and allied tumor like pathologies is largely limited to the external and visible tumors, and there is no clear clinical description available about internal neoplasia except occasional mention of their incurability. As an example, a*rbud* originating at *mahasrotus* (gastrointestinal tract) is considered incurable. Unlike many other diseases described in Ayurveda with a highly specific note upon their etiopathogenesis, localized swellings (including *granthi*, *apachi*, *arbud*, and *galaganda*) do not possess such description in details. Etiological factors have not been clearly described about such diseases in Ayurveda. If there are genetic factors leading to disharmony of *dosha*, *dushya*, and *agni*, having their effect throughout the body, is it difficult to interpret how a specific tissue is getting involved in cancer production? As the same changes are also responsible for the production of various other diseases, what stimulates them developing cancer and not any other pathology? Another question of significance in cancer pathobiology is, "can the mutant cells of cancer be reverted?" We know that cancer cells are immortal, and therefore once it occurs, the only treatment is to kill such cells completely and to eradicate any possibility of their regeneration. How Ayurvedic treatment may help in this condition? Cancer passes through many stages before it reaches to malignant stage. There are no obvious clinical signs to know it clearly that something of this sort is happening in the body. Can Ayurveda help in understanding the subtle signs of upcoming malignancy which has already rooted in the body?

Telomeres, specialized DNA-protein complex present at the termini of all chromosomes, are the guardians of individual 46 chromosomes in human cells. Their maintenance is highly desirable for healthy cells. Their length is maintained by an enzyme—telomerase, which is either absent or is at very low activity in human somatic cells. Genetic instability is caused by telomere attrition and is the hallmark of most cancer types [32]. During neoplastic transformation (cancer formation), telomerase gets activated/upregulated and adds TTAGGGn (telomere repeats) at chromosomal ends. What could be the possible trigger which is perceived by the cell to activate the immortality mechanism and reactivating/upregulating telomerase activity? Essentially this is a threat to die, either by means of external factors causing a direct threat to the cellular survival or an internal mechanism creating a completely unfavorable environment in the milieu leading to a threatened survival of the cells. It is important to understand if removal of any such stress has a possibility of disease reversal, a concept which Ayurveda initially proposed referring to the management of every disease. At least theoretically, it seems possible that if all such factors are removed in order to nullify the cause of telomerase activation/upregulation, possibly that can again be made dormant.

Ayurveda may help understand the cause of cancer in individual cases by carefully observing the breeches in healthy routines. A sustained breech may be linked to *tridoshaja* pathogenesis. A carefully planned reversal from breech to the normality may reverse the pathology at least theoretically. Appropriate studies may therefore be warranted to evaluate disease reversal possibilities through proper adoption of Ayurvedic recommendations [33]. *Rasayana* drugs and *panchakarma* therapy may help keeping the milieu interior in its best functioning state, hence avoiding chronic suppression induced pathogenesis. Observing a code of conduct (good *karma*) may also help in avoiding the development of many diseases including cancer.

References

1. Cancer, Fact sheet, February 2017. http://www.who.int/mediacentre/factsheets/fs297/en/. Last accessed on 12 Nov 2017.
2. Singh RH. Perspectives in innovation in the AYUSH sector. J Ayurveda Integr Med. 2011;2(2):52–4. https://doi.org/10.4103/0975-9476.82516.
3. Union for International Cancer Control. The economics of cancer prevention and control. Data digest. http://issuu.com/uicc.org/docs/wcls2014_economics_of_cancer_final?e=0. Published 2014. Accessed 4 Feb 2015.
4. Carter AJ, Nguyen CN. A comparison of cancer burden and research spending reveals discrepancies in the distribution of research funding. BMC Public Health. 2012;12:526. https://doi.org/10.1186/1471-2458-12-526.
5. Mile stones in Cancer research and discovery. https://www.cancer.gov/research/progress/250-years-milestones. Last accessed on 15 Nov 2017.
6. Govindarajan V, Trimble C. Reverse innovation: create far from home win everywhere. Boston: Harward University Press; 2012.
7. Lancet. Water with sugar and salt. Lancet 1978;312:300–1 (Originally published as Volume 2, 300–301, 1978). [PubMed].
8. Rahaman MM, Aziz KM, Patwari Y, et al. Diarrhoeal mortality in two Bangladeshi villages with and without community-based oral rehydration therapy. Lancet. 1979;2:809–12. [PubMed].
9. Patwardhan B, Vaidya ADB, Chorghade M, Joshi SP. Reverse pharmacology and systems approaches for drug discovery and development. Curr Bioactive Comp. 2008;4:201–12.
10. Gupta AK. Grass roots innovation. New Delhi: Penguin Random House India; 2016.
11. Fridlender M, Kapulnik Y, Koltai H. Plant derived substances with anti-cancer activity: from folklore to practice. Front Plant Sci. 2015;6:799. https://doi.org/10.3389/fpls.2015.00799.
12. Swyngedouw E. Globalisation or 'glocalisation'? Networks, territories and rescaling. Camb Rev Int Aff. 2004;17(1):25–48.
13. Hawking S. On the shoulders of giants. The great works of physics and astronomy (Running Press 2002). ISBN 0-7624-1698-X.

14. https://www.theguardian.com/society/2014/sep/22/cancer-late-diagnosis-half-patients
15. Cancer Prev. http://www.who.int/cancer/prevention/en/. Last accessed on 9 Mar 2018.
16. Sloan FA, Gelband H, editors. Cancer control opportunities in low- and middle-income countries. Institute of Medicine (US) Committee on Cancer Control in Low- and Middle-Income Countries. Washington, DC: National Academies Press (US); 2007.
17. Al-Azri MH. Delay in Cancer diagnosis: causes and possible solutions. Oman Med J. 2016;31(5):325–6. https://doi.org/10.5001/omj.2016.65.
18. Ahmad AS, Ormiston-Smith N, Saseini PD. Trends in the life time risk of developing cancer in great Britain: comparison of risk for those born from 1930 to 1960. Br J Cancer. 2015;112:943–7. https://doi.org/10.1038/bjc.2014.606.
19. Ghodke Y, Joshi K, Patwardhan B. Traditional medicine to modern pharmacogenomics: Ayurveda Prakriti type and CYP2C19 gene polymorphism associated with the metabolic variability. Evid Based Complement Alternat Med. 2011;2011(249528):1.
20. Aggarwal S, Negi S, Jha P, Singh PK, Stobdan T, Pasha MA. Indian genome variation consortium. EGLN1 involvement in high-altitude adaptation revealed through genetic analysis of extreme constitution types defined in Ayurveda. Proc Natl Acad Sci U S A. 2010;107:18961–6.
21. Akoury D. Epigenetics effects of stress influence the genomics, proteomics, metabolomics of addiction and cancer pathways. Adv Genet Eng. 2015;4:122. https://doi.org/10.4172/2169-0111.1000122.
22. Valiathan MS. Ayurvedic Biology: a decadal vision document. Bengaluru: Indian Academy of Science; 2006.
23. Rastogi S. Ayurvedic principles of food and nutrition: translating the theory into evidence based practice. In: Rastogi S, editor. Ayurvedic science of food and nutrition. New York: Springer; 2014.
24. Szymanski J, Jozefczuk S, Nikoloski Z, et al. Stability of metabolic correlations under changing environmental conditions in *Escherichia coli*—a systems approach. PLoS One. 2009;4(10):e7441. https://doi.org/10.1371/journal.pone.0007441.
25. Vousden KH, Xin L. Live or let die: the cell's response to p53. Nat Rev Cancer. 2002;2:594–604. https://doi.org/10.1038/nrc864.
26. Hamada N, Kodama S, Suzuki K, Watanabe M. Gap junctional intercellular communication and cellular response to heat stress. Carcinogenesis. 2003;24(11):1723–8. Epub 2003 Aug 14.
27. Garg P. Awareness that early cancer lump is painless could decrease breast cancer mortality in developing countries. World J Clin Oncol. 2016;7(3):321–3. https://doi.org/10.5306/wjco.v7.i3.321.
28. Hoang JK, Lee WK, Lee M, Johnson D, Farrell S. US features of thyroid malignancy: pearls and pitfalls. Radio Graphics. 2007;27:847–65.
29. Rastogi S, editor. Ayurvedic science of food and nutrition. NewYork: Springer; 2014.
30. Smetana K, Lacina L, Szabo P, Dvorankova B, Broz P, Sedo A. Ageing as an important risk factor for cancer. Anticancer Res. 2016;36(10):5009–17.
31. White MC, Holman DM, Boehm JE, Peipins LA, Grossman M, Henley SJ. Age and cancer risk: a potentially modifiable relationship. Am J Prev Med. 2014;46(3 Suppl 1):S7–15. https://doi.org/10.1016/j.amepre.2013.10.029.
32. Pathak S, Multani AS. Aneuploidy, stem cells and cancer. In: Bignold LP, editor. Cancer: cell structure, carcinogens and genomic instability. Cham: Birkhauser Verlag; 2006. p. 49–64.
33. Singh RH. Reverse innovation and translational studies in AYUSH. Ann Ayurvedic Med. 2012;1(1–2):2–3.

Understanding Diabetes: Uncovering the Leads from Ayurveda

8

Sanjeev Rastogi

8.1 Introduction

The world is observing an unprecedented rise in the diabetes prevalence during the recent decades. The world diabetic population rose exponentially to 422 million in 2014 from 108 million in 1980 [1]. Most importantly and alarmingly, the growth in diabetic population is not uniform around the world but is segmental. There are distinct areas of higher, average, and lower prevalence of diabetes marked with well-defined geographical boundaries. Age-adjusted adult diabetes prevalence in 2014 was lowest in Northwestern Europe and highest in Polynesia and Micronesia, at nearly 25%, followed by Melanesia and the Middle East and North Africa.

A recent rapid increase in the prevalence of diabetes has brought China on the top of countries representing the largest diabetic populations [2]. Diabetic population in China increased phenomenally from 20.4 million (1980) to 102.9 million (2014), a five times rise in three decades. India has followed a similar trend showing a rise from 11.9 million (1980) to 64.5 million (2014) in same time span [3]. China contributes about 25% of the current global diabetic population, whereas India contributes about 15.5% of it. These countries, with their 40% share in net diabetic population of the globe, paradoxically also cradle two most ancient health-care traditions, TCM and Ayurveda. These systems, often known as the oldest living health traditions of the world, are flourishing and practiced in their respective countries of origin and neighborhoods.

With a huge diabetic burden to shoulder upon, this is relevant to see how these countries have responded to the burden so far and how they are utilizing their traditional health-care wisdom to ease out the burden. A literature search aiming to identify the researches done by these countries in the area of concern however has shown a gross mismatch between the disease burden and the share of research aiming to

S. Rastogi
Department of Kaya Chikitsa, State Ayurvedic College and Hospital,
Lucknow University, Lucknow, India

S. Rastogi (ed.), *Translational Ayurveda*, https://doi.org/10.1007/978-981-13-2062-0_8

reduce the burden. Despite their high share in the net diabetic population of the world, their contribution to research in the area is less than 2% [4]. India being endowed with a pluralistic health-care model finds unique encounters of diabetes management. Many diabetic patients here take a respite in alternative medicines collectively referred as AYUSH (Ayurveda, Yoga and Naturopathy, Unani, Siddha, and Homeopathy) pronouncing to have a cure or management for diabetes. While keeping a watch upon conventional health care of diabetes, our concern here is to know and to understand how Ayurveda in particular is affecting diabetic people in India and what realistic role it may play in the future regarding the diabetes understanding and its management strategies.

8.2 Diabetes Research in India

Research on diabetes is still nascent in India. In a citation review for the published literature on diabetes done between 1976 and 2006, it was found that India shared a dismal 1.04% of global research publications on diabetes [5]. The area of these researches was much diverse although the predominant focus was upon pharmaceutical and endocrine research (approx. 35% of Indian publications on diabetes). Areas like nutrition and diet (approx. 5% of Indian publications) found less attention of Indian researcher, despite them being focused in global diabetic research. Indian publications had much share of the global publication done on plant-based diabetes researches (155 from total 314 global publications), which is reflective of Indian rich heritage of plant-based health-care practice of Ayurveda [5]. Research on diabetes also has unequal geographical distribution in India. The major stakeholding in the field was limited to a few places, institutions, or persons. Major research organization involved in research on diabetes in India are All India Institute of Medical Sciences (AIIMS), New Delhi; Diabetes Research Centre (DRC), Chennai; Annamalai University, Annamalai Nagar; Postgraduate Institute of Medical Education and Research (PGIMER), Chandigarh; University of Madras, Chennai; Madras Diabetes Research Foundation (MDRF), Chennai; Jawaharlal Nehru University (JNU), New Delhi; and Central Drug Research Institute (CDRI), Lucknow. There are few more involved sparingly in diabetic research.

8.3 Focus of Indian Research on Diabetes

What is Indian focus in diabetic research? India currently is home to over 60 million adults with diabetes (7.8% of its population), of which more than 30 million are undiagnosed or untreated, thus increasing the risk of developing complications and premature mortality [6]. Our existing experience with the disease shows that there are no promising ways to cure this disease, and hence a comprehensive yet meticulous preventive and management plan may hold the key to success. Despite a huge population being affected by diabetes, its contextual epidemiology, early detection, and possible prevention have rarely been attempted in Indian researches done in the field (Table 8.1).

Table 8.1 Publication in various areas of research on diabetes in India (1976–2014)

Endocrinology and metabolism	612
Medicine, general, and internal	198
Peripheral vascular disease	65
Cardiac and cardiovascular systems	75
Biochemistry and molecular biology	301
Pharmacology and pharmacy	497
Urology and nephrology	144
Plant sciences	155
Ophthalmology	140
Chemistry, medicinal	262
Cell biology	118
Surgery	69
Nutrition and dietetics	148
Medicine, research, and experiment	157
Multidisciplinary sciences	125
Immunology	118
Hematology	26
Biology	114
Biophysics	110

Although relatively higher proportion of plant-based diabetes researches is done in India, its focus remained concentrated upon exploration of the hypoglycemic properties of plant extracts and their active principles. Clinical trials of various combinations of such drugs have also been attempted although sparingly and poorly [7].

8.4 Ayurveda Propositions to Diabetes Understanding

Diabetes has a historical association with human civilization. It was widely known to world through its pathognomonic symptoms like sweetness of urine and progressive weakness. *Prameha*, as the condition is known in Ayurveda, has a vivid description including its etiopathogenesis and individualized management protocols. Diabetes mellitus (*madhumeha*) is considered as an epitome of all *prameha*, and it is warned that all *prameha* may eventually convert into *madhumeha*, if not duly managed. There had also been a number of management plans to treat diabetes in Ayurveda with a clear notion about *madhumeha* that it is a "difficult to be treated" condition, and hence a careful lifetime palliation may be needed. Such prognosis-based classification however is principally based upon the *dosha* culminating into the disease. *Prameha* caused by *kapha* is treatable, whereas of *pitta* and *vata* is difficult to be treated and untreatable, respectively. In a most surprising manner, Sushruta, the iconic surgery legend of India, was able to state the two distinct varieties of diabetes on the basis of their origin and called them *sahaja* (present since birth) and *apathya nimittaja* (caused by inappropriate food not suitable for individual consumption). Today we recognize these conditions as insulin-dependent diabetes mellitus (IDDM) and non-insulin-dependent diabetes mellitus (NIDDM).

8.5 Contemporary Ayurvedic Researches on Diabetes

Contemporary Ayurvedic research on diabetes in India have failed identifying the need of revalidating the Ayurvedic conceptualization about the disease contextual to its etiopathogenesis, early clinical diagnosis, and management. The whole focus of Ayurveda research on diabetes so far remained limited to clinical trials of various herbs, minerals, and their formulations for their possible hypoglycemic roles in diabetics. At the same time, minimal efforts have been made to unearth the basic understanding of diabetes in Ayurveda to design a better and comprehensive cure for the disease.

A systematic review by the Agency for Healthcare Research and Quality (AHRQ) on Ayurvedic clinical researches on diabetes (2001) revealed that most of these researches are composed of poor basic science studies, fewer RCTs, small sample size, poor study plans, limited external validity, and poor data analysis [8]. A concern was also raised about the distinctive use of complex herb combinations against a single or fewer herbs and argued for a genuinely proven data to support any addition of herbs in a formulation against the net cost, efficacy, and possibility of food–herb, herb–herb, or herb–drug interactions. The report highlighted that real-life clinical studies should have been conducted with due involvement of multiple humane approaches adopted in the common households to manage diabetes. An isolated and also a collective effect of all modalities used in diabetes is required to be thoroughly analyzed in order to ensure their collective benefits in the clinical practice. Things did not change much in the last 15 years since this AHRQ review. A recent look at AYUSH Research Portal identified 136 published researches related to diabetes of which only 17 (12.5%) were eligible to come under evidence level A [9].

India is recently observing a vigorous market campaigning for a few chosen Ayurvedic antidiabetic products with unproven claims. Some of these products are said to be based upon a formulation endorsed by the Central Council of Research in Ayurvedic Science (CCRAS), an apex Ayurveda research organization under the Ministry of AYUSH in India. These marketed products are linked back with AYUSH 82, a drug composed of *karela* seeds (*Momordica charantia* Linn.), *Jambu* seeds (*Syzygium cumuni* Linn.), *Amra* seed (*Mangifera indica* Linn.), and *Gudmar* leaves (*Gymnema sylvestre* R. Br.), having been tried clinically on 805 diabetic patients for its effectiveness in glucose control. The results claimed it to be effective in 70% of patients without any significant adversity [10].

This is amazing to see that how an inappropriately done short-term single clinical trial involving a small sample size without a long-term follow-up for a disease like diabetes affecting 7.8% Indian population is leading to OTC marketing for drugs endorsed by the agencies having the responsibility of creating evidences of safety and efficacy based upon rigors of science.

This approach of research and subsequent war-footed marketing under the endorsement of those who are responsible of bringing ethics in research raises a serious concern about the intentions of such researches [11]. This is noteworthy here that US FDA recommends a phase 3 trial for diabetes be done upon at least

2500 subjects with at least 1300–1500 exposed to the investigational product for 1 year or more and at least 300–500 subjects exposed to the investigational product for 18 months or more [12]. A disease of a magnitude of diabetes in an ethnically diverse country which ranks (unfortunately) second in the world in terms of diabetic population, an efficacy claim and subsequent marketing on the basis of a small-sample clinical trial, raises a question against our research concerns, methods and priorities.

This inadvertent marketing of herbal antidiabetics also has created a unique never before situation. In lack of proper information based upon long-term studies, a sizeable number of diabetics stop taking recommended oral hypoglycemic drugs upon the initiation of herbal antidiabetics. Some co-consume it in addition to their recommended conventional medicine with or without the consent of their treating physicians in a hope that addition of herbal drugs may help them reducing the dose of oral hypoglycemics. OTC availability of Ayurvedic antidiabetic drugs has permitted an unmonitored and erratic consumption of such drugs without a close watch upon their immediate and long-term role in diabetes management. In the absence of adequate studies on possible herb–drug interactions for any co-consumption with allopathic drugs, it is easy to arrive at erratic and poor outcomes. One such herb–drug interaction has a sense to be mentioned here. Aqueous extract of the fresh leaves of *Abroma augusta* L. (known as *Ulat Kambal* in Ayurveda, a common ingredient of many Ayurvedic antidiabetic formulations) was found to reduce the metformin hydrochloride absorption due to their mutual interaction [13]. This study warns about coadministration of such combinations for their unexpected results unless these combinations are well studied.

8.6 Contemporary Ayurvedic Practice of Diabetes Management

Indian Ayurvedic drug market is flooded with large number of proprietary drugs claiming to have antidiabetic potentials. Almost every Indian pharmaceutical company dealing with Ayurveda has one or more products listed for diabetes. Besides classical formulations referred in ancient texts of Ayurveda, there are also many novel, experiential, and empirical herbal combinations available as OTC products. Most of such products share a few common ingredients reported to have antidiabetic potential [14]. Unfortunately, the claims of such combinations do not possess any clinical research to substantiate their worthiness.

Another critical issue associated with Ayurvedic management of diabetes is the toxicity of some of its herbo-mineral preparations. A number of Ayurvedic classical formulations of diabetes contain *naga* (lead) [15]. Lead is a known toxic heavy metal having a property of causing cumulative toxicity. Many adversity reports are available in published literature reporting about lead toxicity among people consuming Ayurvedic medicine for their diabetes management [16]. Two things which need urgent attention here are as follows: first, diabetes being a chronic illness requires long-term, often the lifetime, management; therefore, the safety of a drug to treat this condition is of paramount importance. Second, in the absence of overt manifestations, the diabetic patients do not return very often for the follow-up visits to their physicians. In a preconceived assumption that the drugs recommended are sufficient and safe for their illness, the drugs are often continued without proper follow-ups unless something of concern appears. Ignorance of practicing physicians about potential toxicity of a preparation upon its long-term use further magnifies the chances of toxicity in the absence of a clear knowledge of duration of the drug use. Finally, lead being a neurotoxin presenting symptoms strikingly similar to those of diabetic complications, chances are there for missing such symptoms as diabetic complications rather than those of a drug toxicity.

Although never surveyed, contemporary Ayurvedic clinical practice on diabetes is also marked with huge gaps between expectations and deliverance. Diabetology per se is not a specialized branch of study in Ayurveda, and hence the practitioners in the field are self-praised diabetologists, claiming to have an experience-based specialization in that area. Ayurvedic management of diabetes largely focuses upon reduction of blood sugar levels with the help of Ayurvedic herbs and formulations. There had been negligible efforts offering a comprehensive management to diabetes by proposing a rational combination of diet, exercise, avoidance of possible precipitating factors, and supportive therapy. Also, there is a lack of thorough monitoring of the patients in view of their fluctuating blood sugar levels. The physicians are not aware of relative strengths and mechanisms of functioning of their prescribed drugs and hence are not aware if one class of drug fails, what comes next? There are also no clear evidences if Ayurveda may dependably be considered as a stand-alone therapy in diabetes or may be co-prescribed with conventional therapy as an adjunct. In case of co-prescription, mutual interaction of herbs and drugs is of crucial importance to be understood before being recommended for practice.

In lack of clear directives and understanding, this is obvious to see that many diabetics under alternative management may face complications due to erratic management of the disease in the long run. There had also been negligible efforts to screen the proportion of diabetic population under the influence of Ayurveda or other alternative systems in India in order to evaluate the magnitude of the population and impact of the system on their disease management [17].

8.7 Scope of Ayurveda to Contribute into the Current Diabetes Research and Management

There is a common consensus in contemporary medical science about the limitations of drug management of diabetes and its complications [18, 19]. Many barriers hinder the effective translation of diabetes management protocol into realistic outcomes [20]. Such barriers are dominant in countries where literacy is less and cultural ethos is stronger. Improving communication, addressing prevailing misconceptions, and culture-specific strategies are suggested to be useful for improving diabetes management in such situations [20]. This may find a strong relevance here that the culture-specific strategies as suggested for the regionalized management of diabetes should include the traditional health-care knowledge prevalent in a particular culture. This argument is more meaningful for India where Ayurveda is believed to be a safe and effective option for the management of many chronic diseases including diabetes. This further suggests that the Ayurvedic wisdom about diabetes is required to be thoroughly explored and adopted in diabetes management action plans for its possible benefits to a country which is becoming a homeland to diabetics.

There can be multiple areas where Ayurvedic wisdom, after its thorough exploration under the rigor of science, can be of help to understand and to manage the disease in a better way. Such areas can be from the identification of risk factors, possible etiopathogenesis, clinical profile, disease course, and diagnostic and management strategies including its preventive and curative propositions [21].

8.8 Identification of the Risk Factors for Their Possible Association with Diabetes

There are elaborate descriptions in Ayurvedic classics regarding possible causes of *prameha* and its subtypes. Such causes are categorized as per the *dosha* predominance in pathogenesis. Most of such causes enumerated in Ayurveda referring to diabetes fall into categories of diet, eating behavior, lifestyle, and mental state-related factors (Table 8.2).

Ayurveda duly recognizes the multifactorial nature of diabetes and hence identifies a vast array of possible players in the genesis of this disease. Ayurvedic classification of disease on the basis of nutrition brings *prameha* under overnutrition category (*santarpana janya*) contrary to the other category of diseases where undernutrition (*apatarpan janya*) is the principal cause. This understanding of over nourishment in *prameha* is very much similar to what is conventionally understood as the common

Table 8.2 Factors leading to diabetes as per Ayurveda

Category	Subcategory	Ayurvedic description	Contemporary explanation
Food	Food taste	*Amla*	Sour predominant food
		Lavana	Salt predominant food
		Madhur	Sweet predominant food
	Food quality	*Guru*	Complex food taking longer time to get digested
		Snigdha	Oil-rich food
	Food type as per its age	*Navanna*	New grain
		Nava pana	
Lifestyle	Sleep	*Nidra*	Excessive sleep
		Aasya sukhani	Prolonged comfortable sitting
	Exercise	*Tyakta vyaayam*	No exercise
Mental state	Stress	*Chintaanam*	Excessive mental activity
Routine disease preventive activities	Bio-detoxification	*Samshodhanam akurvataam*	No detoxification

cause of diabetes. High-calorie food and no exercise are principal precipitating factors for a poor glucose metabolism eventually terminating as diabetes. In contrast to conventional understanding, however, Ayurveda does not consider sweet taste alone as implicative of diabetes, and on the contrary, excess indulgence to sour and salt is also considered culminative to diabetes (*Charak sutra sthana Chapter 17/ 78–81*). On another note, *Vasant Kusumakar Rasa*, one most acclaimed Ayurvedic drug for diabetes, is found processed with sugarcane juice. Excess of sweet therefore seems finding its way to diabetes through indirect route of causing obesity. Recent observations endorse this observation by noting that moderate amount of sugar intake actually do not have deleterious effects on diabetes management [22].

Regarding the food quality, Ayurveda proposes *guru* food association with diabetes. *Guru* and *laghu* are two functional properties of food distinguished on the basis of time needed for their digestion. *Guru* requires longer time to get digested comparing to *laghu*. By virtue of its properties, *guru* food causes heaviness and satiety for a longer time. New grains, black lentil, curd, and materials processed with lots of ghee and oil are the examples of *guru* food. Although *guru* food is often linked with diabetes on account of them being high on glycemic index, it is not only this which signifies *guru*. *Guru* also stands for a complex food taking longer time to get digested owing to its complex nature. Now due to this complex nature, they get digested slowly and in turn remain a sustained source of glucose delivery in the blood long after the clearance of postprandial rise of blood glucose. This causes a sustained load upon the pancreas to meet with additional demands of glucose level controls.

8.9 *Guru* and *Laghu* Food: Can They Be Understood by Glycemic Index and Glycemic Load

While describing the properties of *laghu* and *guru* food, Ayurveda further states that despite their impacts upon digestibility, they should be taken in the recommended quantity only, a concept which reminds us the idea of glycemic index and glycemic load. Glycemic index at one point indicates the relative rise in blood glucose after the consumption of a given amount of food comparing to the equal amount of sugar; the glycemic load refers to the total quantity of food consumed. It is obvious to see that it is not only the glycemic index but also the glycemic load which determines the rise in blood sugar levels, an idea which was postulated in Ayurveda by stating that ultimately the quantity of the food matters most, no matter if it is *laghu* or *guru* (Fig. 8.1). Ayurveda proposes various instructions to be followed regarding the intake of different food. A few can be taken regularly, whereas a few others only occasionally. The quantity of *guru* food is said to be of amount of 1/2 or 3/4 volume of the stomach only. Ayurveda proposes that the *guru* food should never be eaten to the level of satiety and should never be eaten again once a meal is over. Many clinical conditions are found associated with overconsumption of *guru* food, and on the contrary, although *laghu* food can be taken in a liberal quantity, it may also give rise to the problems of overeating. Such problems of overeating of *laghu* food may however be of lesser intensity comparing to that of the *guru* food (Table 8.3).

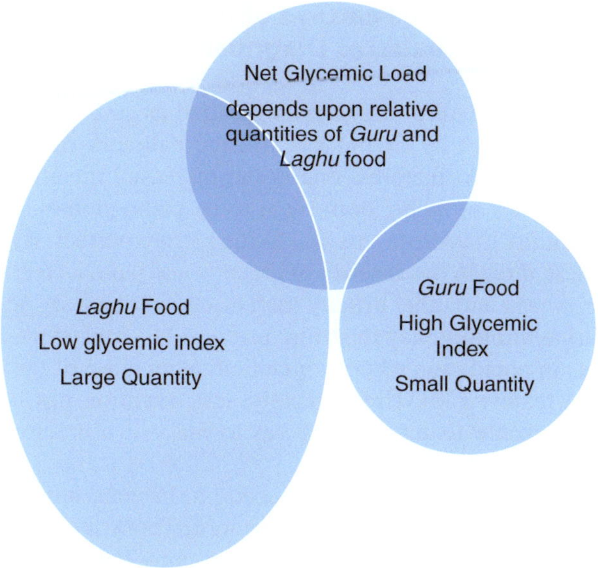

Fig. 8.1 Depiction of quantity of *guru* and *laghu* food in reference to glycemic index and load

Table 8.3 Examples of *guru* and *laghu* foods

Category	Variety	Current interpretation	Ayurvedic recommendation
Laghu	*Shali*	A variety of rice	Eat in appropriate quantity
	Shashti	A variety of rice	Eat in appropriate quantity
	Mudga	Green gram	Eat in appropriate quantity
		Goat, chicken, lamb meat	Eat in appropriate quantity
Guru	*Pishta Vikriti*	Processed food made with paste of wheat flour, black gram flour	Eat in little quantity
	Ikshu Vikriti	Sweets made of cane sugar	Eat in little quantity
	Ksheer Vikriti	Cheese, paneer	Eat in little quantity
	Til	Sesame seeds	Eat in little quantity
	Mash	Black gram	Eat in little quantity
	Tandul	Rice	Eat in little quantity, and don't eat again after finishing the meal
	Prathuka	Rice flakes	Eat in little quantity, and don't eat again after finishing the meal
	Vallur	Dried meat	Don't eat regularly
	Shushka shaka	Dried vegetables	Don't eat regularly
	Kurchika	Sweets made of concentrated milk	Don't eat regularly
	Kilata	Cheese, fresh cheese	Don't eat regularly
	Dadhi	Curd	Don't eat regularly
	Yavaka	A type of *shali* rice	Don't eat regularly
		Pork, beef, buffalo meat, fish	Don't eat regularly

8.10 Clinical Features of *Prameha*: Inspiring Clues for Diabetes Diagnosis and Management

Classical feature of *prameha* recalled as *prabhuta aavila mutrata* (copious and turbid urine) by Charaka is still the hallmark of the disease. *Prabhuta mutrata* signifies two features, one is the increased quantity, and the other is increased frequency of urine; both seem to be pathognomonic to diabetes. An addition of turbidity in urine to this makes the picture perfect. By observing a combination of these three in the absence of urgency and pain, a clear clinical distinction between *prameha* and other urinary tract diseases can easily be made. A simple measure of urine turbidity may therefore prove to be a milestone in rapid screening of diabetes in population where a quantitative increase of the urine is available as a clinical feature [23]. Unfortunately, less attention has been paid to this simple yet remarkable feature of diabetes to make it a precise tool for mass screening of diabetes.

What causes urine of a diabetic to become turbid? We know that, in diabetes, urine can be a mix of multiple abnormal constituents like glucose, albumin, ketone, and blood cells which together can contribute to its turbidity. Most importantly, microalbuminuria, an often ignored condition in diabetes, is found to precede the overt nephropathy in diabetics by 10–14 years [24]. This is obvious to see that this microalbuminuria could be an important reason of turbid urine, and by merely observing it timely, a lot can be saved in terms of management and ensuing complications of diabetes.

Pathogenesis of *prameha* also proposes striking similarities between what is known about diabetes in current science. It proposes that an increased intake of *kapha*-promotive food (*madhura, amla*, and *lavana* are *kapha* promotive) causes a change in nature of *kleda* (interstitial fluid) pertaining to *meda* (fat) and *mamsa* (muscles). Very interestingly, this is observed that in diabetics, pH of the interstitial fluid is found altered and less than normal controls [25]. This alteration in interstitial fluid pH is presumed to be one preceding reason of insulin resistance leading to reduced glucose intake by the skeletal muscles, thereby raising the blood sugar level. This is observed that insulin binding to its receptors is pH dependent and is proportional to the pH of interstitial fluid. An interesting proposition to manage diabetes therefore is to improve the pH of interstitial fluid or *kleda* as is known in Ayurveda.

While talking about the body tissues affected by the diabetes, Ayurveda further elaborates a list of ten *dushya* which gradually get affected by diabetes (Table 8.4). This list is inclusive of three primary body components (*kleda*, *mamsa*, and *meda*) affected by diabetes. It is important to observe that Ayurveda proposes a subsequent and not initial involvement of blood and other components of body like lymph in the pathogenesis of diabetes. A very important inference to this reference is that possibly the pathogenesis of diabetes starts early with the changes in the interstitial fluid (*kleda*) which gradually develops the insulin resistance and subsequently raises the

Table 8.4 *Dosha* and *dushya* of *prameha*

No.	*Dosha*	*Dushya*	Biological correlate
1.	*Vata*	*Meda*	Adipose tissue
2.	*Pitta*	*Rakta*	Blood
3.	*Kapha*	*Shukra*	Semen
4.		*Ambu*	Extracellular fluid
5.		*Vasa*	Muscle fat
6.		*Lasika*	Lymph
7.		*Majja*	Bone marrow
8.		*Rasa*	First product of digestion
9.		*Oja*	
10.		*Mamsa*	Skeletal muscles

blood sugar level. That means even before the prediabetic stage, there can be detectable changes in the *kleda*, and upon their judicious correction, possibly the stage of prediabetes may also be prevented.

8.11 Prediabetes and *Prameha Purvarupa*

A great deal of emphasis has been laid upon prediabetes these days for its potential to be converted as fully manifested diabetes in the future if not prevented. Over 80 million people in India are currently found under the category of prediabetics, having every possibility of being transformed into diabetics if not cared for. Unfortunately there are no clear clinical methods to know if a person is prediabetic, and hence its diagnosis solely depends upon investigations seeking the levels of blood sugar (Table 8.5). Ayurveda here proposes a constellation of symptoms being considered as the alarm for impending diabetes (Table 8.6). This would be very apt to check if the *prameha purvarupa* features as described in Ayurveda, are truly reflected in prediabetic population. Moving a step ahead to what is considered as prediabetic, Ayurveda can help in screening the population at large for their proneness to diabetes by simple clinical observations noticeable by the patients at their own.[1]

---

1 स्वेदोअंगगन्धः शिथिलांगता च शय्यासन स्वप्नसुखे रतिश्च।
हृन्नेत्रजिह्वाश्रवणोपदेहो घनांगता केशनखाति वृद्धिः॥
शीत प्रियत्वम गल तालु शोषो माधुर्यमास्ये कर पाद दाहः।
भविष्यतो मेह गदस्य रूपं मूत्रे अभिधावन्ति पिपीलिकाश्च॥ च.चि. ६/१३-१४.

Excessive sweating, smell from body, fatigue, likening to sit or to sleep, excessive discharges or waste over chest, eyes, tongue, ear, lustrous body, excessive growth of hair and nail, excessive likening of cold, dryness of throat and palate, sweetness of mouth, burning hands and feet and ants associating with the discharged urine are the prodromal features of diabetes.

Charaka Samhita Chikitsaa Sthana 6/13–14.

Table 8.5 Laboratory diagnostic criteria of prediabetes

	A1C	Fasting plasma glucose (FPG)	Oral glucose tolerance test (OGTT)
Normal	Less than 5.7%	Less than 100 mg/dL	Less than 140 mg/dL
Prediabetes	5.8–6.4%	100–125 mg/dL	140–199 mg/dL
Diabetes	More than 6.5%	More than 126 mg/dL	200 mg/dL or higher

8.12 Choosing the Right Therapy in Diabetes: Does Individualization Matter?

Which therapy for which person? This is possibly the trickiest question faced by most physicians in the clinical practice. This is a common observation that a set of medicine effective in one patient do not respond to the other despite a similar clinical presentation. This situation is more observable with conditions like diabetes when treated with Ayurveda. In clinics of Ayurveda, this is a common observation that a few patients under treatment may get a good glycemic control with Ayurvedic drugs alone, a few may require additional allopathic hypoglycemic agents, and a few others do not respond even to the combination. This is also a known fact that one Ayurvedic formulation is not effective to all diabetics, and hence a large range of drugs with variable composition is available in Ayurvedic drug market referring to diabetes. There are compelling evidences to believe that diabetes has a multifactorial etiopathogenesis [26]. This multifactorial pathogenesis paves a way for believing in a heterogeneity of the whole diabetic population where, although the phenotype of the manifestation is same, the genotype of individuals is divisible into distinct subpopulations susceptible more specifically to some etiological factors more than others [27].

It is now believed that diabetes is much more heterogeneous than its present subdivision into types 1 and 2 assumes. These two divisions probably represent extremes of a continuum of diabetic disorders. Diabetes seems to result from an interaction between genes and environment where genetic predisposition establishes its susceptibility and environmental factors explaining the rapid increase in its incidence. With improved characterization of patients with diabetes, the range of diabetic subgroups will possibly become even more diverse in the future [28]. Novel diagnostic markers for diabetes are also proposed to identify heterogeneity within a prediabetic and overt diabetic population [27].

8.13 A Pointer of Latency Period of Diabetes

Ayurvedic proposition of conversion of all *prameha* into *madhumeha* in due course of time with poor management is a pointer toward the latency period of precipitation of overt diabetes. Ayurvedic prodromal features of *madhumeha* also state along the similar lines. This is very clear that the pathogenesis of diabetes starts much earlier than it can be diagnosed through blood sugar levels. This latency period however may be different in different people and may be dependent of a complex interplay of genetic susceptibility and environmental factors. By genetic susceptibility, we can postulate the role of *prakriti* also in the genesis of diabetes. This is obvious to see that if some mechanisms can be developed to predict future diabetics by means of subtle subclinical details, a whole bulk of population may be prevented from getting converted into overt diabetics.

8.14 Possibility of Designing Newer Biomarkers and Diagnostic Tools for Diabetes

Seeing the difficulties associated with invasive blood tests required repeatedly for diagnosis and monitoring in diabetes, this is sincerely thought to develop some non-invasive yet dependable test to detect and to monitor the disease. Glucose monitoring through saliva possibly was the first approach to develop such biomarker to detect the sugar level for some body fluid other than blood. Many studies have subsequently established higher saliva glucose levels in diabetics compared to normal controls [29]. Studies have also suggested a dependable correlation between higher salivary glucose levels and blood glucose levels [30]. This fact was utilized in the development of saliva-based diagnostic techniques to monitor blood glucose levels. Interestingly *madhuryam aasyam* (sweetness in the mouth) as a classical feature of *madhumeha* was described long back in Ayurveda. We can easily presume that *madhuryam aasyam* is nothing but a clinical presentation of high salivary glucose levels. A salivary diagnosis of diabetes therefore could have been the application of this lead of Ayurveda to develop a better diagnostic tool. Unfortunately, India could not utilize this wisdom of Ayurveda to take a lead in this regard.

During conditions of energy surplus, growth hormone (GH), in concert with insulin-like growth factor 1 (IGF-I) and insulin, promotes nitrogen retention [31]. This nitrogen retention is subsequently represented as increase in muscle bulk and body weight. *Ghanangata* (more nourished body parts) as a *purvarupa* feature of diabetes needs a special mention here. This seems that before the diabetes actually sets in, under the influence of positive energy balance, GH stimulates the protein accumulation in the body resulting in *ghanangata*-like features. *Kesh nakhati vriddhi* (excessive growth of the hair and nails) is another classical feature associated as a prodroma to diabetes. The hair and nail are composed of keratin found to have special affinity to glucose. Positive nitrogen retention under the influence of increased GH during the state of energy surplus may also have a direct impact upon growth of the nails and hair resulting in their excessive growth.

This excessive growth and luster of the body tissue however are not sustainable for long in case of sustained hyperglycemia of diabetes. Tissue glycation eventually results in case of prolonged hyperglycemia as a result of bonding of the glucose with proteins. Various tissues in the body have variable affinity to glycation. Ayurveda proposes a few key observations on certain body tissues having a greater affinity to glucose in response to the early glycation before the onset of overt

Table 8.6 Prodromal features of *prameha*[1]

No.	Features	Biological correlates
1.	*Sweda*	Excessive sweating
2.	*Anga gandha*	Smell from body parts
3.	*Shithilangata*	Dullness in the body
4.	*Shayyasana swapnasukhe ratishcha*	Increased liking to sit or to lie
5.	*Hrinnetrajihvashravanopadeho*	Excess waste production over the chest, eyes, tongue, and ear
6.	*Ghanangata*	Apparently more lustrous and nourished body parts
7.	*Kesh nakhati vriddhi*	Excessive growth of the hair and nails
8.	*Sheeta priyatvam*	Increased liking of cold
9.	*Gala talushosha*	Dryness of the throat and palate
11.	*Kar-paada daha*	Burning the hands and feet
12.	*Mutre abhidhavanti pipilikashca*	Ants moving toward the urine

diabetes (Table 8.6). Advanced glycation end products (AGEs) are produced irreversibly in conditions of sustained hyperglycemia, and these are responsible from multiple systemic and structural tissue changes resulting from their premature damage. AGEs are therefore considered as a dependable cause of premature aging, apparent in diabetics, a condition known to be caused by *vata* dominance in *madhumeha* when the disease is fully bloomed. Special affinity of glucose with keratin and irreversibility of AGEs has proposed an idea of considering the hair and nails as possible means of speculating blood glucose. Keratin glycation is found to have a linear relationship sustained over time. Techniques are underway to find mechanisms which can dependably read the blood glucose levels through the examination of the hair or nail clippings in a patient of diabetes [32].

Gala talu shosha (dryness of the throat and palate) is also recommended as one important prodromal feature of diabetes. Such dryness may be a direct reflection of reduced salivary secretions. Studies have revealed qualitative and quantitative differences of salivary secretions in diabetics compared with healthy controls. Diabetic patients are found to secrete significantly less saliva compared to healthy controls. It is also found that the diabetic patients have an increased salivary protein concentration and calcium compared to healthy controls. In contrast, the levels of magnesium, zinc, and potassium are significantly reduced in diabetic saliva compared to the controls. These results indicate that diabetes mellitus leads to marked dysfunction of the secretory capacity of the salivary glands [33]. Such information may also be utilized for developing a new diagnostic tool for detecting diabetes early in time and also for monitoring the progress of the disease or the effects of a therapy in a given case.

Sheeta priyatvam (increased liking of cold), *sweda* (excessive sweating), and *kar-paada daha* (burning the hands and feet) are three important features indicating the initiation of faulty thermoregulation in impending diabetes. Though this is an area of new investigation in science, this is interesting to postulate if sweat can also be considered as a body secretion able to predict blood glucose levels [34]. Studies have suggested its feasibility by suggesting that sweat glucose levels are having a strong correlation with blood glucose, and therefore if the sweat samples can be collected meticulously, they can easily predict blood glucose levels [35, 36].

Anga gandha (specific odor of the body) on the similar grounds can also be a fascinating area of research as a lead to investigate impending diabetes. Body odor is the outcome of bacterial degradation of compounds available on sweat. An excessive glucose in sweat may lead to changes in skin bacterial flora normally available on the skin of a healthy subject. Such bacteria may use glucose as metabolic substrate and may produce a specific odor as an outcome of the process. A changing bacterial flora on the skin therefore possibly is the earliest indication of subtle changes occurring inside the body in terms of tissue glucose levels [37].

Conclusion

Ayurveda presents a highly illustrated description of diabetes rich in almost every segment of its clinical understanding. Unfortunately, researches in Ayurveda on diabetes completely undermined the strength of Ayurvedic clinical understanding of diabetes and, instead, remained limited on exploring hypoglycemic effects of the drugs alone. We may see that a thorough exploration of Ayurvedic literature on diabetes may not only help identifying the disease early in its course but even can help preventing the precipitation of overt diabetes. There are amazing leads in Ayurveda as the telltale of the ongoing erratic glucose metabolism, and there are striking explanations available in the modern literature for many of such descriptions. Unfortunately in the stream of science and Ayurveda, such works are completely independent and ignorant of developments made by each other. In such conditions, the real benefits of research and subsequently generated knowledge are either not reaching to the target population or are reaching so late that it becomes less meaningful. Translating the clues of Ayurveda for their possible exploration under the rigor of science thus seems something urgent to be done. For a disease like diabetes which is gripping the whole world under a common death warrant (diabetes is shifted as third leading cause of death in the USA from its seventh rank earlier reported) [38] at an alarming pace and where still profound leads are almost thoroughly scattered waiting to be explored in the form of traditional wisdom as is evident in Ayurveda, this becomes even more urgent and direly needed.

References[2]

1. NCD Risk Factor Collaboration (NCD-RisC). Worldwide trends in diabetes since 1980: a pooled analysis of 751 population-based studies with 4.4 million participants. Lancet. 2016;387(10027):1513–30.
2. Jia W. Diabetes research in China: making progress. Lancet Diabetes Endocrinol. 2017; 5(1):9–10.

[2] 80 million Indians have pre-diabetes, available at http://www.theweek.in/health/cover/80-million-indians-have-pre-diabetes.html (Last accessed on 16.10.2017).

3. WHO Global report of Diabetes 2016.
4. Arunachalam S, Gunasekaran S. Diabetes research in India and China today: from literature-based mapping to health-care policy. Curr Sci. 2002;82(9):1086–97.
5. Ratnakar A, Satyanarayan K. Diabetes research In India: a citation profile. Indian J Med Res. 2007;125:483–7.
6. Why m Diabetes. Http://Mdiabetes.Nhp.Gov.In/. Last downloaded on 20 Sep 2016.
7. Modak M, Dixit P, Londhe J, Ghaskadbi S, Paul T, Devasagayam A. Indian herbs and herbal drugs used for the treatment of diabetes. J Clin Biochem Nutr. 2007;40:163–73.
8. Ayurvedic interventions for diabetes mellitus: a systematic review. Summary, evidence report/ technology assessment: number 41. AHRQ Publication No. 01-E039, June 2001.
9. Ayush Research Portal.
10. http://www.ccras.nic.in/researchactivities/diabetes.htm. Last accessed on 20 Jan 2017.
11. Patwardhan B. Ayurvedic drugs in case: claims, evidence, regulations and ethics. J Ayurveda Integr Med. 2016;7(3):135–7.
12. Guidance for industry-diabetes mellitus: developing drugs and therapeutic biologics for treatment and prevention. http://www.fda.gov/downloads/Drugs/Guidances/ucm071624.pdf. Last accessed on 20 Jan 2017.
13. Islam T, Rahman A, Islam AU. Effects of aqueous extract of fresh leaves of *Abroma augusta* L. on oral absorption of glucose and metformin hydrochloride in experimental rats. ISRN Pharm. 2012;2012:472586. https://doi.org/10.5402/2012/472586.
14. Ayurvedline. Ayurvedic drug index. 11th ed. Bangalore: 2010. p. 471–78.
15. Rajput DS, Patgiri BJ, Galib R, Prajapati PK. Anti-diabetic formulations of *Nāga bhasma* (lead calx): a brief review. Ancient Sci Life. 2013;33(1):52–9.
16. Guntaru KS, Nagarajan P, Mcphedran P, Goodman TR, Hodsdon ME, Strout MP. Ayurvedic herbal medicine and lead poisoning. J Hematol Oncol. 2011;4:51.
17. Parivallal T, Anjana RM, Mohan V. Frequency of use of Indian systems of Medicine and homeopathy among diabetic patients in Chennai (CURES-80). J Social Health Diabetes. 2015;3(2):125.
18. Mac Lean CD, Littenberg B, Kennedy AG. Limitations of diabetes pharmacotherapy: results from the Vermont Diabetes Information System study. BMC Fam Pract. 2006;7:50.
19. Ritz E. Limitations and future treatment options in type 2 diabetes with renal impairment. Diabetes Care. 2011;34(Suppl 2):S330–4.
20. Sohal T, Sohal P, King Shier KM, Khan NA. Barriers and facilitators for type-2 diabetes management in South Asians: a systematic review. PLoS One. 2015;10(9):e0136202.
21. Banerjee S, Debnath P, Rao PN, Tripathy TB, Adhikari A, Debnath PK. Ayurveda in changing scenario of diabetes management for developing safe and effective treatment choices for the future. J Comp Integr Med. 2015;12(2):101–10.
22. Janket S, Manson JE, Sesso H, Buring JE, Liu S. A prospective study of sugar intake and risk of type 2 diabetes in women. Diabetes Care. 2003;26(4):1008–15.
23. Marsden J, Pickering D. Urine testing for diabetic analysis. Community Eye Health. 2015;28(92):77.
24. Chowta NK, Pant P, Chowta MN. Microalbuminuria in diabetes mellitus: association with age, sex, weight, and creatinine clearance. Indian J Nephrol. 2009;19(2):53–6.
25. Marunaka Y. Roles of interstitial fluid pH in diabetes mellitus: Glycolysis and mitochondrial function. World J Diabetes. 2015;6(1):125–35.
26. Hansen T. Type 2 diabetes mellitus—a multifactorial disease. Ann Univ Mariae Curie Sklodowska Med. 2002;57(1):544–9.
27. Faerch K, Hulmán A, Solomon TP. Heterogeneity of pre-diabetes and type 2 diabetes: implications for prediction, prevention and treatment responsiveness. Curr Diabetes Rev. 2016;12(1):30–41.
28. Tuomi T, Santoro N, Caprio S, Cai M, Weng J, Groop L. The many faces of diabetes: a disease with increasing heterogeneity. Lancet. 2014;383(9922):1084–94. doi: https://doi.org/10.1016/S01406736(13)62219-9. Epub 2013 Dec 3.

29. Jurysta C, Bulur N, Oguzhan B, et al. Salivary glucose concentration and excretion in normal and diabetic subjects. J Biomed Biotechnol. 2009; 2009, Article ID 430426, 6 pages. https://doi.org/10.1155/2009/430426
30. Kumar S, Padmashree S, Jayalekshmi R. Correlation of salivary glucose, blood glucose and oral candidal carriage in the saliva of type 2 diabetics: a case-control study. Contemp Clin Dentist. 2014;5(3):312–7. https://doi.org/10.4103/0976-237X.137925.
31. Møller N, Jørgensen JOL. Effects of growth hormone on glucose, lipid, and protein metabolism in human subjects. Endocr Rev. 2009;30(2):152–77. https://doi.org/10.1210/er.2008-0027.
32. Glycated nail protein suitability for diabetes testing. https://www.avantes.com/applications/application/item/1184-nir-in-diabetes-testing
33. Mata AD, Marques D, Rocha S, Francisco H, Santos C, Mesquita MF, Singh J. Effects of diabetes mellitus on salivary secretion and its composition in the human. Mol Cell Biochem. 2004;261(1–2):137–42.
34. Kenny GP, Sigal RJ, McGinn R. Body temperature regulation in diabetes. Temp Multidiscip Biomed J. 2016;3(1):119–45. https://doi.org/10.1080/23328940.2015.1131506.
35. Moyer J, Wilson DF, inkelshtein I, Wong B, Potts R. Correlation between sweat glucose and blood glucose in subjects with diabetes. Diabetes Technol Ther. 2012;14(5):398–402. doi: https://doi.org/10.1089/dia.2011.0262. Epub 2012 Feb 29.
36. Jadoon S, Karim S, Akram MR, et al. Recent developments in sweat analysis and its applications. Int J Anal Chem. 2015; 2015: Article ID 164974, 7 pages. https://doi.org/10.1155/2015/164974.
37. Grice EA, Segre JA. The skin microbiome. Nat Rev Microbiol. 2011;9(4):244–53. https://doi.org/10.1038/nrmicro2537.
38. Stokes A, Preston SH. Deaths attributable to diabetes in the United States: comparison of data sources and estimation approaches. PLoS One. 2017;12(1):e0170219. https://doi.org/10.1371/journal.pone.0170219.

Integrative Dermatology: Applying Knowledge of Ayurvedic Skin Care and Experience of the Past 20 Years at the Bedside

9

S. R. Narahari, M. G. Aggithaya, and T. J. Ryan

9.1 Introduction

Ryan, a doyen of Oxford dermatology, supports the use of oils for skin care; 'in dermatology, the first commandment is the use of emollients' [1]. The Lancet reported that premature infants massaged with sunflower seed oil were 41% less likely to develop nosocomial infections than untreated controls [2]. The practice of oil massage of neonates is routine throughout the Indian subcontinent. In Bangladesh oil massage was practised by over 96% of surveyed caretakers of new-borns, irrespective of socioeconomic status or place of residence [3]. In Ayurveda emollients are widely used to promote skin health and suppleness. There are a number of traditional Ayurveda practices that contribute to skin hygiene and the maintenance of skin health. Using skin care as the objective for general dermatologic management while looking for specific treatment for conditions such as vitiligo, wound healing, burns management, etc. offers an easier and more available testing ground for Ayurveda treatments. It is mostly low-cost technology, and studies have shown that it is easily adoptable at primary care [4]. Studies using objective outcomes are few, and methodological errors in trials using Ayurvedic medicines are among the major road blocks to achieve wider integration versus mainstream biomedicine [5]. The evaluation of integrative medicine (IM) approaches to the care of the skin requires a flexible and interdisciplinary approach to research, congruent with the principles of Ayurveda therapies, which added biomedical evidence for efficacy and safety [6]. One important tested strategy is the use of full treatment protocols, encompassing all the techniques offered for each individual. They include individual case series, surveys, and modulated questionnaires from both the system of medicine

S. R. Narahari (✉) · M. G. Aggithaya
Institute of Applied Dermatology, Kasaragod, Kerala, India

T. J. Ryan
Emeritus Professor Green Templeton College, Department of Dermatology, Churchill Hospital, Oxford, UK

S. Rastogi (ed.), *Translational Ayurveda*, https://doi.org/10.1007/978-981-13-2062-0_9

well-monitored for over a decade. Interventional trials have described methodology when integrating complementary and alternative medicine with dermatology [7]. This led to a published description of concepts in different therapeutic options in integrative dermatology [8]. Ryan advocates that skin care should be viewed as a pyramid of different levels of delivery for governance with management, teaching and research, financing, and patient empowerment. Skin care of populations with patient empowerment using self-help techniques is at the base of the pyramid. The experts are nearer the top and few in number. Ryan emphasizes that such expertise sited in the upper level has to always inform management and governance at the very top of the pyramid about all that is being advocated for lower levels. Thus, the effective educator knows that there is teaching to be done not only of the patient population but also of those determining funding and governance. This pyramid emphasizes that skin care for commonly occurring diseases should be easily accessible and mostly low-cost technology, easily adaptable as a public health intervention linked with improvements in health-related quality of life adopted for patient management.

During the last decade, usually only studies that used randomized controlled trials were afforded scientific credibility [9]. There is now growing recognition of the value of other forms of study designs, for the successful execution of biomedical and public health research [10] and health-care evidence is exploring observational health data sciences and informatics [11], and consequently treatment methods and data analytics based on all forms of interventional trials will be useful to health-care providers for the treatment of chronic patients. Especially skin care in Ayurveda occupies several levels of 'Ryan's skin care pyramid' [12]. This means, especially in countries where traditional Ayurveda is part of government's health-care delivery system, its medicines can be used in medical practice even though levels of evidence are low using current standards of evaluation.

9.2 Ayurvedic Dermatology

Ayurveda classifies skin diseases under 18 different '*kusta rogas*' [13], and many other skin diseases are described in other chapters on *astanga hridaya* such as *kshudra roga* diseases [14]. Relating them to over 1500 or more biomedically named skin diseases becomes an extremely daunting task. There are no specific treatments described for each of the 18 *kusta*, and they are decided on vitiation of three energy principles (*dosha vaishamya*), which essentially identify patterns in pathology (*vikruthi* especially *sthaneeya vikruthi*) and clinical presentations. This gives liberty to the therapists to select from many available treatment options that are not necessarily described only for *kusta*. *Dosha vaishamya* therefore should be a foundation for comparison with biomedical diagnosis. It has to be stated that defining all skin diseases known to allopathy using Ayurvedic terminology may not be achievable at the present time. It is early days both for clinical evidence and expertise. Recognizing constellations of clinical presentations and a kind of 'syndromic approach' to treatment might make it easier for theoretical translation from one system to another.

Especially important will be to explore a large number of therapeutic options that are available in Ayurvedic dermatology using skin care as the objective for general dermatologic management. Skin care is provided with the focus on the quality of treatments given within the context of the system, including diagnosis, personalization of the treatment, and use of either one or several treatment modalities in accordance with the individual needs of the patient. This evaluates whether a specific treatment platform (e.g. a programme of multiple Ayurvedic, skin therapies) is effective, with acceptance that it may be changed from day to day rather than a specific product, technique, or herb given for a set number of days or weeks. This can be easily achieved when biomedical dermatologists, Ayurveda physicians, and nurses examine patients together. The team should also comprise experts in related disciplines of care.

9.3 Clinical Methods in Ayurvedic Dermatology

There are 16 essential clinical features that should be elicited in patients prior to drug selection for skin diseases. They are the energy principles (*dosha*), patient's biological constitution (*prakruthi*); the status of 'body tissues' and 'process behind excretions' and inferred through energy principle (*dooshya*); the 'habitat' (*desha*); life stage of a patient (*vayas*); body 'measurement' (*pramana*); factors indicating firmness or dominance (*sara*); acquired body 'build' or physique (*samhanana*); seasonal nature and duration of disease (*kala*); exercise tolerance (*vyayamashakti*); digestion process and bowel patterns (*agni* and *kosta*); patterns of human behaviour (*satwa*); assessment of a patient's dietary habits, aspects may be described as 'compatible' or 'incompatible' (*sathmyam*); immunity of the patient to infections (*bala*), disease stage (*rogaavastha*); and clinical pharmacology (*bhaishajya*). The dominance of energy principles calculated through a *sthaneeya vikruthi* table (SVT) decides the indication for a drug. Fifteen other parameters help to determine contraindications for the selected drug, including assessment for likely side effects which should be anticipated by the clinician, disease aggravation, dosage, how much and for how long, and the determination of other constituents of any herbo-mineral treatment cocktail.

9.3.1 Energy Principles *(Dosha)*

There are three types of energy principles, motion (wind (*vata*)), metabolism (*pitta*), and structure (*kapha*). Out of these three energy principles, *pitta* is responsible for the colour and warmth of the skin and especially *bhrajaka pitta*, which is one among the five subtypes of *pitta* [15]. The *bhrajaka pitta* resides in the skin, gives colour to it, and together with the degree of moisturization or dryness (in combination with *vata*) is responsible for the skin radiance. The discolouration results from diminution (*kshaya*) [16] of *bhrajaka pitta*, which may be due to expulsion from its own seat by other vitiated energy principles (known as *ashaya apakarsha*) [17], although *bhrajaka pitta* is in normal state or covering (*avarana*) [18] by other energy principle. If vitiligo patients with *pitta*-dominant biological constitution consume *dhathryadi kashayam*, an herbalized solution, prepared by using *Acacia catechu* (*khadira*), *Emblica officinale* (*amalaki*), and *Psoralea corylifolia* (*bakuchi*) [19], they generally develop bullae or erythema when exposed to sunrays. The *pitta* biological constitution persons have dominant *bhrajaka pitta*, which is represented by warmth of the skin and appearance of moles/freckles (*thilakalaka*) in the body. The depigmentation in vitiligo is due to the *kapha* vitiation, which exhibits its symptoms at the seat of pitta. In this case, if vitiligo is treated with drugs having penetrating potency (*theeksha veerya*), *pitta* vitiation occurs, resulting in bullae and erythema or may worsen the vitiligo.

Health is the state of equilibrium of three energy principles, and disease is the condition of its derangement due to various causes (*nidana*). The impairment of one or more of energy principles may occur due to etiological factors such as poor diet, harmful environment, or psychological factors, thus producing disease. The diseased state is described in Ayurvedic terminology as *vikruthi* or *doshavaishamya* or *roga* [7]. *Vata*-dominant pathology in skin lesions may appear black (*krishna*) and/or exhibit a dusky or dusky red colour (*aruna*), violaceous (*shyava*). Its surface may be xerotic (*ruksha*, *parusha*) and rough/uneven (*khara*). Pitta skin lesions are generally associated with pain and redness (*rakta varna*) or often a yellowish colour (*peethavarna*), burning sensation (*daha*), erythematous (*raga*), and discharging/exuding lesions (*srava*). *Kapha* leads to excessive oily appearance of the skin (*athisnigdha*), white colour (*shwetha*), unctuous (*pichila*), firm like the tip of the nose (*ghana*), pruritus (*kandu*), and cold to touch (*sheetha*). Patients may feel heaviness (*guru*) of the affected part of the body [20]. The skin lesions showing pathology with a combination of two energy principles are difficult to cure and pathology involving all three energy principles at the same time is incurable according to Ayurvedic literature. The skin diseases categorized under 18 *kusta rogas*, which may be due to involvement of single, two, or all three energy principles, can be treated based on energy principle dominance symptoms. The lymphoedema (known as *sleepada*) is a *kapha*-dominant disease, but it should be managed depending on local energy principle dominance. *Nalpamaradi thailam*, a sesame oil preparation including *Ficus arnottiana* stem bark (*plaksa*), *F. benghalensis* stem bark (*nyagrodha*), *F. religiosa* stem bark (*aswatha*), and *F. glomerata* stem bark (*udumbara*) as major ingredients, is used for Indian manual lymph drainage (known as *udwarthana*) in *kapha*-dominant *sthaneeya vikruthi* and *Pinda thailam*, made from the *Madhuca indica* flower (*madhuka*), beeswax (*madhuchchista*), *Shorea robusta* gum resin (*sarja rasa*), and *Hemidesmus indicus* root (*sariva*), in *Pitta*-dominant condition [21]. The *kapha vata* lesions of hypertrophied lichen planus (Fig. 9.1) are not described by any specific name in Ayurveda, but it is possible to treat this disease using *vikruthi* analysis of energy principles. *Mahamanjisthadi kashayam*, *kaishore guggulu* and *mahamarichyadi taila* [22] are used because they involve *pathology* of only two energy principles.

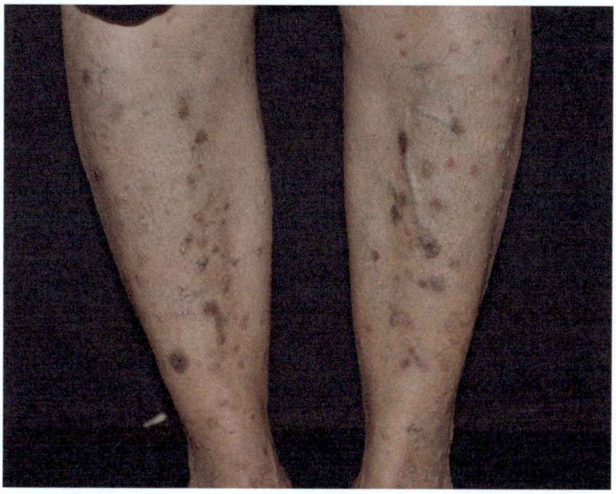

Fig. 9.1 Lichen planus lesions with xerosis on inspection (*ruksha*), xerosis on palpation (*parusha*), uneven surface (*khara*), violaceous (*shyava*) features of *vata* dominance and elevated (*utsedha*), and firm (*ghana*) features of *kapha* dominance. There are erythematous papules (*pidaka*) of *pitta* dominance. Both the lesions associated with severe pruritis, which is also a *kapha* dominance feature. The violaceous, raised with thick plaques, non-oozy lesions are hypertrophic lichen planus. Often such lesions appear initially as erythematous papules and are called lichen rubor planus. Ayurveda describes that both kinds of lesions are due to vitiation of two *dosha* (*dwidosha*)

There are two pathology states of energy principles, augmentation (*vrudhi*) and diminution, assessed through history-taking, inspection, and examination. Augmented *vata* causes hyperpigmentation of the skin along with other generalized symptoms such as emaciation, sleep disturbance, reduced strength, sensory disturbance, abdominal distension secondary to constipation, giddiness, tremor, and incoherent speech. However, in the absence of systemic symptoms, only hyperpigmentations of the skin with xerosis are local manifestations of *vatavikruthi* as in lichen planus pigmentosus. This can be treated with local application of *vata-hara* (*hara* means eliminate) oils such as *bala ashwagandha tailam*. Similarly, augmented *pitta* manifests on the skin and as yellowish discolouration of urine, dusky sclera, along with systemic symptoms of excessive thirst, insomnia, and burning sensation. The augmented *kapha* leads with pale and cold skin with or without breathlessness, cough and excessive sleep. Patients also complain of body 'heaviness' and of feeling 'lazy'. There is no discoloration of the skin during diminution of *vata* and *kapha* energy principles [20]; *pitta* diminution leads to 'lustrelessness' (*prabha hani*). Ayurveda doesn't recommend treatment for diminution of energy principles. The diseases can occur due to the pathology of energy principles singly or and of their 63 combinations. The hypertrophied lichen planus lesions are due to *kapha vata* dominance, whereas violaceous lesions of lichen planus pigmentosus are due to *vata* energy principle vitiation.

9.3.2 Disease Progression *(Shatkriyakala)*

Progression of the disease occurs over the time in six stages (known as *shatkriyakala*) and depends on such different pathologies as accumulates in the energy principles. They are (1) moderate accumulation of pathology in the seat of any energy principle (*sanchaya*), (2) that leading to aggravation of an energy principle in its site of origin (*prakopa*), (3) which displaces the affected energy principle and pushes it to circulate throughout the body (*prasara*), (4) and the circulating energy principle gets localized in another pathological site (*sthana samsraya*). Later it produces (5) manifestation of signs and symptoms (*vyakta*) and, finally if still not treated, leads to (6) the stage of complications (*bheda*). During the circulation of pathological and displaced energy principles, there begins a complex interaction with basic body tissues (*dhathu*) and metabolic products (*mala*) showing premonitory symptoms of the disease (known as *dosha-dooshya sammoorchana*). They include xerosis of the skin, sudden goose bumps without any cause, pruritus, increased perspiration or absence of perspiration, and numbness over the body parts. Generally, patients approach doctors when disease reaches stage 5 or 6.

9.3.3 Biological Constitution (*Prakruthi)*

Prakruthi is the biological constitution of a person, which is determined at the time of conception. It is dependent on season of fertilization, mother's food habits, and habitat during pregnancy. The biological constitution of a person is determined by assessing clinical, mental, behavioural, and nutritional/routine diet parameters. Biological constitution is identified by dominance of single energy principle, which is uncommon, two energy principles having equal dominance, or all three energy principles equal and balanced (*thridoshaja*) which are the usual presentations. Persons with *pitta* as a dominant biological constitution have a fair (*gaura*) or coppery colour (*tamra*). In *kapha*-dominant biological constitution, the skin may show a golden colour (*suvarna*), or a colour of dried *Cynodon dactylon* grass (*durva*). The skin of *vata*-dominant biological constitution persons appears dry and with fissures (*sputitha angaavayava*). In *pitta*-dominant biological constitution persons, the skin exhibits multiple freckles, pigmented spots over the body which resembles sesame seeds (*prabhuta vyanga* similar to junctional nevi), and filiform eruptions (*pidaka* similar to dermatosis papulose nigra lesions), whereas in *kapha*-dominant biological constitution persons, the skin will be shiny on inspection (*snigdhavarna*), soft (*komala*), and smooth (*snigda*) to the touch. *Prakruthi* is used for deciding on contraindications to certain drugs and in prognostic assessment. If a patient's vitiated energy principle and dominant biological constitution are the same, then the disease is considered to be difficult to manage. For example, hypertrophic lichen planus is a *kapha vata*-dominant disease; and a patient of *kapha vata*-dominant biological constitution may not respond to treatments. *Kapha*-dominant biological constitution patients are less prone to skin diseases. We observed that skin diseases are manifested more commonly (63%) in *pitta* biological constitution patients (either *kapha* or *vata* associated).

9.3.4 Local Disease Pathology (*Sthaneeya Vikruthi*)

Sthaneeya (local) *vikruthi* (pathology) is the most important step to elicit the disease and energy principle dominance before prescribing medicines for skin diseases. Local skin pathology is the tissue responses to the pathological processes. Bedsides charting of a table, comprising of Ayurvedic clinical descriptions of *vata*, *pitta*, and *kapha*, energy principle dominance along with its comparable biomedical descriptions gives essential clinical evidence for the multisystem medical (MSM) team to decide on the treatment. In integrative dermatology SVT and other 15 clinical parameters such as the stage of the disease (*roga avastha*), *nidana panchaka*, behavioural patterns, and strength and body measurements identify the suitable medications for a given patient [20]. This assessment is also a process to decide on contraindications for Ayurvedic herbal formulations. In *pitta*-dominant vitiligo lesions, applying *bakuchyadi lepam* is contraindicated because of *pitta* vitiation due to *Psoralea corylifolia*, which results in bullae, burning sensation, and erythema. Currently SVTs for lymphoedema [15], vitiligo [15], lichen planus [22] and hemiplegia [23] have been developed. The process of developing a SVT for any disease is explained in *Narahari* et al. [15]. During bedside examination of patients, several observations of Ayurveda may need to be reclassified or reassigned to different named diseases of biomedicine. The coppery red colour (*tamra varna*), thin (*thanu*), absence of hair in lesional skin (*romavidhwamsa*) in *pitta*-dominant *shwitra* is not vitiligo but should treated as leprosy [24] (Fig. 9.2) while determining nerve thickening and loss of sensation. Once the local pathology is identified, drug selection becomes easier. The management of local features is supported using oral medications directed against other systemic features. Such features are often ignored during biomedical treatment or referred to other specialist doctors.

9.3.5 Digestion Process (*Agni*)

Assessment of digestion process is also done before prescribing for skin diseases. We have described this process in detail elsewhere [20]. The process of assimilation of the 'essences of digestion' (comparable to nutrients) is termed *dhathu agni* (*dhathu* = basic body tissue). There are seven *dhathu agni*, which nourishes the respective basic body tissue. The skin being the product of *rasa dhathu* (comparable to lymph/lymphatic system), a basic body tissue, first receives nourishment from the gut. According to Ayurveda the nourishment of other body tissues follows sequentially later, blood and vascular system (*raktha*), muscle tissue (*mamsa*), adipose tissue (*meda*), bone (*asthi*), bone marrow (*majja*), and semen (*shukra*). If there is no proper digestion, the undigested food turns in to a 'fermented state' (known as *ama* [25]). *Ama* contains harmful substances arising from improper digestion. After its absorption into the body, *ama* gets localized to any pathological sites, leading to the disease (read *shat-kriya kala* above). The extent of the damage caused by *ama* can be determined by assessing the function of basic body tissues because it blocks *dhathu agni* channels, in a sequence. Many lymphoedema patients at IAD, who have the affection of lymph/lymphatic system, also suffered from anaemia indicated

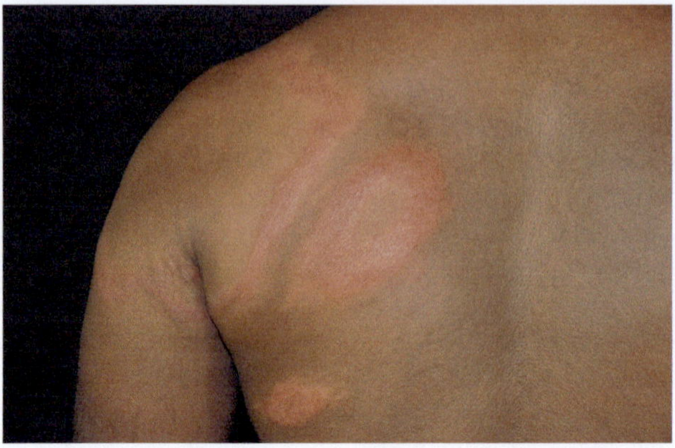

Fig. 9.2 In this picture the lesion has raised borders giving punched out appearance, classical description of borderline multibacillary leprosy. A close observation shows loss of hair compared to the normal skin of the back. Ayurveda literature don't describe such lesions. The *pittaja shwitra* (*aruna shwitra*) is described as coppery red colour (*tamra varna*), absence of hair in lesional skin (*roma vidhwamsa*), and areas of atrophy or thinning (*thanu*). In biomedicine lesions bearing coppery red colour are diagnosed as leprosy. This is caused by mycobacterium and should be treated with standard regimens recommended by national health programmes. In integrated medicine approach to treatment, Ayurveda doctors should be educated to learn these differences and refer such patients to national health programme units. (Also read Chandler D. Integrated care and leprosy in India: a role for Indian systems of medicine and traditional health practice in the eradication of leprosy. Current Science; 2016: 351–355)

by low haemoglobin levels, comparable to *raktha kshaya*. Following the lymphatic block, the next body tissue to become involved is blood. This logic of Ayurveda is substantiated by finding of anaemia in chronic lymphoedema patients. Anaemia of chronic disease is discussed in biomedicine literature, albeit with much less knowledge on its aetiology and treatment. It accounts for low oxygenation and delayed healing.

The clinical recognition of *ama* and its management using drugs to restore bowel movements are discussed in detail [20]. If patient develops *ama* features during the course of the treatment, all medicines should be withdrawn till *ama* features are completely resolved. *Ama* features should be looked for and treated before initiating any treatment for any disease. The bowel patterns also should be corrected before prescribing Ayurvedic medicines. The normalcy in bowel movements are influenced by digestion process, patient's food intake, nature of work, and stress. The continuous intake of spicy food in *mrudu kosta* persons can precipitate *grahani*, a disease which is comparable to irritable bowel syndrome. The diseases are classified based on their site of origin, upper part (GI tract) known as *amashaya* (*ama* = undigested food, *ashaya* = place) and lower part (GI tract) known as *pakwashaya* (*pakwa* = digested food, *ashaya* = place). Developmentally both the skin and the gut are of ectodermal origin [26]. This biomedical knowledge aligns well with the

Ayurvedic treatment principle. Many of our patients either had a constipated bowel or bowel associated presentations that are largely ignored by dermatologists.

Children with *krimikosta* need additional treatment before treating their skin disease. *Vata*-dominant biological constitution patients generally have *krurakosta*. Such patients require mild purgatives on a daily basis (*nithya virechana*). In patients with *mrudu kosta* (if a patient has loose bowels after consuming mild laxatives such as milk), medicines with quickly penetrating (*theekshna)* quality such as *Psoralea corylifolia* (e.g. *dhathryadi kashayam*) are not prescribed. Patients with *pitta* biological constitution generally have *mrudukosta*. If patients have *mandagni* (i.e. digestion takes more than 3 h of food), the herbalized ghee (*ghritha)* is contraindicated. Adding liver tonic to regular vitiligo treatment is beneficial especially for poor responders. *Arogyavardhini vati* and *thiktaka ghritham* is used as an adjunct, both hepatoprotective agents and for vitiligo. Turmeric is gaining credibility in biomedical practice.

9.3.6 Habitat *(Desha)*

There are three habitats where patients live—desert (*janghala*), fertile (*anoopa*), and moderate (*sadharana*)—which are determined through the trees, animals grown in that region, and type of soil. The region with dry soil and with thick evergreen forests with *Acacia catechu* and *Terminalia tomentosa* is a desert habitat. Persons residing in a desert habitat generally exhibit *vata*-dominant biological constitution and are more likely to suffer from diseases of *vata*. The fertile land is generally below the sea level, surrounded by backwaters, ponds, are fertile habitat and patients dominantly have *kapha* biological constitution. They often present with problems related to *kapha*-dominant pathology such as breathlessness. *Sleepada* is endemic in fertile habitat. The habitat plays major role to differentiate *sleepada* from other lymphoedema. A patient's food habits will also depend on habitat, for example, spicy and dry foods are more common in dry regions. Biomedicine has emphasized that a green environment has healing properties [27].

Dooshya refers to the basic body tissues (*dhathu*) and excretions (*mala*: urine, faeces, and sweat). This also produces disease if affected by vitiated energy principle. There are seven basic body tissues. The energy principles may augment or diminish these. In long-standing skin diseases, energy principle may enter different *dhathu* levels in the same sequential pathway as *ama* described above manifesting clinical features suggesting poorer prognosis. This worsening of any skin disease is known as *dhathugathatwa*. It manifests by a set of symptoms indicating the type of the basic body tissue affected. When the energy principle enters into *rasa dhathu* or the skin (*twak*), manifestations include an area of anaesthesia (*sparsahani*), hyperhidrosis (*atisweda*), pruritis (*eshat kandu*), discoloration (*vaivarnya*), skin appears dry (*rukshabhava*), pricking pain (*thoda*), numbness (*twak swapa*), and goose bumps (horripilate, *romaharsha*). Anaesthesia has a wider implication in biomedicine. All causes of loss of sensations should be explored before one should consider only Ayurvedic treatments for this. In basic body

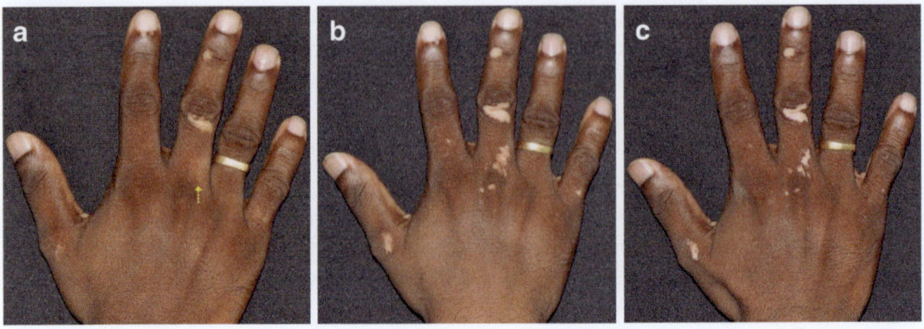

Fig. 9.3 The colour changes in vitiligo lesions representing the dominance of energy principles. The hypopigmented lesions in (**a**) became depigmented within 1 month. (**b**) Change of *vata*-dominant lesion to *kapha* dominance, as the vitiated energy principles enters from blood (*rakta*) to adipose tissue (*meda*) level. (**c**) shows the marginal repigmentation after 1 month of treatment with *dhathryadi kashayam*, a herbalized liquid containing *Emblica officinalis* fruit (*dhatri*), *Acacia catechu* stem (*khadira*), and *Psoralea corylifolia* seed (*avalguja*) used to treat *kapha* pathology

tissues (*dhathu*), diminution of lymph/lymphatic system (*rasa*), blood, and vascular system (*raktha*) reduces skin lustre and radiance [20]. The augmentation of adipose tissue (*meda*) also reduces skin lustre and radiance, due to excessive oiliness, as in diabetes mellitus (*prameha*) [28]. We have described the clinical manifestations of *dhathugathatwa* in [7].

In vitiligo, when the energy principle enters in to different *dhathu* level, the depigmented lesions gradually brighten (Fig. 9.3), without producing other systemic symptoms.

9.3.7 Life Stages (*Vayas*)

Three life stages are described in Ayurveda: childhood (*balya*), the middle age (*madhyama*), and old (*jeerna*). The medicines and dose selected on each life stage of a patient are different. For example, the medicines containing *Psoralea corylifolia* is not indicated for *balya* and *jeerna* patients.

The body 'measurement' (*pramana*), factors indicating firmness or dominance (*sara*), acquired body 'build' or physique (*samhanana*), exercise tolerance (*vyayamashakti*), and immunity of the patient to infections (*bala*) also influence the dosage and medicines given to patients and are less studied by biomedical practitioners.

9.3.8 Seasonal Nature and Duration of Disease (*Kala*)

Some diseases have seasonal variations. The *sheethapitta* (comparable to urticaria) and *mandala kusta* (guttate psoriasis) are aggravated in winter. The duration of the disease is important to determine the prognosis. Similarly human behaviour (*satwa*) also influences treatment concordance and their interaction with environment such as food and allergens.

9.3.9 Disease Stage (*Rogaavastha*)

Different stages of the same disease are treated with different medicines in Ayurveda. The chronic skin diseases and/or diseases with exhibiting all clinical features have poor prognosis. History-taking identifies and helps to determine aetiology, prodromal symptoms, and pathogenesis of the disease. Often Ayurveda's 'trial and error' method of drug administration (*upashaya*) is required to determine the stage of the disease.

9.3.10 Dietary Ecosystem *(Sathmyam)*

The assessment of dietary habit is known as *sathmyam*. A set of dietary advice is listed in core Ayurvedic texts to be followed by every patient. Such a list includes black gram lentils, non-vegetarian items, radishes, and citrus fruits. Food is included in the list of aetiological factors. They include consumption of incompatible food (*virudha*), food which takes longer time to digest (*guru*), non-vegetarian, citrus fruits, spicy foods, sesame (*thila*), sesame oil (*thilathaila*), horse gram (*kulatha*), curd prepared of water buffalo (*mahisha dadhi*), brinjal (*vrinthaka*). The food is considered to be incompatible when it is against the digestion process, food habit or habitual food tolerances (*sathmya*), potency (*veerya*), state of health (*avastha*), diet indications of disease (*parihara*), combination of foods (*samyoga*), ripeness of ingredients (*sampath*), energy principles, quality (*rasa*), season when eating food (*kala*), proportion of ingredients of food (*mathra*), preparation of food (*samskara/karma*), bowel pattern, order (*krama*), cooking (*paka*), whether the patient is frequently consuming food to which he or she has aversions (*hruth*), and the location of the patient's home (habitat). For example, patients with *pitta*-dominant disease consuming spicy food are considered incompatible to their inherent energy principle (*dosha virudha*). Pungent taste (*katu rasa*) dominates spicy foods which vitiates *pitta*.

The personalized medicine concept in Ayurveda focuses on different combinations of medicines, its ingredients, dosage patterns, route of administration, fluid vehicle, etc. An example is that of a medicine by the name *kaishore guggulu*. If consumed along with *mahamanjisthadi kashayam*, it reduces skin ailments associated with *kapha vata* dominance, whereas if along with *varunadi kashayam*, it is helpful to treat diseases related to involvement of adipose tissues (*medohara* action of the drug). The *pitta*-dominant local skin pathology in lymphoedema, presenting with erythema, warmth of limb site, and burning sensation, reduces by using *pinda thailam* for IMLD [15]. Several drugs are used to manage the same pathology occurring in different situations. The combinations of all clinical features elicited using 16 steps described above determine which drugs should be selected in a clinical situation. This training is given to Ayurveda doctors during their 5 years of undergraduate medical education. We have explained a few situations in our earlier publications. Examples are the sesame oil preparations: *chandanadi thailam* reduces *pitta* dominance, *ksheerabala thailam* reduces *vata*, and *nalpamaradi thailam* reduces *kapha*. Drug selection is also made on the basis of pharmacological properties in situations of when pathogenesis of disease is not clear and provisional diagnosis couldn't be arrived at. Here exploratory therapy (*upashaya*) is trialled using a medicinal formulation which is most likely to result in the amelioration of illness. In such cases, the medicine and/or its dosage may change during the course of treatment, and a retrospective diagnosis is made consequent on the therapeutic trial if the response is positive. The provisional diagnosis is made in the absence of laboratory investigations. However, IM protocols use biomedical investigations to support Ayurvedic clinical decisions.

9.4 Establishing a Multisystem Medical Doctors' Team [15]

The first step of developing an integrated clinical management service would be establishing mutual orientation among multiple systems doctors of medicine. Exchanging the cross-medical system dialogues after examining a patient in detail to elicit the clinical presentation will be important for the MSM team. The MSM team is led by a dermatologist in IAD. Original descriptions in Ayurveda are written in Sanskrit. The English translations should use biomedical terms identified in the course of parallel examinations of patients conducted by Ayurvedic physicians and dermatologists. They need not reflect the exact meaning of the Ayurvedic or Sanskrit terminology. The interview protocol used in homoeopathic practice may be used to elicit the most detailed history, because homoeopathy prescribes on the basis of a 'totality of symptoms', knowledge of which is achieved only after lengthy questioning and listening to the patient's story. Counselling of patients is necessary to address their overall needs and to explain the new therapeutic approaches used in IM.

Briefly a structure for developing the integrative treatment protocol for a chronic disease should include the following. There is initially a detailed and time-consuming case history, followed by clinical examinations conducted separately by the members of the MSM team in order to allow team members to arrive at their own conclusions about the disease. The process of reaching these conclusions should follow the standard guidelines in the respective therapeutic disciplines (i.e. pathophysiology in allopathy/biomedicine, *samprapti* in Ayurveda). The terminologies used to describe the disease or treatment and the pathophysiological basis of each treatment are to be presented later using the descriptions native to the respective disciplines (e.g. the biological constitution in this patient is *kapha vataja*, pathology of the disease is *kapha pittaja*, etc.), to adopt biomedical diagnosis and indicators of improvement. A biomedical dermatologist may decide on diagnostic tests to be employed and if and when they are to be repeated to determine how the patient responded to integrative treatment. Diagnosis should be supported by the recording of essential baseline clinical characteristics in biomedicine and in Ayurveda as described above. However, in patients whose clinical presentation is insufficient to determine the disease, skin biopsy and other investigations necessary to confirm the final diagnosis may be carried out wherever indicated. Later, baseline photographs and the clinical notes for each patient examined are pooled to develop the *vikruthi* table. Review of response during follow-up is essential. At this stage, any decisions to change or modify treatments or dosages are made in response to the outcome measures of individual examinations. Thus, if the disease presented in *vata* form and the response to treatment of vitiligo were poor, the Ayurvedic doctor in the MSM team would decide if other *vata*-reducing (*hara*) drugs should be added, the dosage of medicine increased, the patient's dietary ecosystem (*sathmyam*) reassessed, the patient's digestive capacity re-determined, etc. We inform all patients that the integrative regimen doesn't promise cure.

A decade of work beginning from 2000 led to this structured clinical approach using Ayurvedic methods of examination in our IM protocol. This showed a way for routine selection of drugs from a large list of drugs available in many volumes of its standard books. We have now evolved methods for simultaneous use of drugs from

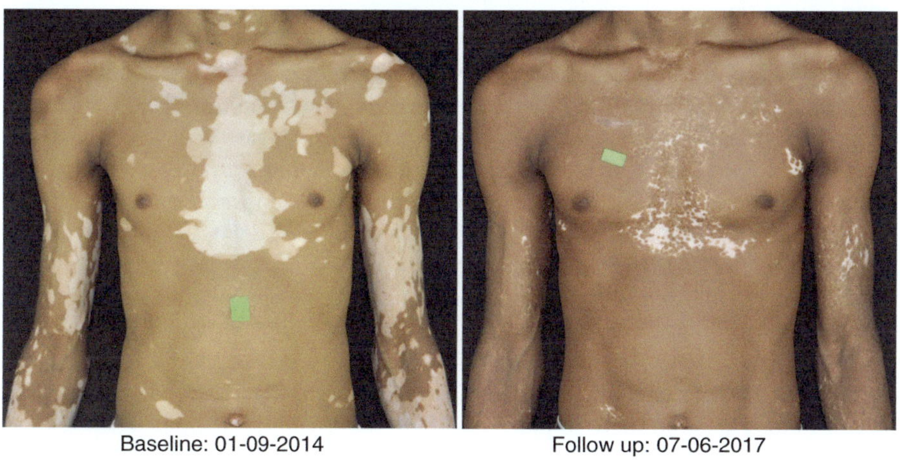

Fig. 9.4 The changes in vitiligo lesions after 3 years of treatment. Integrated medicine regimen included monthly pulses of controlled induced purgation. Several drugs are changed in the course of treatment, and they included *ayaskruthy* and *kakodumbarikadi kashayam*, a herbalized liquid preparation containing *Ficus hispida* stem bark (*kakodumbarika*) as main ingredient and hepatoprotectives such as *arogyavardhini vati* in schedules. Specific diet management to avoid incompatible food was part of the regimen. Analysis of different clinical presentations over the past 3 years and clustering similar responses are likely to define the specific use of large number of drugs available in Ayurveda to treat vitiligo. Also read Narahari et al. A protocol for systematic reviews of Ayurveda treatments. Int. J Ayurveda Research 2010; 1: 192–205

Ayurveda and biomedicine in chronic skin diseases in routine IM practice (Fig. 9.4). We now briefly describe below how management of lymphoedema has changed using IM and that led to patient acceptance of treatment regimens hitherto not treatable in India.

9.5 Patient Care Protocols of Lymphoedema

IM protocol for lymphoedema (known as *sleepada* in Ayurveda) is a complex and demanding self-help regimen that is a burden to the individual and the many who participate in giving their support to the patient at home.

Step 1: Counselling. Patient concordance with this complex IM protocol depends on skilled and time-consuming counselling which is probably in itself therapeutic. Every detail of the proposed therapy is discussed, and an understanding of lymphoedema and its management is tested. Close family members also attend the sessions. That therapy will be lifelong is emphasized.

Step 2: Washing and herbal soaks. Treatment by washing is effective for reducing entry lesions for bacteria. The swollen limb is soaked in an herbal mixture (*phanta* solution) for 20 min. The several herbals prescribed may have antiseptic or anti-inflammatory effects, but at present, they are prescribed according to the Ayurvedic system of diagnosis.

Step 4: Indian Manual Lymphatic Drainage (*IMLD*). Part 1 of IMLD (*unmardhana*) is a type of nonoil massage that requires the masseur to apply a squeezing pressure using both palms and fingers and moving from the tip of the toes to the upper edge of the lymphoedema. This is performed for 10 min with the patient in a supine position. It is a manoeuvre that might be initiating a shift of lymph to and from the initial lymphatics in the upper dermis. The upper dermal lymphatics respond to light touch and movement, while the thickened deep dermis responds to squeezing. Part 2 of MLD (*udwarthana*) is a massage using oil. In this procedure, oil is applied to the skin, and the limb is massaged in the opposite direction for hair growth. The oil is selected according to a local skin pathology table.

Steps 3 and 6: Yoga. There are several types of yoga. At the IAD, it is movement of the tissues synchronized with breathing that is taught. It replaces MLD and relies on self-help. This kind of yoga places the body in obviously advantageous seating or lying positions that enable reduced venous load and improved lymph flow: a straight back and a non-tilted pelvis, for example. Movements include whole body stretching, antigravity positioning, and ankle movements obviously ideal for reducing venous overload. Breathing is coordinated. Breathing coordination with movement is probably ideal for emptying the large veins of the upper chest into which the thoracic duct's lymph has to empty. To leave the large veins well filled and the dilated collecting lymphatics of the trunk equally overfilled when trying to enforce emptying of peripheral lymphatics is obviously without benefit. It is expiratory breathing that is emphasized, synchronized with body movements that shift the lymph. Such synchronized breathing is believed to empty core lymphatic trunks facilitating emptying of the peripheral impeded and overfilled lymphatics. Thus, during the distal to proximal movement in IMLD parts 1 and 2, the patient breathes out slowly or holds the breath after exhalation. The patient takes a sudden and deep inhalation during the pause between the end and beginning of IMLD strokes. IMLD is administered by a masseur who subsequently coaches the patient's home caregiver in the technique. This yoga is done twice each session. The first time, it is done without bandaging, and then later, the movements within support bandaging encourage muscle contraction to work against some resistance when contracting thereby squeezing the tissues, so that lymph exits.

In lymphoedema, especially from filariasis, the long collecting ducts are grossly dilated and overfilled, and they have lost their contractility. The contractility of the vessels is influenced by the autonomic nervous system, also influenced by yoga. Very often the patient is discomforted at first by the procedures. Pain excites the sympathetic nervous system, and the instructor will aim to induce procedures that cause discomfort more slowly, until they are tolerated. Mindfulness as another feature of yoga reduces anxiety. Another feature of lymphoedema is the poor health of the adipose tissue, which is often hypoxic and inflamed but overgrown in lymphoedema. Such loss of lymphatic function and unhealthy adipose tissue responds to expiratory breathing by vasoconstriction (whereas healthy adipose tissue responds by both vasodilation and vasoconstriction).

The patients are taught to breathe through one side of the nose only. With the vagus on the left of the chest, a parasympathetic response to changing intrathoracic pressure, when breathing through the left side of the nose, may be distinguished from right-sided sympathetic responses when breathing through the right side of the nose. A complete list of yoga asanas to be practised before and after IMLD is given in [15].

Step 5: Compression therapy. Biomedicine has a large range of bandages and hosiery. However, short-stretch bandages and well-fitted hosiery are too expensive for the resource-poor village patient unless donated/sponsored by the government. Short-stretch bandages are not available routinely in the Indian market (in

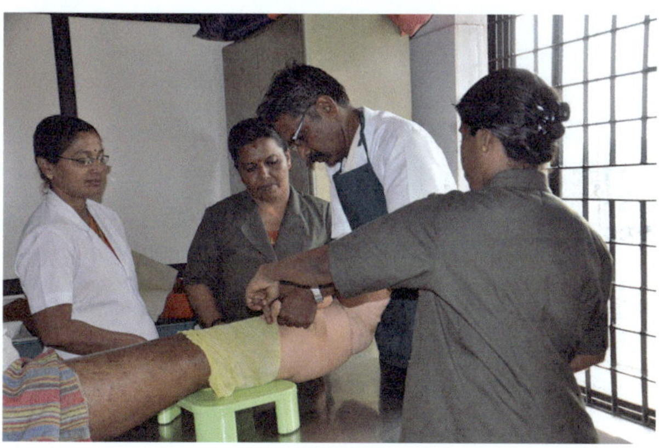

Fig. 9.5 The procedure of compression bandaging to lymphoedematous limb. Here long-stretch compression bandages is applied in a figure of eight manner. Dekinking is to be done using sponge moulds. The compression therapy has many complex systems and should be administered by skilled nurses and therapists

2018 they started appearing the market). Some patients may need at least 20 bandages per week and ample foam rubber materials that help reshape the limb. The life of a bandage becomes short after it has experienced, repeated washing, the heat of the tropics and oils adding to the cost of treatment. Bandaging techniques and monitoring compression therapy is explained in detail by Moffatt [29] (Fig. 9.5).

Step 7: Medicated steam heating of affected limb (Ekanga swedana) is a well-established treatment in Ayurveda. It has both mechanical and biochemical effects. The melting point of fat and the effectiveness of lipases require that fat is not solidified by cooling. Enzymes such as collagenase which remove collagen have an optimal temperature of 37 °C rarely reached in the lymphoedematous periphery. The decreased tissue viscosity and the emptying of fluid from the tissues into the lymphatic system are not so rapidly managed by any other intervention. This treatment is not done in all patients. Those with hardened limbs showing non-pitting oedema ('organized/tight limbs') are given this treatment over the affected limb under medical supervision for the second half of 7 days during supervised treatment regimen for lymphoedema. Herbalized steam made with the roots of ten herbs is passed through a pipe and sprayed directly over the affected area after IMLD-2. An additional layer of oil used for massage in IMLD-2 is applied over the area before steaming. The steam is sprayed until the treated limb shows uniform beads of

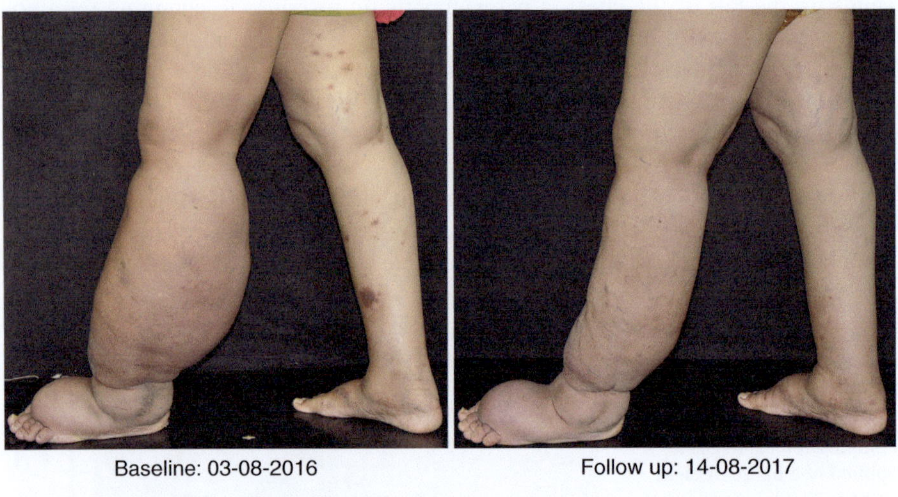

Fig. 9.6 The changes in lymphoedema after 1 year of integrated treatment. Patient also had chronic plaque psoriasis lesions on the left leg at baseline. Psoriatic lesions had *pitta vata* dominance and are reduced during follow-up. The patient consumed *mahamanjisthadi kashayam* and *kanchanar guggulu* as oral medications and *nalpamaradi thailam* for Indian manual lymph drainage

moisture. The process is continued until the patient cannot tolerate the heat any longer. This takes an average of 15–20 min. Pain and temperature sensations are tested before administering this treatment [30].

The outcome of such IM protocol is shown in Fig. 9.6.

This model for integrative dermatology at IAD is now established and recognized by dermatology groups around the world [31]. This evolved over two decades of work built by a small team in an incremental way. Several flagship programmes of IAD in IM are now published. Clinician-led multisystem medical teams with strong mentoring from academic clinicians using the current standards of evidence will offer new patient care IM protocols for many neglected and orphan diseases.

Annexe 1: Biomedical Dermatology's Tips for Recognizing Acute Skin Conditions That Require Urgent Care by Dermatologists

Most skin disease can be recognized clinically; some reflect on internal disease. Experience in clinical dermatology is especially important to spot skin diseases. Histopathology is used when diagnosis is not certain. When the following skin conditions are encountered, refer such patients for acute dermatology care (Table 9.1).

Mucocutaneous Signs of Internal Malignancy

The common presentation is a nodule as indurated plaque of melanoma or adenocarcinomas. Paraneoplastic syndromes present as vasculitis, dermatomyositis, and acanthosis nigricans. They may be associated with tuberous sclerosis or Peutz-Jeghers syndrome. Cutaneous metastasis is characterized by one to multiple nodules. They are firm, indurated, inflammatory, or ulcerated. They are typical patterns of cutaneous involvement by internal malignancy. Examples are well-defined macules or plaques of erythema with actively spreading border (breast and ovarian carcinomas), telangiectatic metastatic carcinoma, sclerodermoid plaques around the chest, and dilated capillaries in erysipelas like plaques or macules. Paget's disease is sharply demarcated in erythema and scaling occurring on the nipple or areola. Large intestine cancers generally manifest over abdomen, perineal area, and head and neck. A pyogenic granuloma over the head and neck could be due to hypernephroma. Sister Mary Joseph nodules, migratory necrolytic erythema tripe palms, Leser-Trelat syndrome, and acquired ichthyosis are other classical examples. Salient features of epidermal precancers and malignancies are briefly listed below:

Table 9.1 Fitzpatrick's 'serious skin signs in sick patients (4 S) table'

Serious skin signs in sick patients	Common examples[a]
Generalized red rash with fever	Viral exanthema Drug eruptions Bacterial toxins
Generalized red rash with blisters and prominent mouth lesions	Erythema multiforme (major) Pemphigus Bullous pemphigoid Drug eruptions
Generalized red rash with pustules	Pustular psoriasis Infected varicella Drug eruptions
Generalized rash with vesicles	Varicella Disseminated herpes zoster Drug eruptions
Generalized red rash with scaling	Exfoliative dermatitis Rule out internal malignancy
Generalized purpura	Drug eruptions Thrombocytopenia Dengue and other causes of disseminated intravascular coagulation Septicaemia
Generalized wheals and soft tissue swelling	Urticaria Angioedema, Vasculitis
Generalized palpable purpura	Vasculitis Bacterial endocarditis
Multiple skin infarcts	Meningococcemia Gonococcemia Disseminated intravascular coagulopathy Toxic epidermal Necrolysis (when generalized)
Localized skin infarcts	Drug eruption (Warfarin necrosis) Atherosclerosis obliterans Connective tissue disorders
Facial inflammatory oedema with fever	Cellulites/erysipelas Herpes zoster Lupus erythematosus
Fever with generalized macular and papules, may be pruritic	Drugs Viral exanthema Systematic lupus erythematosus

[a]See [32] for illustrative examples of this table

- Cutaneous epithelial cancers are known as non-melanoma skin cancers. They originate from keratinocytes or adnexal structures. They are common in fairer skin of white populations.
- Pigmented skin has lesser UV damage and melanomas are rare. Hyperkeratotic papules or plaque are called keratosis and could have dysplastic cells.

- All cutaneous horns should be biopsied by excision. The base of these horns may show benign lesions or invasive squamous cell carcinoma.
- Arsenical keratosis of palms, solar keratosis, pigmented keratosis (spreading), Bowenoid actinic keratosis, and human papillomavirus-induced intraepithelial lesions are precancerous and should be regularly followed up.

References

1. Ryan TJ. The first commandment: oil it! An appreciation of the science underlying water and emollients for skin care. Community Dermatol. 2004;1:3–5.
2. Darmstadt GL, Saha SK, Ahmed AS, et al. Effect of topical treatment with skin barrier-enhancing emollients on nosocomial infections in preterm infants in Bangladesh: a randomised controlled trial. Lancet. 2005;365:1039–45.
3. Darmstadt GL, Saha SK. Traditional practice of oil massage of neonates in Bangladesh. J Health Popul Nutr. 2002;20:184–8.
4. Narahari SR, Bose KS, Aggithaya MG, Swamy GK, Ryan TJ, et al. Community level morbidity control of lymphoedema using self care and integrative treatment in two Lymphatic Filariasis endemic districts of South India a non randomized interventional study. Trans R Soc Trop Med Hyg. 2013;107:566. https://doi.org/10.1093/trstmh/trt054.
5. Narahari SR, Aggithaya MG, Thamban C, Muralidharan K, Kanjarpane AB. How knowledgeable are investigators studying therapies of traditional medicines? Ayu. 2014;35:243–51.
6. Burford G, Bodeker G, Ryan TJ. Skin and wound care: traditional, complementary and alternative medicine in public health dermatology. In: Bodekar G, Burford G, editors. Traditional, complementary and alternative medicine: policy and public health perspectives. London: Imperial College Press; 2007. p. 311–47.
7. Narahari SR, Ryan TJ, Aggithaya GM, Bose KS, Prasanna KS. Evidence based approaches for Ayurvedic traditional herbal formulations: toward an Ayurvedic CONSORT model. J Alter Compl Med. 2008;14:769–76.
8. Norman RA, Shenefelt PD, Rupani RN, editors. Integrative dermatology. Oxford: Oxford University Press; 2014.
9. Savage J. Ethnographic evidence: the value of applied ethnography in healthcare. J Res Nurs. 2006;11:383. https://doi.org/10.1177/1744987106068297.
10. Thiese MS. Observational and interventional study design types; an overview. Biochem Med. 2014;24(2):199–210.
11. Observational Health Data Sciences and Informatics. www.ohdsi.org. Accessed 3 Apr 2018.
12. Ryan TJ. The wow factor as a determinant of funding for disorders of the skin. Military Med Res. 2015;2:14.
13. Vagbhata. Astanga Hrudaya. Kustashwitra krimi nidana Adhyaya. Varanasi: Krishnadas Academy, 2000; verses 7–9.
14. Vagbhata. Astanga Hrudaya. Kshudraroga vijnaneeya Adhyaya. Varanasi: Krishnadas Academy; 2000.
15. Narahari SR, Ryan TJ, Bose KS, Prasanna KS, Aggithaya GM. Integrating modern dermatology and Ayurveda in the treatment of vitiligo and lymphedema in India. Int J Dermatol. 2011;50:310–34.
16. Vagbhata. Astangahrudaya. Doshadi vijnaneeya adhyaya. Varanasi: Chowkhamba Krishnadas Academy; 2000: verse 16.
17. Madhava. Pandurogadi nidanam. Madhava Nidana. Varanasi: Chowkhamba Orientalia; 2001; verse 17.
18. Caraka. Jwara nidana. In: Caraka D, editor. Caraka Samhita. Varanasi: Chowkhamba Sanskrit Series Office; 2002; verse 59.

19. Narahari SR, Aggithaya MG, Prasanna KS, Bose KS. Evidence toward integrated management of vitiligo, combining Ayurveda and homeopathy with modern dermatology. In: Gupta S, Parsad D, Olsson MJ, Lim HM, Pandya A, Geel N, editors. Vitiligo: medical and surgical management. Hoboken, NJ: Wiley; 2018. p. 159–70.
20. Narahari SR, Aggithaya MG, Morrow SE, Ryan TJ. Developing an integrative medicine patient care protocol from the existing practice of Ayurveda dermatology. Curr Sci. 2016;111:302–17.
21. Narahari SR, Aggithaya MG, Prasanna KS, Bose KS. An integrative treatment for lower limb Lymphoedema (elephantiasis) (photoessay). J Alter Compl Med. 2010;16:145–9.
22. Narahari SR, Prasanna KS, Sushma KV. Evidence based integrative dermatology. Indian J Dermatol. 2013;58:127–31.
23. Aggithaya MG, Narahari SR, Vijaya S, Sushma KV, Anil Kumar NP, Prajeesh P. Navarakizhi and Pinda Sweda as muscle-nourishing Ayurveda procedures in hemiplegia: double-blind randomized comparative pilot clinical trial. J Alter Compl Med. 2014;20:57–64.
24. Kar HK, Kumar B, editors. IAL textbook of leprosy. New Delhi: Jaypee Brothers Medical Publishers; 2016.
25. Vagbhata. Doshopakramaneeya Adhyaya. In: Astanga Hrudaya [in Sanskrit]. Varanasi: Krishnadas Academy; 2000, verse 27.
26. Moore KL, Persaud TVN, Torchia MG. The developing human: clinically oriented embryology. 9th ed. Philadelphia: Saunders; 2011.
27. Ryan TJ, Matts PJ, Snyder B, Orr V. A seminar on gardens for health of the skin. Int J Dermatol. 2014;53:593–600.
28. Vagbhata. Astanga Hrudaya. Prameha nidanam. Varanasi: Krishnadas Academy; 2000; verses 9–10, 2.
29. Moffatt C. Compression therapy in practice. Wounds: Trowbridge; 2007.
30. Ryan TJ, Narahari SR. Reporting an alliance using an integrative approach to the management of Lymphedema in India. Int J Lower Extremity Wounds. 2012;11:5–9.
31. Narahari SR, Prasanna KS. Nurture Indian dermatology innovations as man-maximum, machine-minimum research. Indian J Dermatol Venereol Leprol. 2017;83:684–6.
32. Wof K, Johnson RA. Fitz Patrick's color atlas & synopsis of clinical dermatology. 6th ed. New York: The Mc-Graw-Hill Medical; 2009.

Sleep Medicine: What Can Ayurveda Contribute to the Contemporary Health Care?

10

Sanjeev Rastogi and Rajiv Rastogi

10.1 Introduction

Sleep is essential, albeit a much less understood component of life. Current high competitive environment often forms a prelude of considering it unwanted and compromisable in order to accomplish the desired worldly tasks. Many consider sleep as a waste of time and hence feel that the time consumed in sleep should better be utilized to increase productivity. This ideology reflects the workaholic aptitude considering sleep as an evil [1]. Considering a marginal population belonging to physiological "short sleeper" or "long sleeper" classes, we still have a sizable population requiring good amount of sleep to live normally [2].

Sleep is aptly called as a "blessing in disguise," and its importance is felt only when we actually lose it. A normal person on average consumes one third of his life in sleeping. Sleep is one most obvious indicator of health-related quality of life. Sleeping better is found to be associated with better perception and productivity the next day in health and disease alike. It has rejuvenative, reparative, and curative effect on the body being offered through various mechanisms. Considering its high importance, Ayurveda keeps it under the trinity (*trayopastambha*) essential for life, keeping it at par with the other two, namely, *ahara* (food) and *brahmacharya*[1] (good conduct) (Fig. 10.1).

[1] *Brahmacharya* is often wrongly referred as celibacy. By observing *brahmacharya* Ayurveda actually proposes to have a conduct similar to that is proposed in *brahma satva* type of mental trait. This is considered highest among all kind of mental traits described and is characterized by qualities like cleanliness, adherence to truth, self-control, able to do right work at right time, having

S. Rastogi (✉)
Department of Kaya Chikitsa, State Ayurvedic College and Hospital, Lucknow University, Lucknow, India

R. Rastogi
Central Council for Research in Yoga and Naturopathy, New Delhi, India

S. Rastogi (ed.), *Translational Ayurveda*, https://doi.org/10.1007/978-981-13-2062-0_10

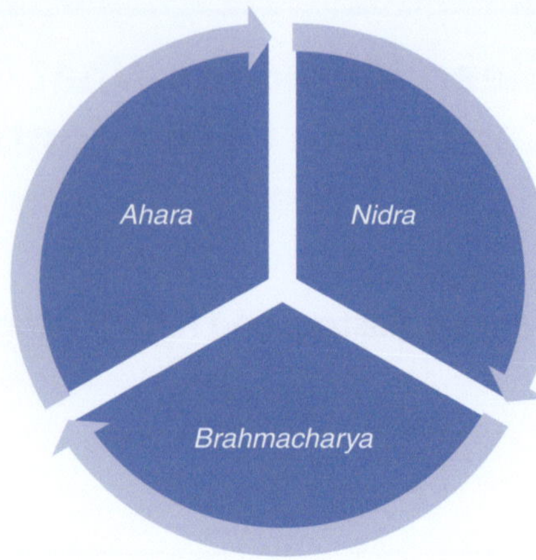

Fig. 10.1 Three foundation pillars of life (*trayopastambha*)

10.2 Why Do We Sleep?

Sleep is a universal phenomenon occurring in every living individual. Irrespective of their being animal or plant, large or small, and simple or complex, sleep is a necessity for everyone. A sleep deprivation is known to cause damage in certain areas in the brain almost instantly. Locus coeruleus (LC) is one such area in the brain which is severely affected by sleep deprivation. LC is the principal area of adrenergic secretion in the brain and hence is important for cognitive functions, memory, stress response, and emotional reactions [3]. Two important observations deserve a mention in this reference. One is that LC functions are mainly the wakeful state functions [4], and second is that LC has a substantially high concentration of copper in its neuronal terminals [5]. Incidentally, copper (*tamra*) in Ayurveda is considered a metal having the properties similar to the Sun and is a strong *pitta* promoter. Both propose for a wakeful state functioning of LC. Does it propose that a forced wakeful state leads to the overactivation of LC eventually self-destroying it? Surprising similarities with the pharmacological actions of copper proposed in Ayurveda can be found to that of LC activities. Copper is proposed to have a strong *lekhana* (scrapping) property which may be considered as an outcome of a pronged wakeful state.

Why do we sleep? As a question, this was tried to be explored since antiquity. Ayurveda proposes it in a simple way by saying that when the mind (brain, for instance) is tired after an eventful day, it gets transiently disconnected with the outer world (with transient inability of the senses to perceive), and this induces

analytic capacity and knowledge, having good memory, not affected by greed, anger, lust, ego, jealousy, and able to see every one as the creation of God. *Charaka Samhita Sharira Sthana Chapter 4 (mahatigarbhaavakrantisharira) verse 36.*

Table 10.1 Systemic effects of sleep

	Effects of good sleep	Effects of bad sleep
1	*Sukha* (pleasure, health)	*Dukha* (misery, illness)
2	*Pushti* (nourishment)	*Karshya* (debility)
3	*Bala* (strength)	*Abala* (loss of strength)
4	*Vrishata* (virility, vigor)	*Kleevata* (impotence, loss of libido)
5	*Gyan* (knowledge, memory)	*Agyan* (ignorance, forgetfulness)
6	*Jeevit* (live)	*Ajeevit* (dead)

sleep.[2] Recent studies have observed that sleep actually provides an opportunity to clean the accumulated waste in the brain produced during the wakeful activities [6]. This scavenging activity, although is operational in the wakeful state too, functions optimally during sleep. It is observed that the cerebrospinal fluid (CSF) acts as a sink for waste which is then headed toward the lymph nodes in the neck through a macroscopic pathway in the central nervous system denoted as the glymphatic system. The whole mechanism is found facilitated by a phenomenon called CSF pulsation produced by the throbbing of the brain. It is interesting to see that Ayurveda proposes a concept of *manovaha srotas* or the conduits for the brain functions. Majority of the mental illnesses manifested through disturbance of cognitive functions are told to be the result of blockade at *manovaha srotas*, and therefore treatment for such conditions is nothing but to offer a clearance to the blocks in the conduit. A process called *sirovirechana* (dredging of brain conduits) is found apt and highly effective for such clogging pathologies pertaining to the brain.

Besides LC acting through adrenergic neuron (AN) system, responsible for wakeful state, there are also the serotonergic neurons (SN) located at raphe nuclei and cholinergic neurons (CN) located at the pons of the brain stem. These three in conjunction regulate the sleep-wake cycle in a person. AN and SN together cause a wakeful state, whereas CN causes a sleep state. Any alteration in their function therefore leads to the disturbance in sleep-wake cycle [7]. Any drug, food, a change in lifestyle, or procedure acting upon the sleep-wake cycle therefore may have a possibility of acting through these pathways. This may be true for Ayurvedic interventions, and we have proposed the role of *tamra* in a similar tune.

10.3 Sleep Benefits

Ayurveda recognizes the systemic effects of sleep and admires the multiple positive and negative health impacts offered by a good or a bad sleep[3] (Table 10.1).

2 यदा तु मनसि क्लान्ते कर्मात्मान: क्ल्मान्विता:।विषयेभ्यो निवर्तन्ते तदा स्वपिति मानव:॥ च.सू.२१/३५.

3 निद्रायतं सुखं दु:खं पुष्टि कार्श्य बलाबलम ।वृषता क्लीवता ज्ञानमज्ञानं जीवितं न च॥ च.सू २१/३६.

10.3.1 Sleep as an Inductor of Sukha-Dukha

Sleep is considered to induce *sukha* and *dukha.* For the common understanding, *sukha* is a perception which is pleasant and desirous. On the contrary *dukha* is unpleasant and undesired. Ayurveda proposes a simple clinical definition to this perception.[4] It says that *sukha* is nothing but the state of *arogya* (a disease-free state), and *dukha* is the state of *vikara* (state of being sick). Sleep in its entirety is being recognized in Ayurveda as the inductor to both *sukha* and *dukha*, i.e., to health and disease. Sleep is a primary indicator of health and healing process. A patient who sleeps well is understood to be in the state of good recovery. Every disease is associated with some form of sleep disturbance either as a cause or as a manifestation. Sleep also has a strong effect upon chronic pain perception. A good sleep offers less intensity of pain the next day, while the reverse offers the contrary [8]. A disturbed sleep relates to the delayed healing process which is demonstrated through many studies. It may delay wound healing, increase the autonomic dysfunction and metabolic disturbances, and increase inflammatory cytokines [9].

While recognizing the importance of sleep in health and disease, Ayurveda also recognizes sleep cycle in reference to the circadian rhythm. Two important aberrant sleep behaviors, namely, *ratriprajagarana* (habitual awakening in night) and *divaswapna* (habitual sleeping during the day), are recognized as the cause to many diseases. Similar to this, forced sleep restriction (*nidravegavarodh*) is also considered as a cause to many diseases (Table 10.2).

10.3.2 Impact of Ratriprajagaran and Divaswapna on Body Physiology

Ayurveda proposes strong physiological impacts of aberrant sleep behavior.[5] A habitual night awakening promotes *ruksha* (roughness and dryness), a feature representing *vata* excess. At the same time, a habitual day sleep promotes *snigdha* (moistness and anointedness), a feature representing excess of *kapha*. Interestingly, napping while sitting (*aseenprachalaayitam*) is not found to be associated with any *dosha* perversion. Now this physiological impact of two common aberrant sleep behaviors is supposed to influence related pathologies pertaining to the rise of *dosha* pertinent to one condition. A night awakening causes increase of *vata* and hence leads to the promotion of *vata*-associated pathologies. Similarly, a daytime sleep leads to increase in *kapha* eventually leading to many *kapha*-dominant pathologies[6] (Table 10.2).

---

4 सुख संज्ञकम आरोग्यम विकारो दु:खमेव चा।.

5 रात्रौ जागरणं रुक्षं स्निग्धं प्रस्वप्नं दिवा।अरुक्षम अनभिष्यन्दि त्वासीन प्रचलायितम॥ च.सू. २१/५०.

6 हलीमक: शिर: शूलं स्तैमित्यं गुरुगात्रता। अंगमर्दो अग्नि नाशश्च प्रलेपो हृदयस्य च॥
शोफारोचक हृल्लास पीनसार्धावभेदका:।कोठाउरु: पिडका: कन्डूस्तन्द्रा कासो गलामया:॥
स्मृति बुद्धि प्रमोहश्च संरोध: स्रोतसां ज्वर:।इन्द्रियाणाम असामर्थ्यम विष वेग प्रवर्तनम ॥.

Table 10.2 Diseases caused by *ratriprajagaran*, *divaswapna*, and *nidravegavarodh*

Ratriprajagaran (habitual awakening in night)	*Divaswapna* (habitual sleeping in day)	*Nidravegavarodh* (forced restriction of sleep)
Vatajwara (fever due to excess *vata*)	*Kapha jwara* (fever due to excess kapha)	*Jrumbha* (excessive sleepiness)
Vata shiroroga (disease of head due to *vata*)	*Pandu* (anemia)	*Angamarda* (body ache)
Urustambha (stiffness of thighs)	*Halimaka* (jaundice)	*Tandra* (drowsiness)
	Staimitya (feeling of being wrapped with wet cloth)	*Shiroroga* (diseases of head)
	Shirah shula (headache)	*Akshigaurva* (heaviness in eyes)
	Guru gatrata (body heaviness)	
	Angamarda (body ache)	
	Agninaasha (loss of metabolic activity)	
	Hrida Pralepa (feeling of being wrapped at the chest)	
	Shopha (swelling)	
	Arochaka (loss of appetite)	
	Hrillasa (nausea)	
	Peenasa (chronic cold)	
	Ardhavabhedak (migraine)	
	Kotha (urticaria)	
	Pidka (pimples)	
	Kandu (itching)	
	Tandra (drowsiness)	
	Kaasa (cough)	
	Galamaya (throat infection)	
	Smriti buddhi pramoha (unclearness of memory and intellect)	
	Srotavarodha (obstructive pathologies)	
	Jwara (fever)	
	Indriyaasaamarthya (inability of the sense organs to perceive)	
	Vishavegapravartan (rapid action of toxins)	
	Kaphaja and sannipataja gulma	
	Kushtha	
	Arsha	
	Urustambha	
	Vaatarakta	

10.3.3 Sleep as an Inductor of Pushti-Karshya

Sleep on the basis of its action through *dosha* is supposed to cause *pushti* (nourishment) and *karshya* (emaciation), respectively. Ayurveda strongly proposes that along with nutrition, sleep also proves to be decisive for *sthaulya* and *karshya*.[7] Those who wish to gain weight are recommended to avoid habitual night awakening.[8] Similarly practicing for not being worried, nutrition and good sleep are also recommended if weight gain is desired.[9]

Current evidences favor the relation of sleep with obesity though in a contrasting way to that of Ayurveda. A sleep deprivation is identified as a cause of obesity in the current literature, and eventually daytime napping is proposed as a remedy to overcome sleep deprivation-induced obesity and associated metabolic syndromes [10]. This opinion seems relevant when we see that the world is currently facing obesity as an epidemic challenge at the same time when the problem of sleep duration and quality is also found rampant. Sleep significantly alters the neuroendocrine functions and glucose metabolism. Sleep loss results in many metabolic and endocrine changes, including decreased glucose tolerance and insulin sensitivity, increased evening concentrations of cortisol, increased levels of ghrelin and leptin, and increased hunger and appetite. Recent evidence confirm the association between sleep loss and increased chances of obesity. The link of obesity and insomnia is found to be associated with sleep duration and eating pattern during the wake period [11]. Taking a note for this, sometimes sleep is recommended as a measure to improve the effects of a weight-loss intervention [12]. A U-shaped relation between sleep duration and obesity is suggested, having a higher risk of obesity linked with both short and long sleep duration [13, 14]. Other sleep patterns including chronotype (i.e., being an evening compared with morning person), daytime napping, and shift work (including night-shift work) are also linked with obesity [15–17]. Interestingly, genetic relations to sleep chronotype and pattern is also tried to be identified recently. Though not conclusive, the study was able to demonstrate a genetic relationship to the sleep pattern [18]. We know that Ayurveda proposes a specific sleep pattern referring to the type of *prakriti*. A *vata* person, by constitution, is supposed to be a poor sleeper in terms of its quality and duration compared to a *kapha* person who is supposed to have a deeper and longer sleep.[10]

10.3.4 Daytime Napping: Who Are Its Qualifiers and Who Are Not?

Daytime napping is described in considerable details in Ayurveda. This is a *kapha*-promoting activity and hence increases the possibility of *kapha*-associated pathologies specially among the people with a preexisting excess of *kapha*. Ayurveda proposes a long list of conditions possible to be provoked by *divaswapna*

---

7 देह वृत्तौ यथा आहारस्तथा स्वप्न: सुखोमत:।स्वप्नाहार समुत्थे च स्थौल्य कार्श्ये विशेपत:॥ च.सू. २१/५१.

8 प्रजागरं व्यवायं च व्यायामं चिन्तनानि च। स्थौल्यम इच्छन परित्यक्तुं क्रमेणाभि प्रवर्धयेत॥ च.सू.२१/२८.

9 अचिन्तनाच्च कार्याणां ध्रुवं सन्तर्पणेन च। स्वप्न प्रसंगाच्च नरो वराह इव पुष्यति ॥ च. सू.२१/३४.

10 जागरूकाश्च भवन्ति' च.वि.८/९८.

(Table 10.2). Interestingly, despite of its evil effects, it is also recommended for some people in some seasons. The season recommended for day nap is summer where a loss of *kapha* and a corresponding increase of *vata* prevail. A small nap in the day therefore makes way to induce the balance. It is however important to observe here that this recommendation is not absolute and is only for the places where there is scorching summer causing dehydration. It is therefore not applicable in temperate or subtropical zones where summer is not intense.

The list of qualifiers for daytime napping[11] includes the people who are exhausted from vocal exercise, study, sexual acts, physical activities, prolonged walking, and carrying of weight. Elderly, infants, and debilitated also come in the category. Certain clinical conditions like excessive thirst, diarrhea, pain, breathlessness, and hiccough are also considered as the qualifiers for day nap. The people who are exhausted from a long-distance travel, involved in a fight, and traumatized or are violent also qualify for this act. The people who are exhausted because of anger, grief, and fear are also recommended for a daytime nap. It is interesting to observe that such people are recommended to have a daytime nap in any season on the basis of prevalence of their acts.

Contrary to the people who are emaciated or exhausted for some mental or physical reasons, daytime nap is absolutely contraindicated among people who are obese, consume oils and fat on a daily basis, are of *kapha* predominance, are having a *kapha* pathology, or are under the influence of a delayed-acting toxin.[12]

10.3.5 Benefits of a Day Nap

For the people to whom a day nap is recommended, it leads to the balance of body tissues and their actions and invigorates them with strength. The *kapha* generated through the process of day nap nourishes the body tissues and makes the person stable and live long.[13] This should however be clearly understood that a day nap is essentially conditional depending upon the prevailing needs. Too much of the nap can reduce the capacity to fall asleep at night and can impair nighttime sleep also [19].

10.3.6 Sleep as an Inductor of Bala-Abala

Sleep is proposed to be a promoter of strength if practiced genuinely. On the contrary this can also lead to debility owing to the erratic practices of sleep. Ayurveda proposes that as sleep improves status of *kapha* in the body, a proper sleep would induce strength in the body. On the contrary, a disturbed or a deficient sleep leads to the promotion of *vata* leading to the loss of strength. *Bala* (strength) from Ayurvedic perspective is considered as of three kinds, *sahaj* (inherent), *kalaj* (seasonal), and *yuktikrita* (procured). Interestingly, a good sleep is supposed to promote all such

11 गीताध्ययन मद्य स्त्री कर्म भाराध्व कर्शिता:।अजीर्णित: क्षता क्षीणा वृद्धा बालास्तथा अबला॥
तृष्णातिसार शूलार्ता: श्वासिनो हिक्किन: कृशा:। पतिता अभिहतोन्मत्ता: क्लान्ता यान प्रजागरे:॥
क्रोध शोक भय क्लान्ता दिवा स्वप्नोचिताश्च ये। सर्व एते दिवा स्वप्नं सेवेरन सार्वकालिकम ॥ च.सू.२१/४१.

12 मेदस्विन: स्नेह नित्या : श्लेष्मला: श्लेष्म रोगिण:।दूषीविषार्ताश्च दिवा न शयीरन कदाचन ॥

13 धातु साम्यं तथा ह्येषां बलं चाप्युपजायते। श्लेष्मा पुष्णाति चांगानि स्थैर्यं भवति चायुष:॥ च.सू.२१/४२.

kind of *bala* through its variable applications as per the requirement. A good parallel has been established with the concept of *bala* and immunity. It is now known that immunity has a circadian and a seasonal variability. A circadian cycle of sleep and wake has its distinctive effect upon immune functions. The nocturnal sleep promotes the production of undifferentiated naïve T cells and pro-inflammatory cytokines, whereas the wakefulness increases the circulating number of immune cells with immediate effecter functions like cytotoxic natural killer cells and anti-inflammatory cytokines [20]. Sleep also has a pronounced effect on immune memory. The people who sleep after active immunization are found to have better protection against diseases compared to the people who do not. Sleep deprivation is also found to have its pronounced effects upon immune function [21].

10.3.7 Sleep as an Inductor of Vrishata-Kleevata

Sleep also has strong effects upon sexual and reproductive functions of a person. Ayurveda proposes sleep as a potent reproductive function modifier. A proper sleep is supposed to enhance the sexual performance, whereas a poor sleep leads to loss of libido and poor sexual performance. New researches have endorsed this proposition of Ayurveda by observing that the male who have a proper sleep have a better chance to impregnate their partners [22]. Another study was able to demonstrate a reduced semen quality among the male suffering with sleep impairment [23]. On the basis of a cohort and a cross-sectional study, an inverse U-shaped association between sleep duration and semen parameters was found and indicated that restricted and excessive sleep both reduce semen quality in terms of sperm count and motility. The potential effect of sleep duration on semen quality deserves attention given the global prevalence of nontraditional sleep schedules and the potential impact on male reproductive health.

Sleep is found to have a direct relationship with the amount of testosterone produced in the body [24]. Plasma testosterone levels show a circadian variation with a peak during sleep and lowest during late afternoon. The testosterone levels are found sleep dependent requiring minimum 3 h of normal sleep to function optimally. Reduced testosterone levels are therefore observable in various sleep disorders disturbances in quality, duration, circadian rhythm, and sleep-disordered breathing.

Sexual desire is typically higher in men than in women, with testosterone thought to account for this difference as well as within-sex variation in desire in both women and men. Few studies have incorporated both hormonal and social or psychological factors in studying sexual desire [25].

Sleep is also recognized as a determinant of women's health and well-being, in the context of the menstrual cycle, pregnancy, and menopause. At present, however, little is known about how fertility is affected by sleep quantity and quality [26]. It may have a large clinical implication if we really know how sleep affects the reproductive function in male and female by and large .

10.3.8 Sleep as an Inductor of Gyan-Agyan

It is a common observation that a non-restorative sleep affects cognitive functions, memory, problem-solving skills, and thought clarity. The people who are sleep deprived are ought to be anxious, agitated, and unable to concentrate compared to the people who sleep well. A positive relation between sleep quality and academic performance has been established recently. A better sleep identified through Pittsburgh Sleep Quality Index (PSQI) was found matching with higher scores obtained in the course exams [27]. Ayurvedic proposition of linking sleep with *gyana* (knowledge) and *agyana* (ignorance) thus gives a valid point when we further see that sleep actually helps in solving the complex natured problems. An overnight sleep with the problem in mind keeps a good possibility of finding its solution next morning [28]. It is interesting to note that such enhanced problem-solving skills are not merely the result of mitigating the interference in concentration in awakened state but is actually related to the mechanism of spreading activation among correlated neurons. This is why sleep helps solve the difficult problems more effectively compared to easy problems where a higher recruitment of neurons may not be required.

Prolonged wakefulness is a commonly observed phenomenon. This can relate either to acute total sleep deprivation (SD) or to chronic partial sleep restriction (SR). Recent experiments suggests a cumulative action of chronic partial sleep restriction below 7 h per night leading to significant daytime cognitive dysfunction comparable to that occurring after severe acute total sleep deprivation [29]. Cognitive performance is affected adversely by both total and partial sleep deprivation. Total SD mainly impairs attention and working memory and also the long-term memory and decision-making. On the other hand, partial SD influences attention and vigilance. Coping with SD is proposed as one mechanism to compensate its ill effects; however, it depends on several factors, especially aging and gender. Inter-individual differences in such responses are also substantial. Ayurveda strongly proposes for such inter-individual differences of responses to sleep deprivation. Methods offering a recovery from ill effects of SD also deserve attention here. Cognitive recovery processes are more difficult in partial sleep restriction than in total SD [30]. As a method to recover cognitive losses due to acute sleep deprivation, Ayurveda recommends a compensatory day nap on the following day. We have seen this recommendation actually working in cases of jet lag where a sleep deprivation due to a change in natural circadian clock is compensated through prolonged daytime sleep for initial days till the recovery takes place.

10.3.9 Sleep as an Inductor of Jeevita-Ajivita

Sleep is essentially a feature of living being. This is a physiological response to the biological clock adjusted chronologically in a living body. Sleep therefore is an essential symbol of functional integrity of an individual.

10.4 Harmonizing the Natural and the Biological Clock

Living beings are accustomed to the natural day and night clock and work accordingly. Daylight is found apt for food procurement and self-defense, whereas its absence offers restoration by cleansing of wakeful accumulation of waste. In order to get accustomed with natural day and night clock, every living cell has developed its own clock working in tune to the natural clock. There are clock genes operational in every cell which respond to the natural clock and get activated to form set of transcription proteins designated for a particular function in the cell [31]. We see that the intensity of light eventually works as the trigger for cascading a series of physiological acts in a living cell synchronizing it with the natural clock. Suprachiasmatic nuclei (SCN) are located at the anterior hypothalamus and actually act as the center of the circadian clock having both photic (glutamatergic) and non-photic (serotonergic) input pathways. A lesion of the SCN disrupts the circadian rhythm of sleep-wake cycle [32].There are number of physiological acts in the human being which have a circadian or ultradian behavior. These acts are essential in order to customize the body as per the requirements of the natural clock (Table 10.3).

More and more evidences are accumulating now to show that a substantial sum of metabolic disorders actually erupt because of disharmony between the natural and the biological clock [33]. Knowing this fact since antiquity, Ayurveda severely discards any attempt to create a disharmony between these two clocks by observing *ratriprajagaran* or a *divaswapna* both of which represent an erratic sleep-wake behavior contrary to the natural clock.

Many things have actually contributed to the epidemic of sleep disturbances. Besides having a competitive environment around compelling to perform outwardly and impacting upon the sleep and its quality, light and sound pollution also have contributed significantly to the problem. Light pollution refers to the excessive, unwanted, and annoying amount of light during night indoors or outdoors and is capable of interfering with normal sleep cycle [34]. Excessive amount of light during night is found to have carcinogenic effects besides its effects upon erratic hormonal secretions in the body regulated by the amount of dark and night in the nature. Environmental noise, especially that caused by transportation means, is also viewed as a significant cause of sleep disturbances [35]. It is not surprising to note that

Table 10.3 Physiological responses as per the natural clock

Name of the hormone	Status in day	Status in night	Physiological effect
Insulin	Increased	Decreased	Glucose metabolism
Leptin	Decreased	Increased	Decreased appetite
Ghrelin	Increased	Decreased	Increased appetite
Testosterone	Decreased	Increased	Sexual desire and performance
Melatonin	Decreased	Increased	Sleep induction
Cortisol	Increased	Decreased	Defense

seeing the ill effects of light and sound upon sleep Ayurveda proposes a pleasing sound and aroma at the sleeping abode and also proposes to irrigate the eyes during night.[14]

10.5 Managing Sleep Disorders: Ayurvedic Wisdom

Sleep loss or poor sleep is considered to be an outcome of excess of *vata*. Similarly an excess of sleep is considered to be the result of excess of *kapha*. On the basis of Ayurvedic contrasting therapy principle, these excess are to be replaced from opposite *doshas*, i.e., *vata* from *kapha* and *kapha* from *vata*. Ayurvedic management of sleep disorders is in strict concordance of this principle.

10.5.1 Insomnia: Ayurvedic Therapy

10.5.1.1 Milk as a Sleep Inducer

Principal interventions recommended for insomnia in Ayurveda are based upon its proposed pathology correction, i.e., reduction of *vata* and increase in *kapha*. It is interesting to see what Ayurveda proposes as the treatment to insomnia is truly based upon this principal. Buffalo milk is proposed as the foremost hypnotic agent from Ayurveda.[15] Sometimes cow milk is also being bestowed with the similar propositions. Current researches have shown milk as a rich source of tryptophan, a precursor to serotonin and of melatonin in turn [36]. How the buffalo milk is better than other milks in terms of its sleep-promoting property may be a matter of interesting research. A recent proposition has come referring to the time of milking and its sleep-inducing properties [37]. We know by convention that the animals are being milked twice in a day, morning and evening. It is observed that the milk derived at night is more hypnotic compared to the milk derived at morning. The impact is because of the amount of dark in the evening which induces melatonin secretion in the animal which in turn is available in the milk also. This proposition however is different than that of Ayurvedic wisdom in this regards which proposes that the morning milk is relatively *guru* (heavy) on account of previous sedentary night. The evening milk should have been *laghu* (lighter) for the animals who kept grazing throughout the day. A higher hypnotic property of buffalo milk in Ayurveda is also proposed to be linked with less active routine of the buffalo compared to that of the cow. The difference of morning and night milk as per Ayurveda however may not be true contemporarily when we see the current trend of animal rearing in the animal farms and that there are no more opportunities for the animals to graze in the open farms throughout the day. Most remarkably we see that having a glass of milk before

14 मनसो अनुगुणा गन्धा: शब्दा: संवाहनानि च।चक्षुषोस्तर्पणम लेप: शिरसो वदनस्य च ॥ च.सू.२१/५२-५४.

15 महिषी क्षीरं स्वप्न जननानां श्रेष्ठ: च.सू.२५/४०.

retiring to the bed is a routine habit in many Indian households. Milk customarily is considered as *rasayana* (rejuvenator) in Ayurveda, and its sleep-inducing property makes it apt to be consumed at night.

10.6 Head and Foot Oil Massage

Another remarkable intervention proposed by Ayurveda for induction of sleep is head and foot massage with oil. Besides many other advantages proposed to be associated with oil head massage, proposing an improved sleep quality and duration through it was something remarkable.[16] There had been many researches putting the evidences for various benefits of the head and body oil massage, but none has absolutely focused upon its impact upon sleep initiation and quality. There are however compelling evidences supporting the idea of improved sleep duration among infants after a body oil massage [38, 39].

10.7 Ancillary Measures in Ayurveda to Improve Sleep Quality

Sleep hygiene is a recently promoted concept which gathers the evidences that avoiding and observing certain measures can help in having a good sleep [40]. This is defined as a set of behavioral and environmental recommendations intended to promote healthy sleep. As an approach to treat mild to moderate insomnia, patients are educated about healthy sleep habits and are encouraged to follow a set of recommendations to improve their sleep (e.g., avoid caffeine, exercise regularly, eliminate noise from the sleeping environment, maintain a regular sleep schedule) [41].

Interestingly, Ayurveda recommends a number of non-pharmacological measures supposed to improve sleep quality[17] (Table 10.4). Out of a good list of such propositions, a few are worth discussing for their realistic impacts upon sleep quality.

10.7.1 *Utsadana* (Rubbing)

Utsadana refers to the body rubbing with dry towel. This is meant to improve the peripheral blood circulation by rubbing the skin. There is a possibility that through this act, blood may be pooled in the peripheral circulation, partially depriving the systemic circulation including of brain. A progressive reduction of cerebral blood flow (CBF) is observed after the onset of sleep till its progress to slow-wave sleep [42]. It is not known if this reduction in CBF precedes the sleep induction and hence

16 निद्रालाभ: सुखं च स्यान मुर्ध्नि तैलनिषेवणात' च.सू.५/८३.

17 अभ्यंगोत्सादनं स्नानं ग्राम्यानूपौदका रसा: । शाल्यन्नं सदधिक्षीरं स्नेहो मद्यं मन:सुखम॥
मनसो अनुगुणा गन्धा: शब्दा: संवाहनानि च। चक्षुषोस्तर्पणम लेप: शिरसो वदनस्य च ॥
स्वास्तीर्ण शयनं वेश्म सुखम कालस्तथोचित:।आनयन्त्य चिरान्निद्रां प्रनष्टा या निमित्त: ॥च.सू.२१/५२-५४.

Table 10.4 Non-pharmacological measures from Ayurveda to improve sleep quality (see Footnote 17)

Ayurvedic non-pharmacological recommendations for sleep	English parallels
Abhyanga	Body massage
Utsaadana	Body rubbing
Snana	Bath
Gramya-aanupa-audaka rasa	Food from water-rich agroclimatic region
Shaalyannasadadhi	Rice with curd
Ksheeram	Milk
Sneha	Oil
Madyam manahsukham	Pleasing alcohol in moderate quantity
Manaso anuguna gandha	Pleasing aroma
Manaso anuguna shabda	Pleasing music/voice
Samvaahanaani	Kneading massage
Cakshutarpana	Wet eye pack/eye irrigation
Shirolepa	Anointing the head
Vadanlepa	Anointing the body
Swaasteernashayana	Well clean and tidy bed
Veshma sukham	Comfortable bed linen
Kaalastathochita	Scheduling for timely and appropriate quantity of sleep

acts as the triggering event to sleep induction. Ayurvedic proposition of *utsadana* therefore presents a possibility of evaluating a hypothesis that if an intervention leading to such differential pooling of blood in the body may somehow help induction of sleep.

10.7.2 *Snana* (Bathing)

Evening bath is customary in many Southeast Asian countries. Its association with sleep induction although is less understood. We commonly observe a custom of taking a bath after a hectic, tiring, and sweaty day. Ayurveda proposes bathing as "*shramharanamshreshta*" (best method to remove the physical fatigue). Very interestingly, this was evaluated scientifically and was found that an immersion bath is able to produce recovery from muscle fatigue [43]. The study revealed a significantly higher skin blood flow after immersion bath. Some recent researchers have identified the beneficial effects of partial bath in inducing sleep [44]. Studies done to identify the hot foot bath effects on sleep could not identify much difference between sleep occurring on bath day and non-bath day [45]. Current studies are in favor of the findings that skin blood flow increases after taking a bath. Does this change in skin blood circulation leads to a peripheral blood pooling and a subsequent decrease in cerebral blood flow? Is still a question to be answered. Not to forget, the basic primary question is still the same, does a reduced cerebral blood flow leads to induction of sleep?

10.7.3 *Gramya-Aanupa-Audaka Rasa* (Food from Water-Rich Agroclimatic Region)

Food is universally accepted as having its impact upon sleep quality and duration. Ayurveda proposes that a food rich in *kapha*-promoting properties is more likely to promote sleep. The food produced in water-rich agroclimatic region is told to be inherently rich in *kapha*-promoting properties. Currently we do not have much scientific information regarding this proposition of Ayurveda. There had been studies reviewing the role of specific food components and their possible impact upon sleep duration, architecture, and quality, but most of these are of preliminary nature and require more serious inquiry before reaching to a conclusion [46]. Ayurvedic proposition of food from water-rich agroclimatic region however have never been enquired, and hence upon enquiry, this may bring some new information about food type and their effects upon nighttime sleep.

10.7.4 *Shalyanna sadadhiksheeram sneho* (Rice with Curd, Milk, and *Ghee*)

Ayurveda proposes a combination of rice and curd or milk or *ghee* (clarified butter) as a promoter of sleep. From Ayurvedic perspective, this looks to be a food combination rich in *kapha*-promoting properties and hence is supposed to promote sleep by virtue of its similarity in nature. Milk, as we know, is a rich source of tryptophan which in turn helps generate serotonin and melatonin playing a major role in sleep genesis and maintenance. Studies have suggested that a high-carbohydrate/low-fat diet is associated with significant reduction in slow-wave sleep (SWS) and an increase in REM compared to low-carbohydrate/high-fat diet which does the contrary [47]. We are aware that SWS offers a deep restorative sleep thus improving the quality of sleep. More recent researches however are able to find a negative impact of dietary fat upon sleep by seeing a positive correlation with sleep latency and a negative correlation to sleep efficiency [48]. There are also reports suggestive of a fatty meal causing daytime sleepiness and hence is recommended to be avoided during daytime [49]. What is required to be understood here is that Ayurvedic proposition of a particular dietary recommendation for sleep promotion cannot simply be equated with dietary fat studies as there are many more micro- and macronutrients in the Ayurvedic food combo which may stand in favor of a good sleep. Besides tryptophan, the casein of the milk is also a good point of evaluation as a slow release protein proposed to offer a quick post-exercise recovery if taken at bedtime [50]. Fermentation products of milk are also found to have strong effects upon sleep quality evident by reduced number of night awakening and improved sleep efficiency [51]. Curd, a fermentation product of milk, is further proposed to have many more properties which may directly or indirectly affect the sleep quality, and this may be the reason of recommending curd as a sleep promoter in Ayurveda.

10.7.5 *Madyam manahsukham* (Alcohol of One's Choice)

Ayurveda proposes an alcoholic drink of one's choice to improve sleep. Current literature is able to differentiate the use of alcohol and its effect upon sleep in occasional drinkers and heavy drinkers. A recent meta-analysis on impact of alcohol on sleep-onset latency and REM latency has shown that the use of alcohol actually does not improve quality [52]. Alcohol reduces the sleep-onset latency among healthy people, but it reduces rapid eye movement (REM) sleep.

10.7.6 *Manaso anuguna gandha shabdaha* (Pleasing Aroma and Sound at Bedtime)

Smell is proposed to have strong effects upon sleep quality. A pleasing smell can promote the sleep quality, whereas an ambient unpleasant smell can do the contrary. The same is found true for the sound also. A pleasing music can be very effective in sleep induction, whereas a noisy ambience can do the contrary. Certain smells are found to have particular effects on sleep. Lavender is shown to decrease heart rate and blood pressure, creating a more relaxed state inductive for sleep [53]. Effects of lavender sniffing during bedtime were monitored through brain wave monitoring, and this was found that such sniffing actually prompts deep and refreshing sleep [54]. In one more study, a bath with lavender-scented water was found to offer deeper sleep and less frequent arousals among infants [55]. Interestingly Ayurveda proposes nasal route of drug application (*nasya*) as a preferred route for diseases pertaining to brain. Among many varieties of *nasya, dhmapana* is the one where a dry powder of the drug is sniffed in the nasal cavity. Among many advantages recommended associated with the use of *nasya*, a better hair growth, better nutrition to head and scalp, and sleep promotion are few enlisted.

Unpleasant environmental nocturnal noise is a known factor leading toward a poor-quality sleep and many associated health hazards [56]. On the contrary, there had been beneficial effects of the sound on sleep. Pleasant music is found to reduce sleep-onset latency and decrease heart rate leading to a more relaxed state [57]. Use of lullabies as a sleep promoter for infants is a universal phenomenon. The effects of lullabies are experienced as calming, quieting, and relaxing to the babies and therefore offer good sleep [58]. This observation has led to the genesis of formal educational programs to educate first-time mothers to make an effective use of this zero-cost tool for improving the quality of sleep of their babies.

Very interestingly, continuous low-tone natural sounds are found to be best inductors of sleep compared to sudden outburst of a sound which immediately responds as an arousal. There had been a distinction between nonthreatening and threatening sound which sets an alarm system in the brain leading to the arousal in wake of a threat. A pleasing sound on the contrary keeps the brain in safe perception leading to improved sleep quality. Listening to light music or to the sound of nature like that of a water flow, raindrops, or wind breeze is a strong facilitator of sleep [59].

10.7.7 *Samvahan* (Non-oil Kneading Massage)

Samvahan is also a customary practice in Indian households where parents are often given a non-oil kneading massage on legs at the time of retiring in night. This act is observed to ease the leg muscle tension and to improve the circulation in order to offer a good night sleep. Such act is anecdotally reported to have sleep benefits; however, systematic studies to explore its role as a sleep promoter have not been done. Massage is proposed to stimulate parasympathetic system, to improve serotonin levels, and to cause relaxation. This in turn may lead to sleep promotion [60].

10.7.8 *Chakkshushtarpana* (Eye Irrigation)

Chakshushatarpan primarily refers to techniques offering relaxation and nutrition to fatigued eyes through irrigation of medicated oil or *ghrita*. This procedure is commonly used for various eye disorders in Ayurveda. How a *ghrita* irrigation to eyes may produce sleep is still a matter of enquiry that needs to be made. One indirect impact *chakshushtarpan* may cause is through a compulsive closing of eyes during the procedure. There are ample evidences that dark promotes sleep, and by closing the eye and covering it with some amount of *ghrita* may possibly reduce the amount of light entering into the eyes substantially, thus perceiving the dark outside. A 30-min procedure may produce a stimulus sufficient to induce sleep. The use of eye mask as a sleep promoter is having evidences of its clinical benefits [61] and hence is promoted for routine patient care for a variety of cases requiring long-term hospital care [62]. Mudpack on the eyes is also promoted for sleep induction for similar reasons [63]. This would be interesting to see if *chakshushtarpan* effects are similar to that of eye masking or are better by virtue of applying medicated *ghrita* upon the eyes. A variability of sleep-onset latency among individuals and its flexibility as per the actual sleep debt is also important to be considered for such studies.

10.7.9 *Swastirna shayanam veshma sukham* (A Tidy Bed and Comfortable Linens)

Ayurveda possibly first time in the history of sleep medicine identified the importance of a clean, well-organized bedding and comfortable linen in the induction of sleep. The fabric used for the bedsheet and linen to cover the body also makes a sense to be evaluated for a good sleep. It is now known that the textile fibers used for bed linen have different thermal properties. It is obvious to think that if such fibers are able to produce an optimal ambient temperature, they eventually help reduce the sleep-onset latency and maintain the sleep. Sleepwears may also be important for sleep induction for similar reasons [64]. A clutter-free and tidy bedroom invites good sleep as clutter is supposed to be a great energy drainer [65]. Foundation of a good sleep also lies deep in a comfortable mattress [66].

10.7.10 *Kaalastathochit* (Timely and Adequate Amount of Sleep)

Sleeping at appropriate time is highly appreciated by Ayurveda. It is for this reason that *divaswapna* is thoroughly discussed and condemned for its possible ill effects upon nighttime sleep, an observation endorsed by current researches also. Sleeping at appropriate time refers to the tuning of the biological clock to a precise sleep-wake cycle. If done precisely, and regularly, it may help having the good sleep in time at the cost of no extra efforts. Although there are not many researches in the area, there is an anecdotal consensus that a regular sleeping habit may actually help getting away with many sleep problems.

Besides a timely sleep, adequate amount of sleep is also crucial. Sleeping less or more than required may eventually invite some sleep-related health issues. We are aware that sleep duration varies greatly among individuals. The physiological basis of this variation is largely unknown although Ayurveda proposes a genetic basis to this by identifying *vata* people as short sleepers and *kapha* people as long sleepers. Sleep duration >9 h is considered to be long, whereas <6 h is considered to be short. Studies have found substantial neuroendocrinal differences between short and long sleepers. There are differences among plasma melatonin and cortisol levels and body temperature within people of two sleep habits. Most interestingly, peak cortisol level and sleepiness are found to have a close relationship to habitual wake-up time. Studies suggest that this occurs approximately 2.5 h later in long sleepers than in short sleepers. It is proposed that sleeping long or short is actually the manifestation of the length of the biological night of the individual. For having a good sleep, this phenomenon should also be respected [2].

10.8 Sleep Medicine in Ayurveda: Translational Possibilities

Ayurveda has a plethora of knowledge collected through centuries which is yet to be explored for its optimal use in health care. Such accumulated knowledge is actually the outcome of a constant research and review process done through centuries upon real patients and with real medicines. The texts of Ayurveda therefore are not merely the recollection of references of previous works but are the summary of the entire philosophy of Ayurveda truly experienced.

A cursory look at Ayurvedic texts often gives an impression of this as being a collection of philosophical thoughts twinned with the health principles though imprecisely. It is for this reason the dogma of Ayurveda is often claimed as unscientific for its incomprehensibility in terms of modern science. It is however only when we start revisiting the Ayurveda and match it with contemporary understanding of science we realize how true this knowledge is in its own and how advanced these ideas might be for being promoted centuries ago, when even the traces of modern science were not visible in the horizon.

Sleep medicine concepts of Ayurveda are full of such principles, applications, and understandings which mesmerize us for their preciseness of interpretations when looked from current perspectives. As sleep is a global problem and a whole lot of people are actually suffering with sleep-associated complications, a review of Ayurvedic dictums about sleep gives us a fresh feel of finding something new to help the ailing community. This exercise is meaningful for two important reasons. One that it endorses the concepts of Ayurveda on terms of current understanding, something although not required but is actually asked repeatedly. It is more important to revalidate Ayurveda for its better acceptance throughout the world. The second has a more appealing value. This reappraisal gives us an opportunity to bring something entirely unknown, from the science of understanding to its practical applications. This is like a reverse pharmacological approach where textual descriptions may be tried afresh with the help of current research tools to find a more precise application leading toward the cure of a disease. We however argue that this approach should not remain limited with applications alone but let it be applicable to the understanding of fundamental science as well, a kind of disease process understanding with the help of what Ayurveda proposes. This understanding may well be related to the prevention of a disease by understanding its causes or also the diagnosis of a disease by knowing the precise clinical descriptions available in Ayurveda. Needless to say, it further proposes a possibility of a real personalized treatment approach with the help of extensive *rog* and *rogi* examination as proposed in Ayurveda.

Beginning with the bedside applications of Ayurvedic wisdom for sleep promotion, there are a number of applications worth trying as a prospective remedy to sleep loss. Buffalo milk seems to be the most promising one. Head and body massages are other methods which are promising their help in sleep loss. A moderate amount of alcohol of one's choice, a pleasing aroma, sound, comfortable bed linen and tidiness of the bedroom, ensuring dark in the room may be with eye cover, sleeping appropriately and adequately, and the food promotive of sleep are all what Ayurveda says for strategic promotion of sleep. This all accounts of Ayurveda although being tried sparingly in clinical researches may be given a robust trial to establish their effects and practical methods of applications. The difficulty in translation of Ayurveda at bedside lies in the compact nature of the Ayurveda *sutras* (phrases or verses). A compact verse often is being interpreted differently at different levels and hence is applied differently in the clinical practice. For exploring its clinical applicability, a precise dose and effect study may be required considering essentially all the variability available within the population and also in the intervention methodologies.

Ayurvedic proposition of day and night sleep and wake cycle is highly admirable. The proposition of multiple health problems associated with disruption of sleep-wake cycle is a common observation now and is more and more realized. This seems that sleep correction should come as the first-line management of all diseases despite of this being reported or not by the patient. We perceive that substantial information is available in Ayurveda regarding the pathophysiology of sleep, its outcomes, and plan of management. What is needed is to make a deeper insight into the leads available in Ayurveda for their dependable application in the clinical setting. This is true for sleep medicine as well as for any other branch of medicine when looked from Ayurvedic perspective.

Some novel approaches like *shirodhara* and *shirovasti* have also been explored recently as promising interventions in sleep loss. These two are actually the applications of classical recommendation of oil massage on the head which is highly praised as a sleep promoter [67]. Although these procedures are proving their effects in sleep loss, it is important to understand that such treatments cannot be recommended as the routine treatment in sleep loss for many reasons. The first and the foremost is the requirement of a specific setting and supervision for such treatments. The cost of the therapy is also one important component which needs to be considered for the success of these treatments. A *shirodhara* procedure happens to be very expensive and hence is not affordable to most people suffering with sleep loss. Some drugs like *sarpagandha* (*Rauwolfia serpentina*), *jatamansi* (*Nardostachys jatamansi*), and *tagar (valerianavelchi)* are also known hypnotics in Ayurveda. Although recommended frequently in Ayurvedic clinics for patients reporting for sleep loss, such drugs have also been devoid of studies identifying their actual indications, doses, and their mechanism of action referring to these cases. In lack of such studies, it is used only empirically and not rationally. Considering the pathophysiology of sleep and roles of adrenergic, serotonergic, and cholinergic neurons in the brain and their impacts upon the sleep-wake cycle, it is important to delineate the role of Ayurvedic interventions to these mechanisms of sleep or to any other possible mechanism which might be leading to the genesis of sleep. It is important to understand here that when we talk of Ayurvedic interventions, we essentially mean the intervention in toto and not in the fragmented form. We had done enough with the extracts of the herbs; now this is the time to do with whole compound, or even a combination of the compounds, to see what they have to offer in sleep.

Acknowledgment Kind help from Prof. M. Singaravel, Ph.D., Chronobiology Lab, Department of Zoology, Institute of Science, Banaras Hindu University, is deeply acknowledged for reviewing the manuscript and for his valuable suggestions.

References

1. https://article.wn.com/view-lemonde/2017/04/09/up_ministers_officials_pant_as_yogi_chants_na_sounga_na/related_news
2. Aeschbach D, Sher L, Postolache TT, Matthews JR, Jackson MA, Wehr TA. A longer biological night in long sleepers than in short sleepers. J Clin Endocrinol Metab. 2003;88(1):26–30.
3. Mather M, Harley CW. The locus coeruleus: essential for maintaining cognitive function and the aging brain. Trends Cogn Sci. 2016;20(3):214–26. https://doi.org/10.1016/j.tics.2016.01.001.
4. Gompf HS, Mathai C, Fuller PM, et al. Locus coeruleus (LC) and anterior cingulate cortex sustain wakefulness in a novel environment. J Neurosci. 2010;30(43):14543–51. https://doi.org/10.1523/JNEUROSCI.3037-10.2010.
5. Sato M, Ohtomo K, Daimon T, Sugiyama T, Iijima K. Localization of copper to afferent terminals in rat locus ceruleus, in contrast to mitochondrial copper in cerebellum. J Histochem Cytochem. 1994;42(12):1585–91.
6. Xie L, Kang H, Xu Q, et al. Sleep drives metabolite clearance from the adult brain. Science (New York, NY). 2013;342(6156):373–7. https://doi.org/10.1126/science.1241224.
7. Hobson JA, Pace-Schott EF. The cognitive neuroscience of sleep: neuronal systems, consciousness and learning. Nat Rev Neurosci. 2002;3(9):679–93. https://doi.org/10.1038/nrn915.

8. Smith MT, Haythornthwaite JA. How do sleep disturbance and chronic pain inter-relate? Insights from the longitudinal and cognitive-behavioral clinical trials literature. Sleep Med Rev. 2004;8(2):119–32.
9. Mullington JM, Simpson NS, Meier-Ewert HK, Haack M. Sleep loss and inflammation. Best Pract Res Clin Endocrinol Metab. 2010;24(5):775–84. https://doi.org/10.1016/j.beem.2010.08.014.
10. Beccuti G, Pannain S. Sleep and obesity. Curr Opin Clin Nutr Metab Care. 2011;14(4):402–12. https://doi.org/10.1097/MCO.0b013e3283479109.
11. Coughlin JW, Smith MT. Sleep, obesity, and weight loss in adults: is there a rationale for providing sleep interventions in the treatment of obesity? Int Rev Psychiatry. 2014;26(2):177–88. https://doi.org/10.3109/09540261.2014.911150.
12. Chaput J-P, Tremblay A. Adequate sleep to improve the treatment of obesity. CMAJ. 2012;184(18):1975–6. https://doi.org/10.1503/cmaj.120876.
13. Cappuccio FP, Taggart FM, Kandala N-B, Currie A, Peile E, Stranges S, Miller MA. Meta-analysis of short sleep duration and obesity in children and adults. Sleep. 2008;31:619–26.
14. Buxton OM, Marcelli E. Short and long sleep are positively associated with obesity, diabetes, hypertension, and cardiovascular disease among adults in the United States. Soc Sci Med. 2010;71:1027–36.
15. Yu JH, Yun C-H, Ahn JH, Suh S, Cho HJ, Lee SK, Yoo HJ, Seo JA, Kim SG, Choi KM, et al. Evening chronotype is associated with metabolic disorders and body composition in middle-aged adults. J Clin Endocrinol Metab. 2015;100:1494–502.
16. Yamada T, Nobuhiro S, Takashi K. Daytime napping, daytime sleepiness and the risk of metabolic diseases: dose-response meta-analysis using restricted cubic spline model. J Am Coll Cardiol. 2016;67:1951.
17. Antunes LC, Levandovski R, Dantas G, Caumo W, Hidalgo MP. Obesity and shift work: chronobiological aspects. Nutr Res Rev. 2010;23:155–68.
18. Jones SE, Tyrrell J, Wood AR, Beaumont RN, Ruth KS, Tuke MA, Yaghootkar H, Hu Y, Teder-laving M, Hayward C, Roenneberg T, Wilson JF, Del Greco F, Hicks AA, Shin C, Yun C, Lee SK, Metspalu A, Byrne EM, Gehrman PR, Tiemeier H, Allebrandt KV, Freathy RM, Murray A, Hinds DA, Frayling TM, Weedon MN, Shi J. Genome-wide association analyses in 128,266 individuals identifies new morningness and sleep duration loci. PLoS Genet. 2016;12(8):e1006125. https://doi.org/10.1371/journal.pgen.1006125.
19. Goldman SE, Hall M, Boudreau R, et al. Association between nighttime sleep and napping in older adults. Sleep. 2008;31(5):733–40.
20. Besedovsky L, Lange T, Born J. Sleep and immune function. Pflugers Archiv. 2012;463(1):121–37. https://doi.org/10.1007/s00424-011-1044-0.
21. Moldofsky H, Lue FA, Davidson JR, Gorczynski R. Effects of sleep deprivation on human immune functions. FASEB J. 1989;3(8):1972–7.
22. Alvarenga TA, Hirotsu C, Mazaro-Costa R, Tufik S, Andersen ML. Impairment of male reproductive function after sleep deprivation. Fertil Steril. 2015;103(5):1355–62.e1. https://doi.org/10.1016/j.fertnstert.2015.02.002. Epub 2015 Mar 4.
23. Chen Q, Yang H, Zhou N, et al. Inverse U-shaped association between sleep duration and semen quality: longitudinal observational study (MARHCS) in Chongqing, China. Sleep. 2016;39(1):79–86. https://doi.org/10.5665/sleep.5322.
24. Wittert G. The relationship between sleep disorders and testosterone in men. Asian J Androl. 2014;16(2):262–5. https://doi.org/10.4103/1008-682X.122586.
25. van Anders SM. Testosterone and sexual desire in healthy women and men. Arch Sex Behav. 2012;41(6):1471–84.
26. Kloss JD, Perlis M, Zamzow J, Culnan E, Gracia C. Sleep, sleep disturbance and fertility in women. Sleep Med Rev. 2015;22:78–87. https://doi.org/10.1016/j.smrv.2014.10.005.
27. Baert S, Omey E, Verhaest D, Vermeir A, Sandman M, Bring me good marks! On the relationship between sleep quality and academic achievement. IZA discussion paper no. 8232. Available at SSRN: https://ssrn.com/abstract=2450423.

28. Sio UN, Monaghan P, Ormerod T. Sleep on it, but only if it is difficult: effects of sleep on problem solving. Mem Cognit. 2013;41(2):159–66. https://doi.org/10.3758/s13421-012-0256-7.
29. Banks S, Dinges DF. Behavioral and physiological consequences of sleep restriction. J Clin Sleep Med. 2007;3(5):519–28.
30. Alhola P, Polo-Kantola P. Sleep deprivation: impact on cognitive performance. Neuropsychiatr Dis Treat. 2007;3(5):553–67.
31. Barclay JL, Husse J, Bode B, Naujokat N, Meyer-Kovac J, et al. Circadian desynchrony promotes metabolic disruption in a mouse model of shiftwork. PLoS One. 2012;7(5):e37150. https://doi.org/10.1371/journal.pone.0037150.
32. Mistlberger RE. Circadian regulation of sleep in mammals: role of the suprachiasmatic nucleus. Brain Res Brain Res Rev. 2005;49(3):429–54.
33. Potter GDM, Skene DJ, Arendt J, Cade JE, Grant PJ, Hardie LJ. Circadian rhythm and sleep disruption: causes, metabolic consequences, and counter measures. Endocr Rev. 2016;37(6):584–608.
34. Chepesiuk R. Missing the dark: health effects of light pollution. Environ Health Perspect. 2009;117(1):A20–7.
35. Halperin D. Environmental noise and sleep disturbances: a threat to health? Sleep Sci. 2014;7(4):209–12. https://doi.org/10.1016/j.slsci.2014.11.003.
36. Richard DM, Dawes MA, Mathias CW, Acheson A, Hill-Kapturczak N, Dougherty DM. L-tryptophan: basic metabolic functions, behavioral research and therapeutic indications. Int J Tryptophan Res. 2009;2:45–60.
37. Valtonen M, Niskanen L, Kangas AP, Koskinen T. Effect of melatonin-rich night-time milk on sleep and activity in elderly institutionalized subjects. Nord J Psychiatry. 2005;59(3):217–21.
38. Yates CC, Mitchell AJ, Booth MY, Williams DK, Lowe LM, Hall RW. The effects of massage therapy to induce sleep in infants born preterm. Pediatr Phys Ther. 2014;26(4):405–10. https://doi.org/10.1097/PEP.0000000000000081.
39. Kulkarni A, Kaushik JS, Gupta P, Sharma H, Agrawal RK. Massage and touch therapy in neonates: the current evidence. Indian Pediatr. 2010;47(9):771–6.
40. Irish LA, Kline CE, Gunn HE, Buysse DJ, Hall MH. The role of sleep hygiene in promoting public health: a review of empirical evidence. Sleep Med Rev. 2015;22:23–36. https://doi.org/10.1016/j.smrv.2014.10.001.
41. Zarcone VP. Sleep hygiene. In: Kryger MH, Roth T, Dement WC, editors. Principles and practice of sleep medicine. 3rd ed. Philadelphia: WB Saunders; 2000. p. 657–61.
42. Klingelhöfer J. Cerebral blood flow velocity in sleep. Perspect Med. 2012;1(1–12):275–84.
43. Lee S, Ishibashi S, Shimomura Y, Katsuura T. Physiological functions of the effects of the different bathing method on recovery from local muscle fatigue. J Physiol Anthropol. 2012;31:26. https://doi.org/10.1186/1880-6805-31-26.
44. Jasmine SE, Lebona GB, Sivamma P, Indira S. Effectiveness of evening partial bath on sleep among hospitalized orthopedic patient. Int J Appl Res. 2017;3(4):444–5.
45. Liao W-C, Chiu M-J, Landis CA. A warm footbath before bedtime and sleep in older Taiwanese with sleep disturbance. Res Nurs Health. 2008;31(5):514–28. https://doi.org/10.1002/nur.20283.
46. St-Onge MP, Mikic A, Pietrolungo CE. Effects of diet on sleep quality. Adv Nutr. 2016;7(5):938–49. https://doi.org/10.3945/an.116.012336.
47. Phillips F, Chen CN, Crisp AH, et al. Isocaloric diet changes and electroencephalographic sleep. Lancet. 1975;2:723–5.
48. Crispim CA, Zimberg IZ, dos Reis BG, et al. Relationship between food intake and sleep pattern in healthy individuals. J Clin Sleep Med. 2011;7:659–64.
49. Panossian LA, Veasey SC. Daytime sleepiness in obesity: mechanisms beyond obstructive sleep apnea—a review. Sleep. 2012;35(5):605–15. https://doi.org/10.5665/sleep.1812.
50. Res PT, Groen B, Pennings B, Beelen M, Wallis GA, Gijsen AP, Senden JM, Van Loon LJ. Protein ingestion before sleep improves postexercise overnight recovery. Med Sci Sports Exerc. 2012;44:1560–9.

51. Yamamura S, Morishima H, Kumano-go T, Suganuma N, Matsumoto H, Adachi H, et al. The effect of lactobacillus helveticus fermented milk on sleep and health perception in elderly subjects. Eur J Clin Nutr. 2009;63:100.
52. Smith, Hannah Lane, "The Impact of Alcohol Consumption on Sleep Onset and REM Latency: A Meta-Analytic Study" (2016).Undergraduate Theses.Paper 135.
53. Goel N, Kim H, Lao RP. An olfactory stimulus modifies nighttime sleep in young men and women. Chronobiol Int. 2005;22(5):889–904.
54. Sayorwan W, Siripornpanich V, Piriyapunyaporn T, Hongratanaworakit T, Kotchabhakdi N, Ruangrungsi N. The effects of lavender oil inhalation on emotional states, autonomic nervous system, and brain electrical activity. J Med Assoc Thail. 2012;95(4):598–606.
55. Rioualen S, Bertelle V, Roué JM, Sizun J. How to improve sleep in a neonatal intensive care unit: a systematic review. Early Hum Dev. 2017;115:1. https://doi.org/10.1016/j.earlhumdev.2017.08.001.
56. Hume KI, Brink M, Basner M. Effects of environmental noise on sleep. Noise Health. 2012;14(61):297–302. https://doi.org/10.4103/1463-1741.104897.
57. Chen YY, Wong AMK. Music therapy effect of music pillow for sleep—preliminary study. In: 3rd Kuala Lumpur international conference on biomedical engineering; 2006. p. 215–8.
58. Baker F, Mackinlay E. Sing, soothe and sleep: a lullaby education programme for first-time mothers. Br J Music Educ. 2006;23(2):147–60. https://doi.org/10.1017/S0265051706006899.
59. Buxton OM, Ellenbogen JM, Wang W, Carballeira A, O'Connor S, Cooper D, Gordhandas AJ, McKinney SM, Solet JM. Sleep disruption due to hospital noises: a prospective evaluation. Ann Intern Med. 2012;157(3):170–9. https://doi.org/10.7326/0003-4819-157-3-201208070-00472.
60. Cutler N. Insomnia, serotonin and massage; Institute for Integrative Healthcare; August 19, 2005. www.integrativehealthcare.org/mt/archives/2005/08/insomnia_seroto.html
61. Babaii A, Adib-Hajbaghery M, Hajibagheri A. Effect of using eye mask on sleep quality in cardiac patients: a randomized controlled trial. Nurs Midwifery Stud. 2015;4(4):eee28332.
62. Le Guen M, Nicolas-Robin A, Lebard C, Arnulf I, Langeron O. Earplugs and eye masks vs routine care prevent sleep impairment in post-anaesthesia care unit: a randomized study. Br J Anaesth. 2014;112:89–95.
63. Rajiv R. Prakritik Chikitsa Paramarsh: Anidra. Agra: Asha Publishing Co.; 2016.
64. Shin M, Halaki M, Swan P, Ireland AH, Chow CM. The effects of fabric for sleepwear and bedding on sleep at ambient temperatures of 17°C and 22°C. Nat Sci Sleep. 2016;8:121–31. https://doi.org/10.2147/NSS.S100271.
65. http://www.sleepcouncil.org.uk/wp-content/uploads/2013/01/Get-a-Good-Nights-Sleep.pdf
66. Lee H, Park S. Quantitative effects of mattress types (comfortable vs. uncomfortable) on sleep quality through polysomnography and skin temperature. Int J Ind Ergon. 2006;36(11):943–9. https://doi.org/10.1016/j.ergon.2006.07.007.
67. Gulia KK, Radhakrishnan A, Kumar VM. Approach to sleep disorders in the traditional school of indian medicine: alternative medicine II. Sleep disorders medicine. New York: Springer. p. 1221–31.

Ayurveda Abroad: Non-native Perspectives and Needs for Translating It to Western Settings

11

Christian Sumith Kessler

11.1 Background

Medical anthropology, sociology, and psychology tell us that no medical tradition is ever static, particularly not when such traditions start to travel abroad [1–6]. While this is evidently so in the case of Ayurveda (alongside other traditional Asian healing systems), it is interesting to reflect on the fact that even within the (sub)specific native cultural contexts of Ayurveda's origin(s) in India/South Asia, developments in the field are (and always have been) highly heterogeneous, multifold, and at times even contradicting. The multifold approaches on many medical questions posed in the "classical" *bṛhat trayī* texts of Caraka, Suśruta, and Vāgbhaṭa [7–9] are prime examples for plurality and diversity that have always been the driving forces of Indian systems of thought and philosophy in general and of traditional Indian medicine (TIM) in particular over millennia [10].

The principle of integrating diverse medical traditions is particularly evident when these traditions travel abroad and marry other medical and/or epistemological traditions, "integrate" with or "complement" local mainstream medicine, "erode" to accommodate wellness/luxury, or even "transform" into new *hybrid Ayurvedas* [3, 11–15] in different settings. In nearly all these cases on Ayurveda's winding roads of whole systems' transmigration to the West, Ayurveda has never remained "the same" as it once might have been in its places of origin. Notably the same is true, for instance, for homeopathy, having migrated in the opposite direction from Europe to India in the past three centuries, or for German anthroposophy that has absorbed timeless Indian philosophy in its (medical) epistemology without necessarily labeling it as such [3, 16–18].

C. S. Kessler
Institute for Social Medicine, Epidemiology and Health Economics,
Charité Medical University, Berlin, Germany

Department for Complementary Medicine, Immanuel Hospital Berlin,
Berlin, Germany

S. Rastogi (ed.), *Translational Ayurveda*, https://doi.org/10.1007/978-981-13-2062-0_11

11.2 The Field

The main driving factors that influence evolution and devolution of such (sub)specific western Ayurveda "realities" in clinical practice and research in the West also influence Westerners receiving Ayurvedic treatment in India:

(a) **Heterogeneity of healthcare regulation**: In most western countries, Ayurveda is not recognized and/or regulated as an independent medical system or as a traditional system of medicine according to WHO guidelines [19, 20]. For example, within Europe, Switzerland is currently the only country with at least one government-acknowledged Ayurveda profession (and a super-qualification for medical doctors in the pipeline) [21]. In all European countries, Ayurveda is part of complementary, alternative, or integrative practices within "universal" healthcare systems; notably it is still not among the top ten CAM practices in the EU [22]. This is unlike India where Ayurveda is a parallel healthcare system and is not categorized as complementary and alternative medicine (CAM) modality but as one of several systems of mainstream medicine [20, 23]; moreover, cross-system practice is not encouraged at large in India to date [24–26].

(b) **Diversity of cultural and historical influences**: The history of interacting with South Asia differs significantly between western countries. European perspectives on India (and thereby on Ayurveda) can be quite heterogeneous from country to country based on different degrees, time spans, and foci of interaction. For instance, the British perspective on India and other commonwealth countries is to a large extent driven by the UK's colonial and postcolonial history in South Asia with a focus on administrative, legal, economical, social, and political aspects, while the German perspective is influenced by a history of academic scholars primarily from linguistics, religious sciences, philosophy, and literature. Since Ayurveda is an absorbent, open-porous traditional whole system of medicine, these regional intercultural and hybridization differences have also impacted on its (sub)specific developments in various "Ayurveda expatriate regions" (for instance, related to legislation, acknowledgment, administration, and perception) (Fig. 11.1).

(c) **Practice as a whole system of medicine**: In most cases, Ayurveda therapy in western countries is characterized by a multimodality whole systems approach of practice (regardless of its therapeutic depth, quality, or "authenticity"). While this might seem trivial on first notion, it is an important issue, because this is in striking contrast to a large fraction of modern mainstream Ayurveda approaches in South Asia, which predominantly or exclusively focus on complex polyherbal treatments and, to a minor degree, on aspects of *pancakarma*. This is also being reflected by the available high-quality preclinical and clinical research data in the field (e.g., [24, 27–30], Fig. 11.2). In western contexts, however, therapists, patients, clients, and observers generally expect Ayurveda treatment to include customized nutritional advice, individual lifestyle and self-effectiveness counseling, Yoga therapy, meditation, and epistemological advice (including philosophical, religious, and spiritual aspects) to be essential parts of

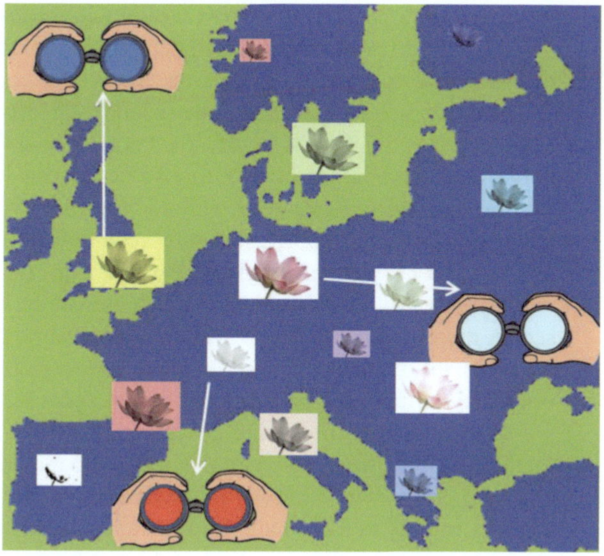

Fig. 11.1 Diversity of cultural perspectives on India and Ayurveda in Europe

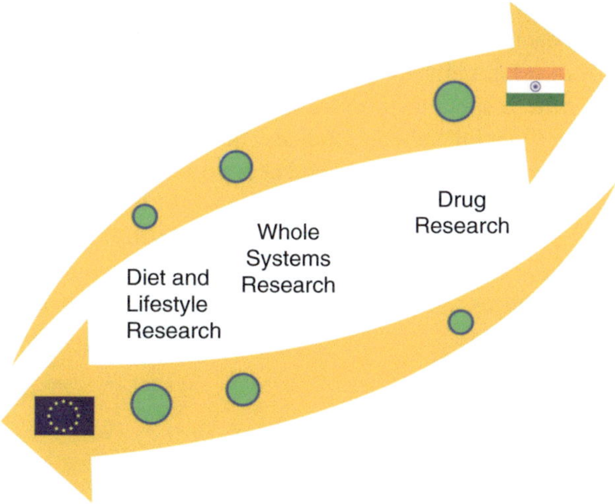

Fig. 11.2 Simplified depiction of Ayurveda research focuses: "East vs. West"

such a whole systems Ayurveda approach, with herbal treatments and *pancakarma* to be just two elements among many others [31–33]. It is a paradox that in a way well-planned and well-performed whole systems Ayurveda in western settings can at times appear to be even more "traditional" than, for instance, the abovementioned quite common Indian interpretations limiting Ayurvedic practice to the administration of herbal preparations [34].

(d) **The Ayurveda wellness paradigm and problem:**
In western countries Ayurveda is perceived, by many and to a large extent, as a form of sophisticated wellness treatment and/or luxury medical wellness [34–

36]. Ever since its arrival in most western countries in the 1980s, the strongest visibility of Ayurveda abroad has been within the context of more or less elaborate massage treatments, *śirodhāra*, Ayurvedic cooking according to heavily simplified *doṣa* concepts, and other (pseudo-)iconic features of Ayurveda. As an example, the number of Ayurveda cookbooks in Germany outnumbers the books on Ayurvedic medical textbooks by far; this is also true for tabloid media coverage where (at least from a more "traditional" South Asian perspective) a heavy imbalance of reporting on Ayurveda in favor of wellness and cooking can be observed [37]. Interestingly, Ayurveda, from its "start" in western countries in the 1980s, has always mainly been located in the high-price out-of-the-pocket sector, thereby making it less available for common people and largely limiting its accessibility to upper middle-class and high-income social strata. This is obviously quite in contrast to most South Asian settings, for example, in India, where Ayurveda is oftentimes perceived as "rural medicine" or "second-class medicine" (e.g., when conventional medicine may not be available due to financial restrictions, etc.). Through the advance of international Ayurveda medical tourism, mainly to Kerala and Sri Lanka, an interesting and rather new phenomenon has emerged: the re-import of Ayurveda as a luxury medicine and a wellness concept to its countries of origin, often in hybrid forms mingling with other traditions and forms of therapies, creating yet other Ayurveda realities in beach resorts, hotels, ashrams, and other places in South Asia (Fig. 11.3). These developments over the last five decades have resulted in significant differences with respect to accessibility, availability, and visibility in different social strata and social spheres and are thus highly relevant for Ayurvedic practice and research on Ayurveda and need to be considered when dealing with Ayurveda in western countries and elsewhere [3, 11, 12, 15, 38].

(e) **Absence of effective funding and lobbying networks:**
Research in complementary and integrative medicine (CAM, CIM) in western countries usually heavily depends on financial support through philanthropic or

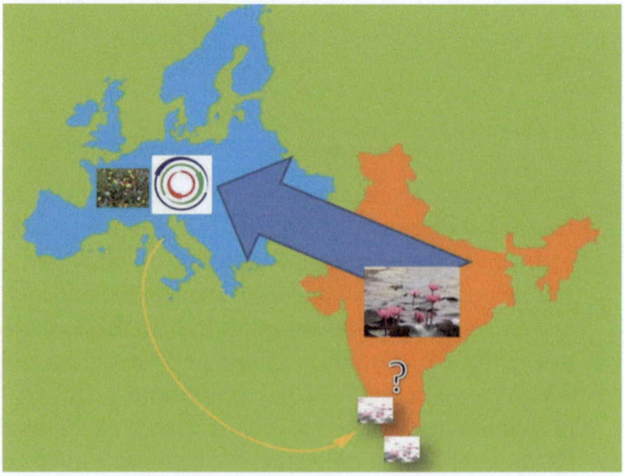

Fig. 11.3 Ayurveda re-import to South Asia: between whole systems and beach resorts

foundation activities. In most cases funds from public research calls (e.g., by health, research, or education ministries) are usually not accessible for non-mainstream, non-conventional medical approaches (which Ayurveda belongs to in all western countries). Or they are not selected for public grants, even if formally suitable (Yoga and mind-body medicine, which have become increasingly mainstream, particularly in the USA, are still the rather rare exception to the rule). For this reason funding options and networks have been built to fill in the gap in other CAM/CIM communities. In Europe, for instance, this is the case for homeopathy, anthroposophy, traditional Chinese medicine, and traditional European medicine [22]. However, for Ayurveda there is still no effective and overarching philanthropic support network, which could enable research, e.g., in the form of large clinical trials, in countries outside of its origin (which is notably in sharp contrast to the fact that Ayurveda is oftentimes being perceived as "luxury medicine" [11, 39] and attracts many decision-makers and influencers as clients or patients in western countries). While a considerable number of Ayurveda associations exist on national levels and supranational levels, e.g., within the European Union and its member states, they remain rather small with very limited visibility in healthcare policy making and, in spite of several attempts by visionaries, pioneers, and mavericks over the last 30 years, have overall not been effective to change regulation in favor of Ayurveda there to date (e.g., EUAA [40], VEAT [41], VSAMT [42], DGA [43], DÄGAM [44], APA [45], NAMA [46], AAPNA [47]). Also, structures of most of these Ayurveda associations are quite heterogeneous. Moreover, interactions and cooperations between most Ayurveda associations are, if at all existent, loose or at times even controversial or adversary; notably, activities for forming an overarching Ayurveda umbrella organization are quite strong in Germany right now, which might be a template for other comparable national or supranational processes in the field.

(f) **The problem with nutritional supplements:**

To date, there are no Ayurvedic products that can officially be purchased as drugs on European markets. For instance, in Germany and all other European countries, all available products belong either to the categories of foods, food supplements, or cosmetics. The manufacturing of Ayurvedic preparations as drugs by German pharmacists is still not practicable, primarily due to economic reasons, based on the legal framework requiring drug manufacturing standards for all raw materials needed for drugs. As rare exceptions to the rule, products authorized as drugs abroad may be imported by international pharmacies based on individual prescriptions by a physician in small quantities. Also, attempts for getting official approval of Ayurveda products as traditional herbal medicine products in the European Union are currently hardly economically feasible because of the high costs involved for manufacturers, and even then, this would only be possible for a few products, most likely single herb preparations. Without amendments to existing regulations in western countries (e.g., of the THMPD in the European Union [48]), Ayurvedic preparations will either remain caught in the abovementioned "nutritional/dietary supplement trap" or will not be available at all in the medium and long term [49]. Another important aspect to consider in this context is the fact that the abundance of Ayurveda formulations, such as is found in India, is not available in western countries due to various reasons, e.g.:

- Varying legal requirements and restrictions from country to country (sometimes even from state to state)
- Lack of general availability of the majority of products in the West due to Ayurveda's overall "exotic status" in those places and therefore missing business incentives in the market segment
- Non-cover or lack of cover by all public and most private health insurance companies due to the products' statuses as foods and nutritional supplements, making it a compulsory out-of-the-pocket treatment

(g) **Sword of Damocles for Ayurveda in the West, heavy metals:**
The whole discussion about heavy metals within the broader context of Ayurveda use and practice is a major handicap for the recognition of Ayurveda in western countries and for its dissemination in their respective healthcare systems. Regardless of whether one is talking about their intentional use within *rasaśāstra* approaches or about the unintentional use of heavy metal-contaminated products through bad manufacturing practice or a mixture of both, the whole heavy metal issue looms like a sword of Damocles over Ayurveda in the West and has led to a number of widely cited publications in impact journals, issuing warnings about Ayurvedic products and therapy ranging from unemotional single case reports of heavy metal intoxications to reports of systematic testing results of available supplements and (sometimes sober, sometimes hysteric) alarms of dangerous herbal therapy, "plumbism," charlatanism, and witchcraft [50–60]. Since the use of Ayurvedic heavy metal products is prohibited in Europe and the USA and convincing clinical data from large randomized trials are missing, let aside the whole highly problematic issue of heavy metal contamination of, by formulation, heavy metal (through lacks of quality and safety both in drug manufacturing exporting countries and receiving importing countries), these products should not enter western markets at this time, particularly not under the less regulated categories of foods or food supplements.

11.3 Ayurveda Research in Western Countries: A Rough Status Quo

11.3.1 Where Is It Happening and in Which Academic Disciplines?

In several EU countries, particularly in Germany (e.g., Berlin, Essen, Heidelberg, Bielefeld), Italy (e.g., Milan), Latvia (e.g., Riga), Hungary (e.g., Debrecen), and the USA (e.g., San Francisco, Albuquerque, Baltimore), research on Ayurveda is being or has been performed during the last decades and centuries in some cases. Ayurveda as a whole system of medicine (and system of thought) has been more or less influenced by Indian systems of philosophy (particularly *Sāṃkhya*, *Yoga*, *Nyāya*,

Vaiśeṣika, *Vedānta*) and religion (predominantly Hinduism and Buddhism), not to forget overlaps to other (aspects of) traditional healing systems (e.g., Siddha, Unani, Greek medicine, Tibetan medicine) [2, 10]. Therefore research on Ayurveda abroad has never been limited to medical research. While western medical research activities in the field of Ayurveda have significantly increased over recent years, several other academic disciplines have also been researching on Ayurveda, e.g., indology, linguistics, religious sciences, philosophy, sociology, and psychology. For instance, indological and linguistic research has a long history in European countries, with the extensive works of the eminent Jan Meulenbeld being a prime example related most directly to Ayurveda [2].

It would go beyond the scope of this chapter to name all academic disciplines and institutes performing research on Ayurveda in western countries. While transdisciplinary research is much needed in order to cover all aspects of the multifaceted Ayurveda cosmos [26, 61], the focus here lies on a depiction of Ayurveda-related medical research outside of South Asia, since the author is primarily from the medical community. The following institutions are currently engaged in clinical or preclinical research with publication visibility in PubMed [62]:

- Germany
  - Charité Medical University Berlin/Immanuel Hospital Berlin [63] (research focuses: whole medical systems, trial methodology, transdisciplinary aspects, qualitative research, diagnostic studies, case reporting, integrative medicine)
  - University of Essen-Duisburg/Knappschafts-Krankenhaus Essen [64] (research focuses: psychosomatic diseases, musculoskeletal diseases, gastroenterology, dermatology, systematic reviews)
  - University of Bochum/Evangelisches Krankenhaus Hattingen [65] (research focuses: neurology, psychiatry, microbiomics)
  - European Academy of Ayurveda, Birstein [66] (research focuses: case reporting, Indology, epistemology)
- Latvia
  - University of Latvia, Riga [67] (diabetes, diabetic foot syndrome, reverse pharmacology, integrative medicine)
- Italy
  - University of Milan/Ayurvedic Point, Milan [68, 69] (research focuses: neurology, translational research, mental health, well-being)
- Hungary
  - University of Debrecen (research focuses: metabolic syndrome, *prakriti* mapping, nutrition, *panchakarma*)
- USA
  - University of California, San Francisco [70] (research focuses: whole medical system, diagnostic research, qualitative research, phytotherapy, oncology)
  - University of California, Los Angeles [71] (research focuses: rheumatology, phytopharmacology, placebo research)

- UK
  – Middlesex University [72] (research focuses: guidelines, case reporting, medical history)
- Australia
  – Swinburne University [73] (research focuses: systematic reviews)
  – University of Adelaide [74] (research focuses: systematic reviews)

11.4 Outlook: What Are the Next Steps?

(a) Ayurveda is a stand-alone, traditional, and highly complex whole system of medicine. For this reason identifying and developing appropriate research designs are necessary in order to analyze Ayurveda as what it is. Over the last decade, the discipline of whole systems research (WSR) has evolved, targeting to assess the complexity of whole system therapies—like Ayurveda—as system-level phenomena, in contrast to single-agent or pauci-dimensional effects (as often performed in "standard" efficacy RCTs). A centrality of WSR philosophy is addressing the need to include the unique healing theories and contexts into customized research methodology when assessing complex healthcare interventions, which Ayurveda embodies. Decision-makers in clinical research on Ayurveda should encourage (and enable financing of such) WMS research projects in order to scientifically advance the understanding of Ayurveda's individualized, multimodality approaches to diagnosis and treatment ([10, 75–78], Fig. 11.4).

(b) Hand in hand with whole systems research goes the need for mixed methods approaches and transdisciplinary/interdisciplinary research concepts in order to adequately address scientific questions regarding clinical Ayurveda practice in western countries. Looking at how Ayurveda is actually being practiced "abroad," this will need to include hybridization research and the inclusion of spiritual, religious, and psycho-emotional aspects, which are usually embedded into such Ayurveda care deliveries, but usually not covered by "standard" quantitative research methods (in spite of the fact that these aspects might have significant therapeutic effects!). Such interdisciplinary research approaches can involve teams including psychologists, sociologists, anthropologist, indologists, etc. alongside researchers with medical background, both Ayurvedic and conventional [26, 32, 33, 61].

Fig. 11.4 Efficacy-effectiveness continuum in Ayurveda research

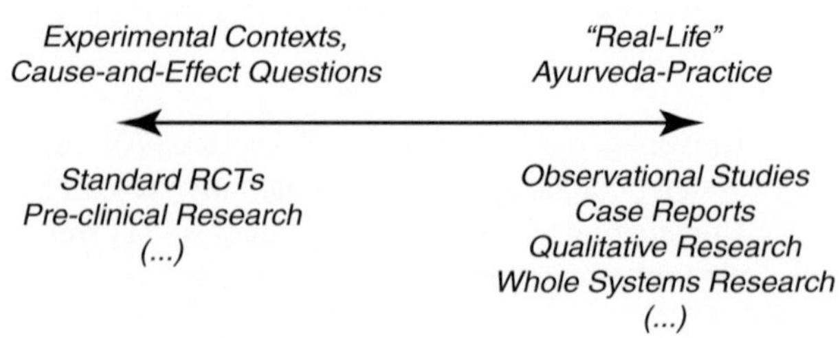

(c) A further "evolution" of (reverse) phytopharmacological complexity research and placebo methodology according to the specific needs and requirements of Ayurveda (as template for whole system of medicine) is warranted in order to demonstrate and prove that the pharmacological realm of Ayurveda can be well analyzed according to the principles of evidence-based medicine and RCT methodology [27, 28]. Based on the still very few but high-quality studies already existing in this field, a growing body of evidence will be a cornerstone in order to strengthen acceptance and availability of Ayurvedic herbal drugs in western countries. Here, a long-term goal could also be the establishment of Ayurvedic herbal drugs outside of South Asia as what they actually are: drugs and not (at least not in the majority of cases) "nutritional supplements," "superfoods," or "nutraceuticals," in order to guide western Ayurvedic phytotherapy out of the "supplement trap" [48, 49].

(d) Looking at the amount of ongoing clinical research projects and published papers in countries outside of South Asia the whole area is still in an infant stage. Also, as outlined before, effective funding and philanthropy networks are not yet (well) established for Ayurveda. For all these reasons, intensified case reporting in peer-reviewed medical mainstream journal (for instance, according to the CARE criteria) is an effective and rather low-cost way to generate awareness for the effectiveness of Ayurveda in the medical research community and among non-Ayurvedic healthcare providers. It will also facilitate to generate hypotheses for subsequent projects and can serve as a basis for brainstorming on which areas might be most promising to conduct clinical trials in. An increasing body of easily retrievable evidence in the form of case reports or case series will increase likelihoods for public funding in later stages. Eventually, Ayurveda case registries will need to be set up for these purposes in order to encourage, systematize, and synergize individual case reporting by medical professionals [79–81].

(e) Cost-effectiveness studies, pragmatic trials, and community-based research projects including patient-centered outcomes should be performed in order to demonstrate that Ayurveda is not only an effective system of medicine but can also be a cost-effective treatment approach when compared to mainstream medicine. Results from such studies will form an excellent basis for initiating discussions with insurance companies and other healthcare policy makers on issues related to costs, reimbursement, and regulation of Ayurvedic care delivery and, ultimately, the integration of elements of Ayurveda into public western healthcare settings [33, 82–85].

(f) Innovative basic, preclinical, and translational approaches, including omics research, based on already existing innovative research approaches from India and elsewhere, adapted to local resources and requirements are warranted as proof-of-principle approaches and to explain and translate Ayurvedic paradigms and epistemology into western medical language and thinking modes [24, 26, 29, 30, 86–92].

(g) It is essential to form effective national and supranational professional Ayurveda networks in order to adequately address and inform clinicians, healthcare policy makers, media and public, academicians, patients, and philanthropist/supporters of Ayurveda. Efforts by such organizations, particularly roof organizations, including university networks, therapeutic networks, patient support groups, and (most of all) medical professional organizations, will increase the visibility of Ayurveda in the West, shift its perception “from wellness to medicine,” and will be very helpful to pave its way into academics and research including scientific conferences, symposia, and CME-certified training options. In this context the advancement of Ayurveda in countries outside of South Asia also requires increased country-tailored AYUSH support, taking into account and respecting local, regional, and national regulatory frameworks. For this purpose outside the norm and unconventional solutions might be necessary in order to establish, e.g., Ayurveda professorships/chairs or international research collaboration cells at medical faculties outside of India. The same accounts for post-doctoral programs, research exchange programs, and public-private research funding initiatives for traditional Indian medicine.

(h) Ayurveda will need to become a more visible part of integrative medicine in western countries. So far it has been rather part of the “alternative” reality of CAM than part of “complementary” or “integrative” medicine. On an important side note, it needs mention that concepts of integrative medicine differ quite significantly between India and western countries when it comes to the integration of Ayurveda—currently, integrative medicine in India relates more to the integration of different systems by means of creating teams of experts from different medical systems rather than encouraging medical integration on the level of the individual medical professional (cross-system practice). While such individual integration might currently not be encouraged in India and Sri Lanka, it attracts many medical professionals in western countries and is certainly one of the main gateways to nurture and establish Ayurveda in countries outside of South Asia and should not be opposed in the West. Here, potential conflicts of interest between South Asian perspectives versus western perspectives on the integration of medical systems need to be put aside in order to nurture Ayurveda in western countries [10, 25, 38, 93, 94–101].

(i) So far, it is largely being taken for granted that Ayurvedic phytotherapy in western countries is performed by using drugs imported from South Asia. However, looking at the emphasis Ayurveda puts on regional and seasonal aspects in the context of foods and medicinal plants, a necessity arises to classify, cultivate, and ultimately use, for instance, European herbs within the paradigms of Ayurveda when practicing it in Europe, in order to make maximum use of local availabilities and “field symbioses,” not to forget ecological aspects and intellectual property issues [102–104].

(j) Measures to step up quality and safety of Ayurvedic care, particularly of Ayurvedic drugs, need to be taken at large. The whole chain of stakeholders—from farmers and producers via exporters and importers to sellers, pharmacies, and prescribers—needs to take utmost care that Ayurvedic care delivery and the administration of Ayurvedic herbals fully comply with local legal and regulatory requirements in western countries. Heavy metal-containing products must categorically not enter western markets at this point of time due to a number of reasons: (1) lack of clinical research according to the principles of EbM, (2) lack of experience in the usage of these products in western countries, (3) enormous resistance among medical professionals and the public against heavy metal-containing product based on (increasing) sporadic case reports on intoxications through such preparations in western patients, and most of all (4) the fact that import and prescription of heavy metal-containing drugs are illegal, e.g., in the EU and the USA. Anything else will cause colossal damage to the reputation and development of Ayurveda in western countries.

(k) Ultimately, Ayurveda guidelines, adapted to local structures, availabilities, and regulatory frameworks, should be adapted to serve Ayurveda care providers and researchers for informed decision-making as a form of twenty-first-century "evidence-based Ayurveda" in western contexts. Moreover, it would be of great strategic value to carry evidence-based elements of Ayurveda into conventional guidelines for chronic diseases in order to increase the visibility of Ayurveda in global medicine.

11.5 Epilogue

Lastly, considering all the abovementioned aspects and specificities of Ayurveda practices and perceptions abroad, it requires transcultural thinking modes and empathy for views and needs that might significantly differ from what one would probably expect to be a "traditional Indian" perspective on Ayurveda. Particularly in the research arena, it needs maximum transparency in communication and collaboration in order to achieve genuine understanding of each other's views and needs. In order to carefully nurture the rapidly growing but still fragile plant of Ayurveda outside its countries of origin, mutual respect for all involved traditions, both for the incoming and the hosting traditions/settings, is required, alongside genuine experimental openness and patience. Much can be done in the emerging field of Ayurveda's globalization if we all join hands in the spirit of *ācārya* Caraka, with India caringly and tolerantly driving the agenda: *kṛtsno hi loko buddhimātāmācārya—for the wise the whole world is a teacher* [7].

Acknowledgments I would like to express my sincere thanks to Dania Schumann and Dr. Vijayendra Murthy for editing this chapter for language and for their valuable advice. Thanks to Prof. Andreas Michalsen and Prof. Claudia Witt for having guided me in clinical research over the last decade. Big thanks also to my friend and colleague Elmar Stapelfeldt for always being a great source of inspiration. I am also most thankful to all my Ayurveda teachers near and far over the past 20 years. Thanks to my parents Carmen and Manfred for their lifelong support. Last but not least, the biggest thanks go to my wife Lea and our sons Noah and Jonah who are always with me with the most valuable thing on earth: love.

References

1. Meulenbeld GJ. The many faces of Ayurveda. Anc Sci Life. 1992;11(3–4):106–13.
2. Meulenbeld GJ. A history of Indian medical literature, vol. 2. Groningen: Egbert Forsten; 2000.
3. Frank R, Stollberg G. Conceptualizing hybridization on the diffusion of Asian medical knowledge to Germany. Int Sociol. 2004;19(1):71–88.
4. Hsu E. The transmission of Chinese medicine, vol. 7. Cambridge: Cambridge University Press; 1999. https://books.google.de/books?hl=de&lr=&id=c-L2pzRvt88C&oi=fnd&pg=PR8&dq=The+Transmission+of+Chinese+Medicine.+Cambridge:+University+Press.+&ots=XYBYg-CRzw&sig=pzDM8pk61cvurMNkhQimIelfCjg.
5. Alter JS. Yoga in modern India: the body between science and philosophy. Princeton: Princeton University Press; 2004. https://books.google.de/books?hl=de&lr=&id=o6anlz6i71oC&oi=fnd&pg=PR11&dq=joseph+alter+yoga+in+modern+india&ots=cSxlysRnnj&sig=9lYJbPXEcMFVr9u9pZ1FvKs7yYk.
6. Leslie CM, Young A. Paths to Asian medical knowledge, vol. 32. California: University of California Press; 1992. https://books.google.de/books?hl=de&lr=&id=yCusL4oT3OoC&oi=fnd&pg=PP11&dq=Epidemiological+issues+and+changing+legitimation:+traditional+medicine+in+the+twentieth+century&ots=xV0nbVr0wC&sig=bd9q8DjFZ70H21t7KFi_cWAC1CU.
7. Caraka, Agnivesa, Cakrapanidatta, Sarma RK, Dash B. Agnivesa's Caraka samhita: text with English translation & critical exposition based on Cakrapani Datta's Ayurveda dipika. Vimanasthana VIII.14. Chowkhamba Sanskrit Series Office; 2002.
8. Sharma PV (transl.). Sushruta samhita. English translation. Reprint 2010. Sutrasthana (Su.) 15.41. Varanasi: Chaukhambha Visvabharati; 2010.
9. Srikantha Murthy KR. Vaghbata astanga hrdayam. Śārīra sthāna. 3, 83; 2007.
10. Kessler C, Michalsen A. The role of whole medical systems in global medicine. Forsch Komplementärmed. 2012;19(2):65–6.
11. Frank R, Stollberg G. Ayurvedic patients in Germany. Anthropol Med. 2002;9(3):223–44.
12. Frank R, Stollberg G. German medical doctors' motives for practising homeopathy, acupuncture or ayurveda. In: Johannesen H, Lazar I, editors. Multiple medical realities patients healer biomedical alternative and traditional medicine. London: Berghahn Books; 2006. p. 72–88.
13. Naraindas H. Of relics, body parts and laser beams: the German Heilpraktiker and his Ayurvedic spa. Anthropol Med. 2011;18(1):67–86.
14. Naraindas H. Of spineless babies and folic acid: evidence and efficacy in biomedicine and Ayurvedic medicine. Soc Sci Med. 2006;62(11):2658–69.
15. Naraindas H, Quack J, Sax WS. asymmetrical conversations: contestations, circumventions, and the blurring of therapeutic boundaries, vol. 14. London: Berghahn Books; 2014. https://books.google.de/books?hl=de&lr=&id=rnAXAwAAQBAJ&oi=fnd&pg=PP5&dq=naraindas+ayurveda&ots=6EcEMGBC91&sig=ngGTvzcV8b9CBf11eOiFcoXNLz0.
16. Hausman GJ. Making medicine indigenous: homeopathy in South India. Soc Hist Med. 2002;15(2):303–22.
17. Dinges M. Medical pluralism and homoeopathy in India and Germany (1810–2010). Stuttg Steiner [Internet]. 2013. http://www.steiner-verlag.de/programm/fachbuch/akademien-und-wissenschaftliche-gesellschaften/reihen/view/titel/59911/print.html.
18. Hammer O. Claiming knowledge: strategies of epistemology from theosophy to the new age, vol. 90. The Netherland: Brill; 2003. https://books.google.de/books?hl=de&lr=&id=EZYsPQgBNioC&oi=fnd&pg=PR13&dq=claiming+knowledge+strategies+of+epistemologies&ots=Q8eLIXdMO8&sig=mDWLhJ2oCph4ClHFgruCIHUleGg.
19. WHO. Benchmarks for training in Ayurveda. Switzerland: WHO Press; 2010. http://www.who.int/medicines/areas/traditional/BenchmarksforTraininginAyurveda.pdf.
20. World Health Organization. WHO traditional medicine strategy: 2014-2023. Switzerland: WHO Press. 2013 [cited 2015 Oct 9]. http://apps.who.int/iris/bitstream/10665/92455/1/9789241506090_eng.pdf.

21. Organisation der Arbeitswelt KomplementärTherapie Organisation der Arbeitswelt KomplementärTherapie [Internet]. [cited 2017 Sep 22]. https://www.oda-kt.ch/.
22. Anonymous. CAMbrella European research network for complementary and alternative medicine [Internet]. 2015. http://www.cambrella.eu/home.php.
23. Katoch D, Sharma JS, Banerjee S, Biswas R, Das B, Goswami D, et al. Government policies and initiatives for development of Ayurveda. J Ethnopharmacol. 2017;197:25–31.
24. Chaturvedi S, Patwardhan B. Building bridges for integrative medicine. Lancet Psychiatry. 2016;3(8):705–6.
25. Manohar PR, Morandi A, Fave AD. The integration quagmire: why we need to watch our steps. Anc Sci Life. 2015;34(3):123–5.
26. Shankar D, Patwardhan B. AYUSH for new India: vision and strategy. J Ayurveda Integr Med. 2017;8(3):137–9.
27. Furst DE, Venkatraman MM, McGann M, Manohar PR, Booth-LaForce C, Sarin R, et al. Double-blind, randomized, controlled, pilot study comparing classic ayurvedic medicine, methotrexate, and their combination in rheumatoid arthritis. J Clin Rheumatol. 2011;17(4):185–92.
28. Furst DE, Venkatraman MM, Krishna Swamy BG, McGann M, Booth-Laforce C, Ram Manohar P, et al. Well controlled, double-blind, placebo-controlled trials of classical Ayurvedic treatment are possible in rheumatoid arthritis. Ann Rheum Dis. 2011;70(2):392–3.
29. Patwardhan B. Time for evidence-based Ayurveda: a clarion call for action. J Ayurveda Integr Med. 2013;4(2):63–6.
30. Patwardhan B, Bodeker G. Ayurvedic genomics: establishing a genetic basis for mind-body typologies. J Altern Complement Med. 2008;14(5):571–6.
31. Kessler C, Wischnewsky M, Michalsen A, Eisenmann C, Melzer J. Ayurveda: between religion, spirituality, and medicine. Evid Based Complement Altern Med. 2013;2013:952432.
32. Kessler CS, Eisenmann C, Oberzaucher F, Forster M, Steckhan N, Meier L, et al. Ayurvedic versus conventional dietary and lifestyle counseling for mothers with burnout-syndrome: a randomized controlled pilot study including a qualitative evaluation. Complement Ther Med. 2017;34:57–65. http://www.sciencedirect.com/science/article/pii/S0965229917300122.
33. Witt CM, Michalsen A, Roll S, Morandi A, Gupta S, Rosenberg M, et al. Comparative effectiveness of a complex Ayurvedic treatment and conventional standard care in osteoarthritis of the knee--study protocol for a randomized controlled trial. Trials. 2013;14:149.
34. Kessler C, Stapelfeldt E. Der lange Weg nach Westen. Dtsch Heilprakt-Z. 2016;11(4):62–5.
35. O'Cathail S, Stebbing J. Ayurveda: alternative or complementary? Lancet Oncol. 2012;13(9):865.
36. New age orientalism: Ayurvedic "wellness and spa culture": Health Sociol Rev. 21(2) [Internet]. [cited 2017 Sep 10]. http://www.tandfonline.com/doi/abs/10.5172/hesr.2012.21.2.220.
37. Suchergebnis auf Amazon.de für: ayurveda [Internet]. [cited 2017 Sep 25]. https://www.amazon.de/s/ref=nb_sb_noss?__mk_de_DE=%C3%85M%C3%85%C5%BD%C3%95%C3%91&url=search-alias%3Daps&field-keywords=ayurveda.
38. Sujatha V. What could "integrative" medicine mean? Social science perspectives on contemporary Ayurveda. J Ayurveda Integr Med. 2011;2(3):115–23.
39. Frank R, Stollberg G. [Are patients of Asian medicine active consumers?] Forsch Komplementarmed Klass Naturheilkd. 2004;11(2):83–92.
40. European Ayurveda Association. European Ayurveda Association [Internet]. 2015. http://www.euroayurveda.eu/.
41. http://www.ayurveda-verband.eu [Internet]. [cited 2017 Sep 25]. https://www.ayurveda-verband.eu/.
42. Schweizer Ayurveda Verband | Verband Schweizer Ayurveda -Mediziner und -Therapeuten [Internet]. [cited 2017 Sep 25]. http://www.vsamt.ch/de/home/.
43. Home [Internet]. [cited 2017 Sep 25]. http://www.ayurveda.de/.
44. Deutsche Ärztegesellschaft für Ayurveda-Medizin. Deutsche Ärztegesellschaft für Ayurveda-Medizin [Internet]. 2015. [cited 2015 Oct 9]. www.daegam.de
45. Ayurvedic Professionals Association—Representing Ayurvedic Practitioners throughout the United Kingdom [Internet]. [cited 2017 Nov 7]. http://apa.uk.com/.

46. National Ayurvedic Medical Association. National Ayurvedic Medical Association [Internet]. 2015. [cited 2015 Oct 9]. http://www.ayurvedanama.org/.
47. AAPNA | Association of Ayurvedic Professionals of North America, Inc. [Internet]. Association of Ayurvedic Professionals of North America. [cited 2017 Sep 25]. http://aapna.org/.
48. Herbal medicinal products—Public Health—European Commission [Internet]. Public Health. [cited 2017 Sep 10]. /health/human-use/herbal-medicines_en.
49. Israelsen L, Lampe F. Three myths about dietary supplements … and how knowing the right answers is good for your integrative medicine practice. Integr Med (Encinitas). 2016;15(3):20–4.
50. Budnik LT, Baur X, Harth V, Hahn A. Alternative drugs go global: possible lead and/or mercury intoxication from imported natural health products and a need for scientifically evaluated poisoning monitoring from environmental exposures. J Occup Med Toxicol. 2016;11:49.
51. Douros A, Bronder E, Andersohn F, Klimpel A, Kreutz R, Garbe E, et al. Herb-induced liver injury in the Berlin case-control surveillance study. Int J Mol Sci. 2016;17(1):114.
52. Saper RB, Phillips RS, Sehgal A, Khouri N, Davis RB, Paquin J, et al. Lead, mercury, and arsenic in US- and Indian-manufactured Ayurvedic medicines sold via the internet. JAMA. 2008;300(8):915–23.
53. Raviraja A, Vishal Babu GN, Sehgal A, Saper RB, Jayawardene I, Amarasiriwardena CJ, et al. Three cases of lead toxicity associated with consumption of ayurvedic medicines. Indian J Clin Biochem. 2010;25(3):326–9.
54. Gupta HH. Ayurveda und Schwermetalle–Versuch einer Aufklärung. Z Für Komplementärmed. 2016;8(03):54–8.
55. Mehta V, Midha V, Mahajan R, Narang V, Wander P, Sood R, et al. Lead intoxication due to ayurvedic medications as a cause of abdominal pain in adults. Clin Toxicol (Phila). 2017;55(2):97–101.
56. Breyre A, Green-McKenzie J. Case of acute lead toxicity associated with Ayurvedic supplements. BMJ Case Rep. 2016;30:2016.
57. Sadler M, Bell S. Ayurvedic plumbism. Intern Med J. 2017;47(7):823–5.
58. Orchard GR, Hielscher KA, Wilke AD, Thomae MKB, Presneill JJ. Lead poisoning in Australia associated with privately imported Ayurvedic complementary medicine. Anaesth Intensive Care. 2015;43(5):669–70.
59. Tsutsui RS, Van Schalkwyk J, Spriggs D. Lead poisoning from Ayurvedic medicines. N Z Med J. 2013;126(1374):80–3.
60. Spriewald BM, Rascu A, Schaller KH, Angerer J, Kalden JR, Harrer T. Lead induced anaemia due to traditional Indian medicine: a case report. Occup Environ Med. 1999;56(4):282–3.
61. Bode M, Shankar P. Ayurvedic college education, reifying biomedicine and the need for reflexivity. Anthropol Med. 2017;16:1–14.
62. pubmeddev. Home - PubMed - NCBI [Internet]. [cited 2017 Oct 1]. https://www.ncbi.nlm.nih.gov/pubmed/.
63. Naturheilkunde in Berlin am Immanuel Krankenhaus—Home [Internet]. [cited 2017 Oct 1]. http://naturheilkunde.immanuel.de/home/.
64. Kliniken Essen-Mitte: Home [Internet]. [cited 2017 Oct 1]. http://www.kliniken-essen-mitte.de/naturheilkunde.
65. Ev. Krankenhaus Hattingen | Komplementärmedizin [Internet]. [cited 2017 Oct 1]. https://www.augusta-bochum.de/evk/evk_komplementaer.html.
66. Ayurveda-Ausbildung und -Weiterbildung | Europäische Akademie für Ayurveda [Internet]. [cited 2017 Oct 1]. https://www.ayurveda-akademie.org/home/.
67. Internal Medicine Department—University of Latvia [Internet]. [cited 2017 Oct 1]. Available from: https://www.lu.lv/eng/faculties/fm/structural-units/internal-medicine-department/
68. Dipartimento di Fisiopatologia Medico-Chirurgica e dei Trapianti—Università degli Studi di Milano [Internet]. [cited 2017 Oct 1]. http://www.unimi.it/chiedove/schedaStrutturaXML.jsp?codice=6588.
69. Ayurvedic Point [Internet]. [cited 2017 Oct 1]. http://www.ayurvedicpoint.it/.

70. Osher Center for Integrative Medicine [Internet]. [cited 2017 Oct 1]. https://www.osher.ucsf.edu/.
71. UCLA Health—Los Angeles, CA [Internet]. [cited 2017 Oct 1]. https://www.uclahealth.org/.
72. Home | Middlesex University London [Internet]. [cited 2017 Oct 1]. http://www.mdx.ac.uk/.
73. Centre for Human Psychopharmacology | Swinburne University | Melbourne [Internet]. [cited 2017 Oct 1]. http://www.swinburne.edu.au/research/human-psychopharmacology/.
74. Facebook, Twitter, LinkedIn, YouTube, Google+, Rss, et al. Faculty of Health Sciences | Faculty of Health and Medical Sciences [Internet]. [cited 2017 Oct 1]. https://health.adelaide.edu.au/admissions/interview/help/.
75. Ritenbaugh C, Aickin M, Bradley R, Caspi O, Grimsgaard S, Musial F. Whole systems research becomes real: new results and next steps. J Altern Complement Med. 2010;16(1):131–7.
76. Ritenbaugh C, Verhoef M, Fleishman S, Boon H, Leis A. Whole systems research: a discipline for studying complementary and alternative medicine. Altern Ther Health Med. 2003;9(4):32–6.
77. Elder C, Aickin M, Bell IR, Fønnebø V, Lewith GT, Ritenbaugh C, et al. Methodological challenges in whole systems research. J Altern Complement Med. 2006;12(9):843–50.
78. Lachance LL, Hawthorne V, Brien S, Hyland ME, Lewith GT, Verhoef MJ, et al. Delphi-derived development of a common core for measuring complementary and alternative medicine prevalence. J Altern Complement Med. 2009;15(5):489–94.
79. Gagnier JJ, Kienle G, Altman DG, Moher D, Sox H, Riley D. The CARE guidelines: consensus-based clinical case reporting guideline development. BMJ Case Rep [Internet]. 2013;2013. https://www.ncbi.nlm.nih.gov/pmc/articles/PMC3822203/.
80. Kessler C, Stapelfeldt E, Michalsen A, Kowalcek I, Kronpaß L, Dhruva A. The effect of a complex multi-modality Ayurvedic treatment in a case of unknown female infertility. Forsch Komplementarmed. 2015;22(4):251–8.
81. Rastogi S. Low-pressure, low-flow voiding dysfunction in an elderly male treated through Ayurveda: a case report. J Evid Based Complement Altern Med. 2017;22(4):846–50. https://doi.org/10.1177/2156587217712764.
82. Witt CM, Manheimer E, Hammerschlag R, Lüdtke R, Lao L, Tunis SR, et al. How well do randomized trials inform decision making: systematic review using comparative effectiveness research measures on acupuncture for back pain. PLoS One. 2012;7(2):e32399. https://www.ncbi.nlm.nih.gov/pmc/articles/PMC3289651/.
83. Witt CM, Aickin M, Baca T, Cherkin D, Haan MN, Hammerschlag R, et al. Effectiveness guidance document (EGD) for acupuncture research - a consensus document for conducting trials. BMC Complement Altern Med. 2012;12:148.
84. Witt CM, Rafferty Withers S, Grant S, Lauer MS, Tunis S, Berman BM. What can comparative effectiveness research contribute to integrative health in international perspective? J Altern Complement Med. 2014;20(11):874–80.
85. Loudon K, Zwarenstein M, Sullivan F, Donnan P, Treweek S. Making clinical trials more relevant: improving and validating the PRECIS tool for matching trial design decisions to trial purpose. Trials. 2013;14:115.
86. Prasher B, Varma B, Kumar A, Khuntia BK, Pandey R, Narang A, et al. Ayurgenomics for stratified medicine: TRISUTRA consortium initiative across ethnically and geographically diverse Indian populations. J Ethnopharmacol. 2017;197:274–93.
87. Tiwari P, Kutum R, Sethi T, Shrivastava A, Girase B, Aggarwal S, et al. Recapitulation of Ayurveda constitution types by machine learning of phenotypic traits. PLoS One. 2017;12(10):e0185380.
88. Stranieri A, Butler-Henderson K, Sahama T, Perera PK, Da Silva JL, Pelonio D, et al. A visual grid to digitally record an Ayurvedic Prakriti assessment; a first step toward integrated electronic health records. J Tradit Complement Med. 2017;7(2):264–8.
89. Bhalerao S, Patwardhan K. Prakriti-based research: good reporting practices. J Ayurveda Integr Med. 2016;7(1):69–72.
90. Kurande V, Bilgrau AE, Waagepetersen R, Toft E, Prasad R. Interrater reliability of diagnostic methods in traditional Indian ayurvedic medicine. Evid Based Complement Altern Med. 2013;2013:658275.

91. Kurande VH, Waagepetersen R, Toft E, Prasad R. Reliability studies of diagnostic methods in Indian traditional Ayurveda medicine: an overview. J Ayurveda Integr Med. 2013;4(2):67–76.
92. Delle Fave A, Negri L, Manohar PR, Morandi A, Bassi M. The Ayurveda concept of Prakṛti and the western construct of personality: a comparative pilot study. Eur J Integr Med. 2015;7(4):396–408.
93. Hegyi G, Petri RP, Roberti di Sarsina P, Niemtzow RC. Overview of integrative medicine practices and policies in NATO participant countries. Med Acupunct. 2015;27(5):318–27.
94. Fischer FH, Lewith G, Witt CM, Linde K, von Ammon K, Cardini F, et al. High prevalence but limited evidence in complementary and alternative medicine: guidelines for future research. BMC Complement Altern Med. 2014;14:46.
95. Reiter B, Baumhöfener F, Dlaboha M, Odde Madsen J, Regenfelder S, Weidenhammer W. Building a sustainable complementary and alternative medicine research network in Europe. Forsch Komplementarmedizin 2006. 2012;19(Suppl 2):61–8.
96. Weidenhammer W, Brinkhaus B. CAMbrella--a pan-European research network for complementary and alternative medicine: from the beginnings up to first results. Forsch Komplementarmed. 2012;19(Suppl 2):3–5.
97. Josyula KL, Sheikh K, Nambiar D, Narayan VV, Sathyanarayana TN, Porter JDH. "Getting the water-carrier to light the lamps": Discrepant role perceptions of traditional, complementary, and alternative medical practitioners in government health facilities in India. Soc Sci Med. 2016;166:214–22.
98. Morandi A, Tosto C. Ayurvedic point: the Italian way to Ayurveda. J Ayurveda Integr Med. 2010;1(2):141–5.
99. Morandi A, Narayanan Nambi AN. An integrated view of health and well-being. Berlin: Springer; 2013 [cited 2017 Feb 24]. http://link.springer.com/content/pdf/10.1007/978-94-007-6689-1.pdf.
100. Niemi M, Ståhle G. The use of ayurvedic medicine in the context of health promotion—a mixed methods case study of an ayurvedic centre in Sweden. BMC Complement Altern Med. 2016;16:62. https://www.ncbi.nlm.nih.gov/pmc/articles/PMC4756420/.
101. Hu X-Y, Lorenc A, Kemper K, Liu J-P, Adams J, Robinson N. Defining integrative medicine in narrative and systematic reviews: a suggested checklist for reporting. Eur J Integr Med. 2015;7(1):76–84.
102. Schrott E, Ammon HPT. Heilpflanzen der ayurvedischen und der westlichen Medizin. Berlin: Springer; 2012.
103. Schrott E. Weihrauch: seine au\s sergewöhnliche Heilwirkung neu entdeckt;[sanfte, natürliche und wirksame Hilfe bei: Rheuma, Allergien, Hauterkrankungen und Darmentzündungen]. Aurum-Verlag in J. Kamphausen Verlag; 2003.
104. Chaudhary A, Singh N. Intellectual property rights and patents in perspective of Ayurveda. Ayu. 2012;33(1):20–6.

12 Dreaming of Health for All in an Unequal World: Finding a Fit for Traditional Health Care Exemplified Through Ayurveda

Sanjeev Rastogi and Arindam Bhattacharya

12.1 Introduction

We live in a diverse and unequal world. There are diversities by virtue of nature making some places more resourceful than the others. There are man-made inequalities too widening the gap between the resource-rich and resource-poor communities on the opposing poles of a socioeconomic globe. Historically, natural resources backed with technological advances supported the economical growth of some parts of the world to the extent that it lead to economic revolution marked with improved buying power and subsequent living standards of their inhabitants. Such socioeconomic differences have their definitive impacts on the "nutrition-health-disease" trio obviously seen in various parts of the world. Originating through their intimate micro- and macroenvironment, the health-care problems of resource-poor economy are found grossly different than that of resource-rich economy. Obviously, the problems originating through different routes require a differential treatment too. "One shoe does not fit all" seems highly applicable in global health-care scenario with emergent regional problems requiring indigenous solutions suiting to such regional needs. It is in this background, the question of health for all required a thorough revisit in light of differential health-care needs of the people and finding their effective and sustainable solutions fitting suitably to the socioethnic and economic background of the addressed people.

Arindam Bhattacharya is from Indian Foreign Service (2004) and had worked for 5 years as Special Secretary, to Government of Uttar Pradesh, India, in the Department of Medical Education and AYUSH.

S. Rastogi (✉)
Department of Kaya Chikitsa, State Ayurvedic College and Hospital, Lucknow University, Lucknow, India

A. Bhattacharya
Government of Uttar Pradesh, Lucknow, India

S. Rastogi (ed.), *Translational Ayurveda*, https://doi.org/10.1007/978-981-13-2062-0_12

Effective utilization of the traditional health-care wisdom prevalent in various parts of the globe on the lanes of mainstream medicine could be one pragmatic way of reaching the dream goal of health for all. Such health-care systems, for the very purpose of their effective utilization in health-care delivery, are initially required to be thoroughly explored and investigated for their possible roles in an affirmative way. Once realistically identified on evidence-based lines, the goal should be to determine and to fix every alternative health-care system with clearly defined responsibilities to be taken up for coming decades with equally clear and defined deliverables. Plans are required to be made accordingly, and an execution framework should be designed in a way that such identified goals can be met positively within a stipulated time frame.

12.2 From "Health for All" to "Leaving No One Behind": The Dream and the Reality

"Health for all" was an idealistic proposal made at Alma-Ata (1978) during the WHO International Conference on Primary Health Care. This congress clearly declared that:

> *An acceptable level of health for all the people of the world by the year 2000 can be attained through a fuller and better use of the world's resources, a considerable part of which is now spent on armaments and military conflicts. A genuine policy of independence, peace, détente and disarmament could and should release additional resources that could well be devoted to peaceful aims and in particular to the acceleration of social and economic development of which primary health care, as an essential part, should be allotted its proper share.* [1]

The focus of Alma-Ata declaration was on better resource utilization through drifting it in a constructive way while keeping the primary health care as an essential mechanism to achieve the goal of health for all. Three years later to this declaration, in 1981, Halfdan Mahler, Director General (1973–1983) of the WHO, defined and expanded the phrase "health for all" as follows:

> *Health For All means that health is to be brought within reach of everyone in a given country. And by "health" is meant a personal state of well being, not just the availability of health services—a state of health that enables a person to lead a socially and economically productive life. Health For All implies the removal of the obstacles to health—that is to say, the elimination of malnutrition, ignorance, contaminated drinking water and unhygienic housing—quite as much as it does the solution of purely medical problems such as a lack of doctors, hospital beds, drugs and vaccines* [2].

Halfdan, through his expansion of the phrase, actually proposed health for all as ensuring universal accessibility to all available means needed to achieve good health. These means may essentially relate to preventive, promotive, and curative methods of disowning the disease and owning the health. With this definition of health for all by Halfdan, we find that traditional health-care systems convincingly find a perfect fit into the context for their straightforward roles in preventive and promotive health care, besides acting adjunctly at curative health-care front.

Looking back at the debate of health for all, we see that after about four decades farther of the Alma-Ata declaration, the initial goal of bringing "an acceptable level of health for all the people of the world by the year 2000" is still far from sight. Still the dream is the same although the phrase has changed to "leave no one behind" in the current Sustainable Development Goals (SDG) declaration of 2015. The utopian goal of health for all, upon facing the practical difficulties, got gradually transformed into the Millennium Development Goal (MDG) in 2000 having a 15-year timeline to arrive at determined millennium goals. In 2015, upon the completion of MDG, this was taken over by Sustainable Development Goals (SDG) for another term of 15 years with an objective of reaching the specified goals by 2030. What we had in MDG and what we have now in SDG, in the essence, are same as what was actually meant at Alma-Ata. The question is still the same with only a little progress to show on many fronts in past four decades [3].

In this long relay race aiming to achieve the ultimate objective of health for all, while changing the baton every time through changing the plans every 15 years, what missed was to take an account of preventive and promotive health care where traditional health wisdom could have emerged as a major stakeholder for their own strengths. A regional peculiarity in terms of local needs and resources has also not been taken much into account while addressing the policy. While the objectives and the goals might be the same for every country referring to the ultimate aim of reaching health for all, we strongly argue that the means of its arrival may be different depending upon the available strengths, resources, immediate and ultimate health-care requirements of the country, and most importantly the indigenous knowledge sources which can help its smooth arrival. The argument is more crucial for the countries like India and China which have a strong traditional health-care knowledge base capable of meeting the health-care needs of their people to a large extent. The argument here is to define the health-care goals as per the global standards but with all liberty to choose the ways which are most suiting to the native situations.

In the year 2000 when MDG was launched, out of its eight focused goals which 191 UN member states agreed to achieve by 2015, at least three had a clear notion of being linked with health. These were to reduce child mortality, to improve maternal health, and to combat HIV/AIDS, malaria, and other diseases. Besides these three, others were interdependent and influential to health and vice versa [4]. SDG, coming next in the row, launched from 1 January 2016 had 17 goals which were broader and more ambitious than the MDGs, keeping a central agenda of "leaving no one behind" a slogan much akin to "health for all" of Alma-Ata.

What we are able to see through recent history of such movements aiming at equitable, affordable, and accessible health care to everyone is that their focus is gradually shifting toward curative health care with a dominating attention on a few conditions while leaving others behind. Preventive health care has also been narrowed to vaccination and immunization alone, and finally the concept of promotive health care is seen largely missing in the scenario. Most importantly and sadly, so far, the health-care knowledge prevalent indigenously in many countries could not truly find a respectable place in mainstream health-care plans aiming to dream of "health for all" for their countrymen. Unfortunately, for this reason, health for all is wrongly equated with increase in number of health-care facilities focusing upon curative health care without taking a note of the steps which might curtail the actual curative need in many instances.

12.3 Traditional Health-Care Wisdom: Why This Shouldn't Be Ignored?

Past few decades have added tremendously to the human understanding of disease and health. A few landmark discoveries in the field of biology have made it easy to look deep into the cellular and molecular intricacies of causes of diseases and their remedies. Rapid advances in the field of chemistry and physics in tune with biology through disciplines like biochemistry and biophysics have made extraordinary efforts to develop tools able to find fine mechanistic details of human biology helping immensely in the disease diagnosis, the prognosis, and the progress of a biological process leading to recovery or decay. Although, this glittering growth of science makes one feel that it is only a recent phenomenon and had never been attempted or thought before, the truth is however contrary. Opposing to this often prevailing thought, an effortful look into the past may show us glorious glimpses of the science flourished in the earlier times, which had kept humanity surviving and moving ahead before the dawn of new age science. Human civilization is older than four millennia, whereas the phase of current scientific boom accounts only for less than 200 years. What has been done through past many centuries to make human life comfortable was no less important for the reason that it formed the foundation of what is being celebrated now. Previous discoveries in the field of science which have been the turning points of human civilization like that of fire, wheel, metallurgy, and architecture have been the marvels of their time possibly more crucial than many of noble winning discoveries of present. Genuinely, if we are running ahead in the race, it is only because we have been handed over a legacy to carry forward.

Although important from many perspectives of traditional wisdom in many diverse areas, traditional health-care wisdom needs a particular attention. We have strong reasons for not ignoring what we have learned in the past because still we don't have the replies to all our miseries related to health and diseases. Proposal of five proto-elements (*panchamahabhuta*) theory of Ayurveda and its transition into *tridosha* theory was a beautiful convergence of a pure physicochemical entity entering into a dynamic biological understanding. Linking the macrocosm with the microcosm (universe with the living body = *lok purusha samya* theory) was the epitome of this theory which explained beautifully how the nature through five proto-elements affects the life and vice versa. Invention of nanotechnology in Ayurveda in order to design more succinct and effective formulations requiring lesser doses and time to act was a remarkable breakthrough made in the early part of this millennium. This was actually the practical merger of life science and metallurgy science which was flourishing to its peak during that period. This discipline, better known as *rasa shastra* (the science of mercury and other metals), was no less important than that of antibiosis theory of modern science. Many other alternative health-care models like that of homeopathy also stand apart by virtue of their merits and distinct theoretical excellence. Unfortunately, although we see many of such systems working excellently on selected patients, we still could not develop the technical know-how to look deep into the fine details of such applications, and hence their generalization remained extremely limited. This reminds us of a saying of Nicola Tesla [5] stating:

> *It is paradoxical, yet true, to say, that the more we know, the more ignorant we become in the absolute sense, for it is only through enlightenment that we become conscious of our limitations. Precisely one of the most gratifying results of intellectual evolution is the continuous opening up of new and greater prospects.*

Accepting the limitations of one's perception yet admiring the observational truth despite being unaware of their "how" and "why" actually opens up a completely unvisited vista of progress by generating curiosity to know the unknown. It is important to understand here that the applications of the observation often do not require the meticulous explanations of how and why, and if at all the applications are waited till we understand the phenomenon, we would simply be keeping ourselves away from the benefits of natural truth. The cost of defying the truth owing to the ignorance of few sometimes requires to be paid back through nose for keeping the whole generation away from the bounty of benefits available at the doorsteps. Cost of ignoring the mother's milk in early 1970s is one critical example of the same where a scientific ignorance has led to the propagation of a wrong message about mother's milk speaking of its inferiority compared to the formula milk. We now know that for over two decades, the babies had to be deprived of the breast feeding just because of this wrong perception and misled science [6]. The debate is still on, and now this is for beneficial versus adverse effects of consuming milk and *ghee* [7]. *Ghee*, particularly the one made of cow milk, has long been promoted in Ayurveda for its *rasayana* (rejuvenative) and antiaging benefits. It is also presumed to be an *agni* promoter (metabolic enhancer) and hence is recommended for its routine consumption on daily basis for its sustained tissue nourishing *rasayana* effects (*ksheera ghrita abhyasa* = daily practice of consuming milk and *ghrita*). Unfortunately, linking fat in general with obesity, cardiovascular diseases, and diabetes [8] has created a global anti-wave against the use of all sorts of fat including *ghee* without discriminating between the good and the bad fat. Ayurveda, in particular, recommends many distinct medicinal usage of *ghee*. For most psychiatric and neurological disorders, *ghee* is a preferred vehicle to enhance the properties of the herbs besides acting as a strong medicine by itself in such conditions. There are evidences that contrary to the cardiovascular risk hype about *ghee* consumption, it actually lowers the cardiovascular risk in a significant proportion [9]. In such conditions, ignoring a knowledge on the basis of lack of clarity or misappropriation may be a gross loss to the society as a whole [10].

Similar is the negative hype about safety of Ayurvedic drugs. There are plenty of retrospective case reports speculating the adversities caused by consumption of different Ayurvedic drugs. Higher levels of heavy metals in Ayurvedic formulations are often attributed to the adversities in all such cases [11]. Unfortunately despite such scary reporting of adversities, we did not find any serious attempt anywhere in the world where a prospective development of such adversities has ever been demonstrated. On the contrary we find the reports showing the clinical improvements in cases of compromised vitals where the use of Ayurvedic formulations known to contain mercury which is otherwise incriminated as causing heavy metal toxicity [12]. Although such cases are less in number in published literature, contemporary Ayurvedic clinical practice has plenty of such examples where the people given up by conventional medicine responded well by Ayurvedic therapy which may or may not be consisting of formulations having heavy metals [13]. Although this cannot be denied that a few Ayurvedic drugs might be causing adversities to few people, at the same time, beneficial effects of the same drugs on a larger population should also not be underestimated, and hence a judicious inference about "what causes adversity in whom" referring to Ayurvedic drugs should be carefully established. This will help us in identifying the defined subpopulation which might get adversely affected with a class of drug whereas sparing others to enjoy the benefits. A scientific research may subsequently probe into making better approaches to make the drugs completely safe for the entire population.

Yet another reason which makes traditional health care a perfect fit in "health for all" scenario is its economy. Economy of such health care comes through two important converging pathways. One is that it relies largely upon local resources which are undoubtedly cheaper and available nearby hence not requiring much of the transportation cost. Second is that, in many cases, in the absence of standard care requiring a sophisticated health-care setting, it keeps open the options of practical care where a similar care may be provided at home without a significant dilution of treatment efficacy. A few procedures of *panchakarma* give an excellent example of this where the patients or the care giver may be given an opportunity to learn home-based care initially which can easily be done at home without coming to the hospital. Such examples are also there with drugs and formulations where number of such preparations can actually be made or prepared fresh at home for better result than obtainable from the medicine bought from the hospital. Preparations of various decoctions (*kwath*) and extracts (*swarasa*) at home are such examples which are extensively used in Ayurvedic clinical practice in various states in India.

Now if we can find a combination of efficacy along with economy even for certain conditions through Ayurveda, naturally this should be chosen as the frontline care at least for that matter.

12.4 Ayurveda: What It Promises to Offer?

To make the world a healthier place to live and to make its inhabitant healthier as a prelude to "health for all," traditional health-care wisdom can be shared with greater responsibilities. Initially, to understand where Ayurveda can join as dependable and accountable stakeholder in the domain of health, it is important to understand what it actually promises and what it actually offers in a concurrent sense. Subsequently, if the gaps are visualized between the promises and the practices, the reasons of such gaps may be delineated and filled to ensure a better delivery.

Such promises of Ayurveda, in the fundamental sense, are wide spectrum, covering broad areas directly or indirectly influencing the health. Beginning from a vivid description of individual code of conduct contextual to societal norms and eco-preservation, it reaches farther into individual affliction of diseases by observation of improper conduct or mass affliction like that in cases of endemic, epidemic, or pandemic occurring due to a gross misconduct of the society or due to an environmental malpresentation. By proposing an intimate, dynamic, and reciprocal relationship between microcosm and macrocosm, Ayurveda puts a large stress upon balancing both to keep them mutually supportive.

Ayurveda promises to act on all fronts of health care like preventive, promotive, supportive, palliative, and curative. At all these fronts, however, it has some of its merits and demerits. The merits are that Ayurvedic approaches in all these segments are collective, comprehensive, and inclusive of every factor that might be playing a role in that matter. Linking health with various associated factors like nutrition, safe drinking water, pollution, and stress besides the direct causes of disease and proposing their remedies was attempted by Ayurveda millenniums before it was thought and conceived as health-related MDG and SDG of recent times. Adding further to this, Ayurveda meticulously attempted the development of guidelines and protocols on various issues directly and indirectly relating to health. Most notable among such contributions are development of a comprehensive protocol related to methods of food consumption (*ahara vidhi visheshayatan*), dietary incompatibility (*virudddha ahara*), and identification of disease promotive and disease suppressive (*pathya* and *apathya*) foods. Besides this a comprehensive protocol of dos and don'ts in order to remain healthy incorporating almost everything mattering to human life is a unique contribution of Ayurveda. Classification of human population on the basis of the biological specifications and subsequently finding its pharmacogenomics-based clinical application is something which was approached in Ayurveda thousands of years before the current thought of personalized medicine [14].

Rasayana therapy and *panchakarma* are two unique approaches of Ayurveda toward health promotion. *Rasayana* by means of certain drugs, foods, and health-promotive activities proposes to minimize the aging effect both physically and physiologically. This is one praiseworthy science embedded in Ayurveda which principally ensures optimal productivity of an individual by ensuring the intactness of his/her functional capabilities suiting to the age. Besides adding to the productivity, eventually this also helps reducing the cost of the burden being created due to inappropriate functional losses not justifiable by the chronological aging. *Panchakarma*, on the other hand, is a novel bio-physico purification protocol, aiming at micro-cleaning at cellular level. The cleaning invoked by *panchakarma* is more pervasive and subtle compared to the gross cleaning observed during the routine excretory process. By adopting a scientifically designed protocol for specific *panchakarma* procedure, it mobilizes the biowaste accumulated in the conduits, cells, and tissues, conventionally unapproachable by routine cleansing process.

A carefully done *panchakarma* results in enhanced biological activity of the tissues, organs, and systems resulting in their better efficiency and performance.

Likewise, there are many more advantages associated with Ayurveda which are novel and unique to this system and which can substantially help in the health keeping both at individual and at community level. The problem however with such promises is that these have not been tested in the field and the classical protocols have not been clearly translated in tune to the contemporary needs along with the justification for each and every step recommended to be followed eventually to obtain a specific set of benefits.

12.5 Frontline Care from Ayurveda: The Areas and the Concerns?

What are the areas where Ayurveda can be equated to conventional therapy in terms of outcomes? What are the areas where Ayurveda can help in improving the net outcome as a supportive therapy? What are the areas where after the primary treatment given from conventional medicine, Ayurveda can take over for the maintenance therapy? And finally, what are the areas where Ayurveda can be considered as a stand-alone therapy at its own with proven benefits? These are the questions which are required to be answered honestly if we wish to crystallize and prioritize the role of Ayurveda in the purview of health for all.

Considering Ayurveda as primary and stand-alone intervention in certain areas which are completely unique to it and which do not exist in conventional medicine looks like a promising avenue to work on. There can be many such areas, but to begin with, a few most important ones among them can be listed as *rasayana* and *panchakarma*. *Rasayana*, for its postulated benefits of delaying the degenerative pathologies as a result of aging process, seems valuable to improve the quality of life of the aging population and also to reduce the burden of degenerative diseases prevalent in growing population. India is consistently rising in terms of its elderly population, and by the year 2050, it is expected to comprise 19% of total Indian population compared to its 8% share currently. In numbers this is expected to be tripled by reaching 300 million compared to 100 million as of now [15]. By proposing generic *rasayana*, Ayurveda recommends a few formulations having their effects on overall aging process, and also by proposing tissue-/organ-/system-specific *rasayana*, it proposes specific formulations intending to improve certain specific functions. There can be many feasible applications to such interventions in order to prevent or delay the onset of degenerative pathologies, eventually to ensure the optimal functioning and hence the optimal productivity for extended period and at the same time reduction of the cost supposed to be paid for care of such pathologies besides a loss of productivity. Any such ambitious plan however needs to have some basic ground work before it can be taken to the phase of execution. Researches to screen fine details of such applications in terms of identifying the beneficiaries, the benefits, and exhaustive details of the plan of the interventions are required to be seriously attempted before such pragmatic plans may be taken on ground. If found consistent with what it promises, *rasayana* may find an easy place among school-going children through existing schemes like "midday meal" aiming to prevent malnutrition among children [16].

Preventive *panchakarma* can be another explorable example of utilizing Ayurvedic wisdom as frontline care. Ayurveda proposes seasonal detoxification among healthy people to prevent certain class of illnesses related to the accumulation of particular toxins or pathogens. On a high note, Ayurveda proposes that if a routine elimination of such disease-causing elements is done seasonally, these may be prevented. This note is highly important seeing the seasonal epidemics occurring in India every year with a huge claim on public and private expenditure, resources, and quality of life. Ranging from common cold, allergies, respiratory infections, asthma, and fever to jaundice, such clinical conditions represent a wide spectrum of diseases theoretically preventable through Ayurvedic preventive *panchakarma* if a suitable and tested protocol to execute the same may be evolved through a process of continuous research and practice.

Ayurvedic *panchakarma* may also be initially employed to clean the biological systems to optimize their functions. This possibility eventually proposes a hypothesis of reduced dose requirements of conventional medication to offer the same action due to their better absorption and quick reach to the target tissue. Although still a hypothesis, it is worth exploring for; in least of its possibilities, it may ease out the therapeutic options to a large extent. Besides having large-scale economic implications, it may have multiple therapeutic implications in the form of lesser adversities due to dose reduction.

There can also be plenty of situations where Ayurveda can be adopted as complimentary to conventional medicine in an integrative model. Adding herbs in conventional formulations to add cutting edge advantages in the existing formula is a highly promising avenue of integration. Ayurvedic herbs for their possible role as bioenhancer have been researched, and their combinations along with synthetic medicine were brought in the market. Adding piperine, an alkaloid from *Piper longum* (*pippali*) with rifampicin, was found to enhance the therapeutic efficacy and bioavailability of the latter to the extent that the same therapeutic effects were observable with about 50% reduced doses. Such integration seems highly valued as it offers the dose reduction hence lesser possibility of drug adversity along with substantial reduction in the cost of the therapy [17].

What are the concerns of putting Ayurveda as the preferred system of medicine in a specific domain of health care? There shall not be many, if Ayurveda adopts a way similar to the one adopted by conventional medicine. The primary concern in fixing the responsibility of Ayurveda for certain cause at policy level is about genuine evidences for the claims promulgated as the advantage of certain interventions of Ayurveda. Safety and clarity of the protocols along with a clear depiction of deliverable are another area of concern. Finally, quality check on services including those offered by the physicians and by ancillary health-care team as well as on drugs and formulation is of prime importance to develop a trust upon a system. There can be two ways of bringing the change, downstream or upstream in the form of policy adoption and in the form of popular practices, respectively. It is commonly observed that the latter way always remains stronger and effective owing to its arrival from something already believed and practiced.

Integration of Ayurveda with conventional systems of health has its own set of concerns. The most important among these is the possibility of a drug herb interaction if two systems of medicine are simultaneously employed on the same patient. The second concern of such approach is to identify the role of one system of medicine in conjunction with another. Whether they need to go hand in hand or if either of them has to take the independent charge requires a clear understanding in order to define individual role in specific care and to avoid additional cost of integration at a stage where it may not add any additional benefits.

12.6 Fixing the Responsibilities: Exemplifying Ayurveda

A much debated crucial difference between Ayurveda and conventional health care consisting of allopathic medicine lies in their approaches. Ayurveda seems holistic and inclusive compared to allopathy which is focused and exclusive. The holistic nature of Ayurveda, although has a novelty and superiority over other systems, has its own set of issues too. The holistic principles and practices of Ayurveda are culturally so deeply ingrained in oriental psyche that they seem part of oriental lifestyle without being noticed and crediting to Ayurveda. When conceived as a limitation of Ayurveda, this comes with the advocacy to develop drug-based Ayurveda in tune to modern science having its thorough specialization on certain specified ailments. A nonconclusive listing of such clinical conditions may include arthritis, degenerative diseases, rehabilitation in certain neuromusculoskeletal conditions, skin diseases, and hepatobiliary diseases besides many others yet to be explored.

Besides this approach of developing a strong evidence basis for Ayurvedic interventions focused upon the ailments where it has its proven strength, Ayurveda can actually go much beyond this by strengthening its core strength of prevention. This is one area where the focus of conventional health care has either been largely missing or minimally explored limited to prevention through avoidance of known causes and through immunization. The core Ayurvedic concept of *swasthasya swasthya rakshanam* (preserving the health of a healthy person) has never been actually exemplified suitably and hence never been brought into the practice despite the fact of it having a greater impact creation possibility compared to the curative component of health care. How the principles of healthy living are depicted in Ayurveda may be brought under the scientific scanner to create evidences so that such principles may authoritatively be promoted for their adoption by the society? Obviously, the conventional short-term clinical research protocols may not suffice to generate sufficient evidence referring to disease preventive impacts of a given Ayurvedic regime. There, however, can be novel study designs to explore this in long term. The simplest of the studies could be the cohort studies choosing a cohort adopting an absolute Ayurvedic lifestyle compared with the one on the contrary. The outcome in terms of average life span, average disease encounters, and average expenditure made against the curative health care, for a defined period, may come out as robust evidence explaining what might be obtained through such practices. Breaking the whole lifestyle recommendations of Ayurveda into small, interpretable, and isolated components may help in understanding each individual component in its own integrity. Such components may be sleep, *pathya*, *rasayana*, food choice and eating practices, seasonal *panchakarma*, avoidance of suppressible urges and non-avoidance of non-suppressible urges, dietary incompatibility, and maintenance of routine in tune to the individual *prakriti* and *achara rasayana*. All these components may, collectively and individually, be observed for what they might be offering to add to the health. As Ayurvedic health-promotive principles are supposed to add disease-free quality years in the life, a workable research to explore this can be a retrospective analysis of lifestyles adopted by elderly who are running in their healthy aging stage. A person who is healthy and who has crossed the average life span in a given context may be enquired for what he did in the past years to keep him healthy.

An interesting proposal in this regard is to look at Ayurveda community at large to observe their health status in general [18]. Do Ayurveda practitioners differ from general population in terms of parameters of health? How practical and feasible do they feel about Ayurvedic postulates of lifestyle recommendations to remain healthy? What do they find as the practical difficulties to observe such recommendations and how do they feel for meeting such difficulties?

12.7 Making It Work Economically

In the above sections, an attempt has been made to position traditional systems of medicine—in particular *Ayurveda*—in the context of efforts toward achieving health for all. Apart from its role as a source of curative medicine, the possibilities of using Ayurveda as a source of preventive, promotive, restorative, or rehabilitative and complementary medicine have been suggested. This section explores the various parameters which need to be considered to ensure that these functions of Ayurvedic medicine may be provided to the community in an efficient and sustainable manner.

Any model of health-care delivery must necessarily consider the economics and the financial aspects of the various agents—the physicians, the drug manufacturing companies, the regulatory agencies, the hospital firms, and even the patients. If we consider health-care delivery as an economic activity which results in the production of health, then these agents may be considered as the *economic agents* in that process; the financial aspect would then refer to the *microeconomic* aspects, while the economic aspect would refer to the *macroeconomic* aspect of health-care delivery.

It may be argued that *traditional systems* of medicine, when thought of as a health-care delivery model, do not conform to such an economic model; for example, if a patient is advised to do *yoga* daily, which results in a better control of certain comorbidities like hypertension, there is no *perceptible economic* or *financial* activity in such a production of health. But this argument is not entirely acceptable for two reasons. One, the time and effort spent in doing yoga are an economic input, and an individual's time and effort are valuable resources which have to be allocated and utilized; it is just that these resources do not have a "market." Doing yoga or following a dietary regime therefore is an example of *nonmarket activity*, but definitely an economic activity. Second, behavioral science is now increasingly a part of mainstream economics; it is now accepted that human beings take decisions and invest resources in decisions which need not seem to be *rational*; thus, if a particular community wishes to stick to its traditional system of medicine based purely on its faith, rather than scientific evidence, such a behavior may be considered unscientific by a certain section, but it is definitely a form of economic behavior. In the 1970s, parallel to the health for all movement in the international health community, the field of economics saw the growth of two major ideas which seem to be more akin to the concepts of traditional systems of medicine, than the modern systems in which they were conceived. One was the influential Grossman's model of health, where health was thought of as a form of capital; the other was Gary Becker's work on the role of the family as a unit which took economic decisions to invest resources in education and health. Traditional systems of medicine have always been emphasizing these ideas—that health is a form of capital which can be used to produce other things and that health-related decisions are almost never taken by an individual alone and are taken in the context of his or her family.

The discourse today on "health for all" is heavily colored by terms like health-care financing or health-care economics. The overwhelming focus today is on ideas like cost containment or cost-effective analysis or QALYs; this is so because starting from the 1990s, modern medicine has become very, very expensive. This was not the case when the bold declarations of Alma-Ata were made or when the barefoot doctors in China were making their remarkable strides in achieving universal health care. This has also not been the case at any point in the long histories of traditional systems of medicine—whether in India, China, or other Asian or African regions. It may have been difficult to source a particular rare herb or animal part or conduct a particular production process which involved precious metals, but traditional systems of medicine almost never faced questions like "Is this particular treatment cost-effective for this class of patients?"

The current obsession with cost-effectiveness is dangerous for two reasons. One, it often denies patients hope and mental support. Second, it provides a basis for insurance companies or other financiers to deny funding for treatment, thereby undercutting at the very root of the idea of health for all. Traditional systems of medicine have never subscribed to this idea and must resist this relatively recent trend of being measured by governments and insurance agencies on parameters like cost-effectiveness and QALYs.

Instead of merely a narrow focus on cost containment or cost-efficiency, the larger field of economics offers many other powerful tools for practitioners of traditional medicine. Some of these tools help us analyze individual decision-making behavior, like health-care seeking; others help us to fine-tune the regulatory interventions which governments seek to make; yet others allow us to process data and see useful patterns. A full description of such tools and models is outside the scope of this work. However the following points must be emphasized—traditional systems of medicine are a "better fit" than modern systems of medicine in "economically producing" health for all; but governments and agencies must resist measuring Ayurveda or TCM in narrow terms of financing and insurance. Instead there has to be a concerted intellectual effort to harness the latest tools available in the field of economics to provide a model for bringing in Ayurveda in our modern medical lives in a sustainable way.

Conclusion

The WHO has declared "Universal Health Coverage: Every One, Every Where" as the theme for World Health Day 2018. This is a reminder of Alma-Ata health for all declaration and an acceptance that despite passing four decades since the declaration we are still far away from what we targeted to achieve [19]. By now it is clear that health needs are different in different perspectives, and eventually the methods of their procurement also ought to be different. There can't be one pill to cure all, and hence a rational region-based strategy is required to be adopted to meet the objectives. It is important to stress that this strategy essentially requires to be derived contextual to the regional culture, beliefs, and resources. Traditional health-care systems may prove to be much useful in the obtainment of the ultimate objective of making this world a healthier place to live and making its inhabitants healthier. We admit that there are initial hiccoughs translating traditional concepts of health care into practically utilizable format but at the same time believe that once such hiccoughs are resolved, we would soon be sailing into a completely different world, the world where one may be more caring toward retaining the health rather than becoming sick and crying for the remedies. Ayurveda can intervene here as an essential and handy tool to bring this into reality.

References

1. Declaration of Alma-Ata International Conference on Primary Health Care, Alma-Ata, USSR, 6–12 September 1978. http://www.who.int/publications/almaata_declaration_en.pdf?ua=1.
2. Halfdan M. The meaning of 'Health for All by the Year 2000'. World Health Forum. 1981;2(1):5–22.
3. World health statistics 2017: monitoring health for the SDGs, sustainable development goals. Geneva: World Health Organization; 2017. Licence: CC BY-NC-SA 3.0 IGO.
4. Millenium Development Goals. http://www.who.int/topics/millennium_development_goals/about/en/. Accessed 9 Apr 2018.
5. https://www.britannica.com/biography/Nikola-Tesla.
6. Stevens EE, Patrick TE, Pickler R. A history of infant feeding. J Perinat Educ. 2009;18(2):32–9. https://doi.org/10.1624/105812409X426314.
7. Mittal TK. Modern understanding of cardiovascular prevention: ayurvedic root with a modern shoot. Ann Ayurvedic Med. 2016;5(1–2):12–6.
8. Krauss RM, Deckelbaum RJ, Ernst N, Fisher E, Howard BV, Knopp RH, et al. Dietary guidelines for healthy American adults: a statement for health professionals from the Nutrition Committee, American Heart Association. Circulation. 1996;94(7):1795–800. https://doi.org/10.1161/01.CIR.94.7.1795.

9. Vyas S, Manna S, Kumar J, Sharma HB. Association of ghee consumption with lowered CHD history: a study in urban north Indian adults. Ann Ayurvedic Med. 2017;6(1–2):10–22.
10. Rastogi S, Rastogi R, Singh RH. What are we losing by ignoring Ayurveda? New Approaches Med Health. 2006;14(1):26–9.
11. Philips CA, Paramaguru R, Joy AK, Antony KL, Augustine P. Clinical outcomes, histopathological patterns, and chemical analysis of Ayurveda and herbal medicine associated with severe liver injury—a single-center experience from southern India. Indian J Gastroenterol. 2018;37(1):9–17. https://doi.org/10.1007/s12664-017-0815-8.
12. Rastogi S, Srivastav PS. Ayurveda in critical care: illustrating Ayurvedic intervention in a case of hepatic encephalopathy. Ayu. 2011;32(3):345–8. https://doi.org/10.4103/0974-8520.93911.
13. Rastogi S. Low pressure low flow voiding dysfunction in an elderly male treated through Ayurveda: a case report. J Evid Based Complement Altern Med. 2017;22(4):846–50.
14. Lurie D. Ayurveda and pharmacogenomics. Ann Ayurvedic Med. 2012;1(4):126–8.
15. United Nations Population Fund. 'Caring for our elders: early responses' - India ageing reports 2017. New Delhi, India: UNFPA; 2017.
16. Mid day meal. http://mdm.nic.in/. Accessed 5 Apr 2018.
17. Atal N, Bedi KL. Bioenhancers: revolutionary concept to the market. J Ayurveda Integr Med. 2010;1(2):96–9. https://doi.org/10.4103/0975-9476.65073.
18. O'Mahong S. Do doctor's die better than philosophers? Lancet. 2018;391:1474–5.
19. Patwardhan B, Tillu G. Universal health coverage and AYUSH systems. J Ayurveda Integr Med. 2018;9(1):1–2. https://doi.org/10.1016/j.jaim.2018.03.001.

MIX
Papier aus verantwortungsvollen Quellen
Paper from responsible sources
FSC® C105338

If you have any concerns about our products,
you can contact us on
ProductSafety@springernature.com

In case Publisher is established outside the EU,
the EU authorized representative is:
Springer Nature Customer Service Center GmbH
Europaplatz 3, 69115 Heidelberg, Germany

Printed by Libri Plureos GmbH
in Hamburg, Germany